Sports Medicine and Rehabilitation: A Sport-Specific Approach

Sports Medicine and Rehabilitation: A Sport-Specific Approach

Edited by

Ralph M. Buschbacher, MD

Clinical Assistant Professor
Department of Physical Medicine and Rehabilitation
Indiana University Medical Center
Indianapolis, Indiana

Randall L. Braddom, MD, MS

Professor and Chairman
Department of Physical Medicine and Rehabilitation
Indiana University Medical Center
Indianapolis, Indiana

HANLEY & BELFUS, INC./ Philadelphia
MOSBY/ St. Louis • Baltimore • Boston • Chicago • London
   Philadelphia • Sydney • Toronto

Publisher: HANLEY & BELFUS, INC.
                        210 S. 13th Street
                        Philadelphia, PA 19107
                        (215) 546-7293
                        FAX (215) 790-9330

North American and worldwide sales and distribution:

                        MOSBY
                        11830 Westline Industrial Drive
                        St. Louis, MO 63146

In Canada: Times Mirror Professional Publishing, Ltd.
                        130 Flaska Drive
                        Markham, Ontario L6G 1B8
                        Canada

Library of Congress Cataloging–in–Publication Data

Sports medicine and rehabilitation : a sport-specific approach /
    [editors], Ralph Buschbacher, Randall L. Braddom.
        p.   cm.
    Includes bibliographical references and index.
    ISBN 1-56053-133-9
    1. Sports Injuries–Patients–Rehabilitation.
    2. Sports physical therapy.   I. Buschbacher, Ralph M.   II. Braddom, Randall L.
    [DNLM: 1. Sports medicine.   2. Athletic Injuries–rehabilitation.
    3. Exercise. QT 260 S76315 1994]
    RD97.S747 1994
    617.1'027–dc20
    DNLM/DLC
    for Library of Congress   94-17
                                                                                     CIP

Sports Medicine and Rehabilitation:
A Sport-Specific Approach   ISBN 1-56053-133-9

Last digit is the print number: 9 8 7 6 5 4 3 2 1

CONTENTS

CONTRIBUTORS

STEVEN J. ANDERSON, MD
Clinical Associate Professor of Pediatrics, University of Washington School of Medicine, Seattle, Washington

JAMES R. ANDREWS, MD
Clinical Professor, Department of Orthopedics and Sports Medicine, University of Virginia Medical School, Charlottesville, Virginia: Medical Director, American Sports Medicine Institute, Birmingham, Alabama

RICHARD P. BONFIGLIO, MD
Clinical Assistant Professor, Department of Rehabilitation Medicine, Jefferson Medical College of Thomas Jefferson University, Philadelphia, Pennsylvania; Medical Director, Bryn Mawr Rehab, Malvern Pennsylvania

RANDALL L. BRADDOM, MD, MS
Professor and Chairman, Department of Physical Medicine and Rehabilitation, Indiana University School of Medicine, Indianapolis; Medical Director, Hook Rehabilitation Center, Indianapolis, Indiana

DAVID K. BRENNAN MED
Assistant Professor, Department of Physical Medicine and Rehabilitation, Baylor College of Medicine, Houston; President, Houston International Running Center, Houston, Texas

PHILLIP R. BRYANT, DO
Assistant Clinical Professor, Department of Orthopaedics and Rehabilitation, University of Tennessee College of Medicine, Chattanooga Unit; Medical Director of Pediatric Rehabilitation, and Associate Program Director, Physical Medicine and Rehabilitation Residency Training Program, Siskin Hospital for Physical Rehabiliation, Chattanooga, Tennessee

LOIS P. BUSCHBACHER, MD
Clinical Assistant Professor, Department of Physical Medicine and Rehabilitation, Indiana University School of Medicine, Indianapolis, Indiana

RALPH M. BUSCHBACHER, MD
Clinical Assistant Professor, Department of Physical Medicine and Rehabilitation, Indiana University School of Medicine, Indianapolis, Indiana

MICHAEL F. DILLINGHAM, MD
Clinical Professor, Department of Orthopedics, Stanford University School of Medicine, Stanford, California

SUSAN LEE HUBBELL, MD, MS
Clinical Assistant Professor, Department of Physical Medicine and Rehabilitation, The Ohio State University College of Medicine, Columbus, Ohio, and Medical College of Ohio, Toledo, Ohio; Chief, Department of Physical Medicine, St. Rita's Medical Center, Lima, Ohio

BARBARA M. KOCH, MD
Private Practitioner, Rockville, Maryland; Consultant, Fairfax Hospital, Shady Grove Hospital, and Holy Cross Hospital

SANFORD S. KUNKEL, MD
Clinical Assistant Professor, Department of Orthopedics, Indiana University School of Medicine, Indianapolis, Indiana

EDWARD R. LASKOWSKI, MD
Co-director, Sports Medicine Center, Mayo Clinic; Assistant Professor, Department of Physical Medicine and Rehabilitation, Mayo Medical School, Rochester, Minnesota

ANTHONY J. MARGHERITA, MD
Assistant Professor, Department of Rehabilitation Medicine, University of Washington School of Medicine, Seattle; Attending Physiatrist and Co-director, Harborview Medical Center Sports Medicine Clinic, Seattle, Washington

DOUGLAS B. McKEAG, MD, MS
Professor of Family Practice, Associate Chair for Education, and Coordinator of Sports Medicine, Department of Family Practice, Michigan State University College of Human Medicine, East Lansing, Michigan

ROBERT S. MILLARD, MD
Sports Orthopedics and Rehabilitation Medicine Associates, Menlo Park, California

JOEL M. PRESS, MD
Medical Director, Center for Spine, Sports, and Occupational Rehabilitation, Rehabilitation Institute of Chicago; Clinical Assistant Professor, Department of Physical Medicine and Rehabilitation, Northwestern University Medical School, Chicago, Illinois

JOHN C. PRITCHARD, MD
Director of Orthopedic Sports Medicine, Orthopedics Northeast, Ft. Wayne, Indiana

MARGOT PUTUKIAN, MD
Formerly, Fellow in Primary Care Sports Medicine, Michigan State University, East Lansing, Michigan; Currently, Team Physician, Pennsylvania State University; Assistant Professor, Departments of Internal Medicine and Orthopedics, Pennsylvania State University, Hershey Medical Center, State College, Pennsylvania

BENJAMIN D. RUBIN, MD
Assistant Clinical Professor, Department of Orthopaedic Surgery, University of California, Irvine, Orange, California

JOEL S. SAAL, MD
Clinical Instructor in Functional Restoration, Stanford University School of Medicine, Stanford, California

LESLIE K. SCHULTZ, MD
Clinical Assistant Professor, Department of Physical Medicine and Rehabilitation, Indiana University School of Medicine, Indianapolis, Indiana

FRANK Y. WEI, MD
Fairview Southdale Hospital, Edina, Minnesota

JAMES A. WHITESIDE, MD
Clinical Associate Professor, Department of Orthopaedics and Sports Medicine, University of Virginia Medical School, Charlottesville, Virginia; Director, Medical Aspects of Sports, Alabama Sports Medicine and Orthopaedic Center, Birmingham, Alabama

ROBERT P. WILDER, MD
Director, Sports Rehabilitation Services, Department of Physical Medicine and Rehabilitation, Baylor University, The Tom Landry Sports Medicine and Research Center, Dallas, Texas; Medical Director, Houston International Running Center

KEVIN E. WILK, PT
Clinical Instructor, Department of Physical Therapy, Louisiana State University, Baton Rouge and New Orleans, Louisiana; National Director of Research and Clinical Education, and Associate Clinical Director, HealthSouth Sports Medicine and Rehabilitation, Birmingham, Alabama

JEFFREY L. YOUNG, MD, MA
Director, Spine and Sports Fellowship, Rehabilitation Institute of Chicago; Assistant Professor, Department of Physical Medicine and Rehabilitation, Northwestern University Medical School, Chicago, Illinois

WILHELM A. ZUELZER, MD
Associate Professor, Department of Orthopedics, Medical College of Virginia, Richmond, Virginia

FOREWORD

Therapeutic exercise is the common pathway to recovery from virtually all sports injuries. Because the starting point of rehabilitation is the athlete's current level of function and the goal of therapy is return to the level of function necessary for specific sports performance, this type of rehabilitation may be called "functional treatment." Functional treatment is symptom guided, injury specific, and sport specific. It should be initiated as soon as possible following injury, immobilization, and/or surgery. It hastens safe return to play and minimizes deconditioning, the detrimental effects of immobilization, and recovery time.

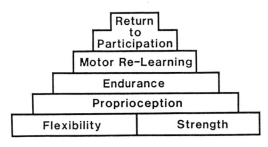

PYRAMID OF RECOVERY
(Therapeutic Exercise)

Several years ago, we assembled the specific components of functional rehabilitation into a Pyramid of Recovery, noting that each component represents a "therapeutic exercise building block" toward the goal of return to play.

After a foundation of flexibility and strength is reestablished in the injured athlete, programs of proprioception and endurance training are instituted in an overlapping manner. The athlete progresses to sport-specific motor relearning and finally returns to participation based on functional testing related to the individual sport. Important adjuncts to this care include relative rest, crutches, taping and bracing, nonsteroidal anti-inflammatory drugs, ice, and other physical modalities.

Drs. Buschbacher and Braddom have developed an excellent volume that applies the functional approach to many popular sports. In addition to the chapters on individual sports, several chapters focus on important rehabilitation issues such as the tissue aspects of injury and healing, hydrotherapy, and the appropriate role of bracing. Three chapters focus on exercise in particular populations: women, individuals with preexisting illness, and healthy individuals desiring to use exercise to prevent illness. Rounding out the functional approach is an excellent chapter on preparticipation evaluation. Here it is appropriate to note that what may be rehabilitation in the injured athlete may be rightly considered "prehabilitation" in the athlete beginning an exercise program or athletic season.

This book is a logical, well-written work that focuses on the similarities and differences in the rehabilitation needs of athletes performing in a variety of sports.

Morris B. Mellion, MD
Guy L. Shelton, MA, PT, ATC
Omaha, Nebraska

ix

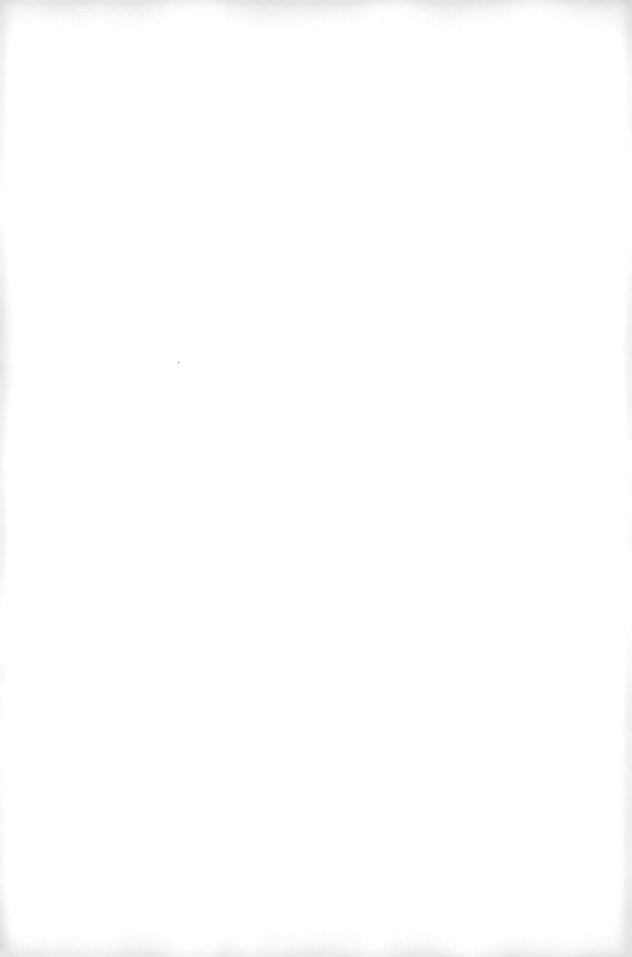

PREFACE

With all the excellent sports medicine texts available, why did we feel the need to add yet another book to the list? First, we wanted to offer a book that emphasizes the *rehabilitation* of athletic injuries. All too often the rehabilitation phase of recovery is neglected, and this neglect may lead to an unsafe return to activity. Second, we wanted a book that would be enjoyable and easy to read. Reading a book about anatomic-specific disorders (i.e., the shoulder, the elbow, the wrist, etc.) can be very dry, even if well written. Consequently, we organized our chapters around a sports-specific approach. This approach is designed to keep the reader involved with the material to a much greater extent. We also included chapters usually excluded or only cursorily mentioned in other texts, including women's issues, wheelchair athletics, tissue injury and healing, exercise in persons with medical illness, knee and ankle bracing, strength and flexibility training, and hydro exercise. We feel that each of the contributing authors did an excellent job on their respective topics, and we hope that our readers will appreciate the quality of their work as well.

Ralph M. Buschbacher, MD
Randall L. Braddom, MD, MS

Chapter 1

THE PREPARTICIPATION PHYSICAL EXAMINATION

Margot Putukian, MD, and Douglas B. McKeag, MD

To qualify for organized athletics, a young athlete usually undergoes a preparticipation physical examination. Similarly, older individuals sometimes seek a preparticipation physical examination because of the common warning: "Consult a physician prior to beginning an exercise program." In both situations the objectives are the same, but the examination will be different for the 14-year-old boy about to start high-school basketball and the 48-year-old diabetic woman initiating a walking program. Factors such as age, gender, contemplated activity, and the personal goals of the individual must be considered in tailoring the preparticipation physical examination. This chapter discusses the core objectives of the preparticipation examination, identifies some of the factors important in tailoring the examination to the individual, and outlines elements of the history and physical examination that help to ensure safe involvement of any individual in an exercise program.

USEFULNESS AND VALIDITY

Much of the data surrounding the usefulness of the preparticipation examination come from studies of adolescent athletes (Table 1). In these studies, there is only a 0.2 to 1.3% incidence of findings that disqualify an athlete or limit participation. Such small numbers among thousands of athletes call into question cost-effectiveness. In a study of 557 athletes,[46] the cost of identifying three adolescents with significant abnormalities was

estimated at \$4,357 per athlete. Some of the identified conditions, however, can be associated with sudden cardiac death or significant medical disease. Consequently, the detection of even one such abnormality seems philosophically valid and cost-justified.

Three areas of the preparticipation examination need to be stressed: the cardiovascular, musculoskeletal, and neurologic systems. Several authors[14,17,20,49] have suggested a limitation of the examination to as few as 4 to 6 questions that address these areas. If an athlete regularly receives comprehensive physical examinations, this approach is reasonable. However, for many young athletes, the preparticipation examination is their only exposure to a physician; thus, additional areas of special importance *should be included,* such as the pulmonary system, thermoregulation, nutrition, weight changes, and drug use. These areas can be addressed in the history without prolonging the examination excessively. Even if the athlete does not feel comfortable discussing certain issues at the initial examination, their inclusion in the history usually draws the athlete's attention to them and may enhance communication on a subsequent visit. In an older individual, the comprehensive physical examination sometimes *includes* a clearance to participate in exercise. If it does not, a preparticipation physical examination may be necessary. It should be emphasized that this examination cannot replace the comprehensive physical.

There are two different methods for implementing the preparticipation physical examination: the station technique and the individ-

TABLE 1. Preparticipation Screening Studies

	No. of Athletes	Temporary Disqualification Pending Referral (%)	Permanent Disqualification (%)
Goldberg, 1980[22]	701	7.8	1.3
Linder, 1981[30]	1268	5.0	0.2
Thompson, 1982[53]	2670	1.2	
Tennant, 1981[51]	2719	9.2	1.2
Hough and McKeag, 1982[25]	989	10.0	1.1
Risser, 1985[47]	2114	3.4	0.3
Magnes, 1992[32]	10540	10.6	0.4

TABLE 2. Comparison of Preparticipation Physical Examination Methods

	Station Technique	Private Office-Based
Past medical history known	No	Yes
Motivation assessed	No	Yes
Sensitive issues discussed	No	Yes
Continuity of care	No	Yes
Teamwork approach with potential use of subspecialists	Yes	No
Consistency among physicians	Yes	No
Cost-effective	Yes	No
Familiarity with demands of sport	Usually	Variable

ual office-based evaluation. In the station technique, different parts of the examination are performed by different health care providers as the individual moves from one station to the next. This method is often used for schools with a large group of young athletes who require evaluation prior to participation in organized school athletics. The individual office-based examination is usually performed by the individual's primary-care provider in his or her office. The advantages and disadvantages to each method are summarized in Table 2. Regardless of the method, as long as the examination is performed in an orderly and objective fashion with emphasis on the salient features, most individuals will be competently assessed.

OBJECTIVES

Seven objectives of the preparticipation examination have been identified: The most obvious are (1) to detect abnormalities or conditions that would make participation dangerous or predispose to injury, (2) to assess general health, and (3) to provide health maintenance. Lombardo[31] has proposed that the preparticipation examination (4) fulfills legal and insurance requirements for organized athletic programs and (5) evaluates the size and level of maturation of younger athletes. For many individuals, the preparticipation examination is (6) an introduction to the health care system and (7) an opportunity for the athlete to become educated about health issues. This last objective may well be the most important because it can establish a physician–patient relationship that leads to better long-term health care delivery. Although some of the goals may be more applicable in younger athletes, most are relevant to all individuals.

IMPORTANT FACTORS

The preparticipation examination must be modified according to the age and sex of the individual, preexisting medical conditions, the contemplated type of exercise, and the individual's goals. Although an examination form cannot cover all these factors perfectly, protocols are described below. Maturational changes and conditions that occur with different ages need to be considered on an individual basis to facilitate a more thorough and directed examination.

Maturational Changes

In terms of maturational changes, it is helpful to separate athletes into:
1. Prepubescent (6–10 yrs),
2. Pubescent (11–15 yrs),
3. Postpubescent/young adult (16–30 yrs),
4. Adult (31–65 yrs), and
5. Elderly (older than 65 yrs).

(The chronological years supplied here are approximate and intended only as a helpful guide.) Through consideration of each maturational stage and the characteristics of each age group, the preparticipation examination can be better tailored to address the appropriate concerns.

For the *prepubescent* age group, the emphasis has shifted recently from spontaneous play to more organized athletics. It is not uncommon to see *prepubescent* youngsters involved in organized soccer, baseball, hockey, swimming, and other sports. The motivation for this age group is fun and participation. Martens[38] outlined the most common reasons for nonparticipation in sports (in order of frequency): (1) not getting the opportunity to play; (2) negative reinforcement; (3) mismatching; (4) psychological stress; (5) failure; and (6) overorganization. In a survey of prepubertal youngsters in organized sports programs, Henschen and Griffin[24] discovered that 95% of their respondents felt that the most important aspect of sports was *having fun,* not winning; 75% said that they would rather *play* on a "loser" than sit on a "winning" team. One of the most important considerations in the examination of this age group is to rule out previously undiagnosed congenital abnormalities.

The *pubescent* athlete is undergoing rapid growth as well as changes in both psychological and sexual development. Puberty is a period of rapid social development, with emphasis on issues of sexuality, drug use, and body image. Athletics in this age group are typically heavily organized, and it is important to establish exercise as part of a healthy lifestyle and as a lifelong activity. Anderson[1] studied alcohol and drug use in college athletes and found that 55% to 65% began use of "social" recreational drugs in high school. Questions about drug and alcohol as well as social and sexual development send a message to the athlete that these are important issues.

For the *postpubescent* or *young adult,* the reasons for exercising are as varied as the skill level of the athletes involved. For this age group the preparticipation physical examination should be individualized to accommodate both the level of intensity as well as the specific anticipated activity. Previous injuries, inadequate rehabilitation, and other medical conditions must be identified. Drug use is again important to consider in this age group. Recommendations should be as sport-specific as possible.

Exercise for the *adult* population is mostly recreational, but intensity and frequency of activity vary greatly. This age group accounts for most of the acute "weekend warrior" injuries as well as many of the overuse injuries. It is uncommon for the adult population to seek a preparticipation examination; it is much more common for the first office visit to occur only after an acute injury.

The *elderly* have learned that exercise can improve general quality of life as well as provide an opportunity for social interaction. Exercise has become a increasingly valuable part of many rehabilitation programs for the elderly, especially in therapeutic regimens for chronic disease (e.g., diabetes mellitus, depression, cerebrovascular accidents, and myocardial infarctions). Fiatarone et al.[16] have shown that 8 weeks of high-intensity strength resistance training in nonagenarians resulted in significant gains in muscle strength, muscle size, and functional mobility. The preparticipation examination for the elderly can be complicated and may serve as only part of a comprehensive physical examination. The physician must carefully appraise the prospective exerciser for coexisting medical conditions, suggest realistic exercise goals, and advise caution to those at risk for falls or injury.

Gender

A second factor to be considered in the preparticipation examination is the gender of the patient. Recently the term *female triad* (disordered eating, amenorrhea, and osteoporosis) has been used in regard to women's athletic issues.[2] Although pathologic eating patterns can occur in all athletes, they are more common in women. Rosen et al.[48] studied 187 female college athletes and demonstrated dangerous weight-control behaviors in 32%, including self-induced vomiting, binges more than twice weekly, and use of laxatives, diet pills, and/or diuretics. Alarmingly, 70% of these athletes felt that their behavior was not harmful. In a study of younger athletes, Dummer et al.[13] studied eating behaviors in 487 female and 468 male swimmers aged 9 to 18 years. They reported eating dysfunction in 15.4% of the girls (24.8% of postmenarcheal girls) and 3.6% of the boys. Disordered eating behavior seems to be most common in sports that emphasize low body weight or involve competition by weight class (e.g., dance, gymnastics, boxing, and wrestling).

Abnormalities in the menstrual cycle are often encountered in intense athletics, and require early assessment. Recent research[4,8,9,18,19] has discussed the relationship between the menstrual cycle, body weight, intensity of exercise, and nutrition, all of which should be considered in evaluating the female athlete. It is important to assess each case for general causes of amenorrhea or oligomenorrhea and not to assume that physical activity is the only possible cause.

The relationship of amenorrhea, bone mineral content, and the risk for osteoporosis and subsequent stress fractures has been examined in several recent studies.[3,10–12,28,29,43] The preparticipation examination provides an opportunity to educate the athlete on the importance of proper nutrition for long-term bone health as well as optimal performance. Johnson[27] recently suggested a supplemental health history questionnaire for the female athlete. Table 3 provides examples of some additional questions useful in addressing special issues of the female athlete.

The use of performance-enhancing drugs can also be gender-specific, as evidenced by a study of college athletes.[1] Steroids and smokeless tobacco were used primarily by male athletes, whereas weight-loss medications were more commonly used by female athletes.

Contemplated Exercise Activity

A third factor that affects the direction of the preparticipation examination is the contemplated activity. The demands of weightlifting are quite different from the demands of marathon running. The major types of

---

TABLE 3.   Supplemental History for the Female Athlete

1. At what age did you have your first menstrual period? _____
2. How many days does your menstrual bleeding last? _____
3. How many days are there between cycles? _____
4. How many periods have you had in the past 12 months? _____
5. What is the date of your last menstrual period? _____
6. Do you ever have cramping with your period? _____
   If so, what do you do? _____
7. Have you ever had "irregular" cycles (shorter than 21 days or with more than 35 days between cycles)? _____
8. Have you ever had heavy bleeding? _____
9. Have you ever stopped having a period? _____
   If so for how long? _____
10. Have you ever had a stress fracture? _____
    If so, please list sites and dates _____
11. When was your last pelvic exam? _____
12. Have you ever had an abnormal pelvic exam or Pap smear? _____
    If so, please explain, _____
13. Do you take birth control pills or hormones? _____
14. Has a physician ever told you that you had anemia? _____
15. What is your present weight? _____
16. Are you happy with your present weight? _____
    If not, what is your desired weight? _____
17. What have you eaten in the last 2 days? _____
18. How many meals do you eat each day? _____
19. Do you refuse to eat certain foods (e.g., meats, breads, dairy products)? _____
20. Do you diet regularly? _____
21. Have you ever tried to control your weight by vomiting? _____
    Laxatives? _____   Diuretics? _____   Diet pills? _____
22. Have you ever been diagnosed as having an eating disorder? _____
23. Do you take vitamins or supplements? _____

exercise are (1) aerobic, (2) anaerobic, and (3) combined aerobic/anaerobic. The long-duration, low-power output of aerobic exercise uses energy obtained through oxidative phosphorylation. It includes activities such as swimming, running, and bicycling. Anaerobic exercise is characterized by short-duration, high-energy bursts that require energy generated by glycolysis. Examples include sprinting and weight-lifting. Combined aerobic/anaerobic activity is characterized by activities that require a combination of both energy systems. Examples include soccer, basketball, lacrosse, and hockey. Figure 1 indicates the relative contribution of the aerobic and anaerobic systems to various activities.

Sports can also be classified according to the amount of contact or collision that occurs with participation (Table 4). If an athlete has a condition that would be adversely affected by contact, classification systems can act as general guidelines for individualized recommendations.

Motivation

The final component in personalizing the preparticipation examination is to discover the motivation and goals of the potential athlete. "Why do you want to exercise?" For younger athletes, goals may include playing for their school or university. For older athletes, goals may be to improve overall health and self-image or to gain social opportunities. For others, exercise may represent part of a therapeutic regimen for treating illness or injury. Determining the goals for the individual athlete is an important aid in making proper exercise recommendations.

IMPLEMENTATION

Implementation of the preparticipation examination requires an organized approach, an understanding of the essential parts of the examination, and a knowledge of the common physical findings in athletes. The station technique and the office-based methods, as discussed earlier, have different advantages and disadvantages, yet both can provide competent results. The locker-room technique, which involves mass examination of athletes within one staging area, is no longer an appropriate method of implementation.

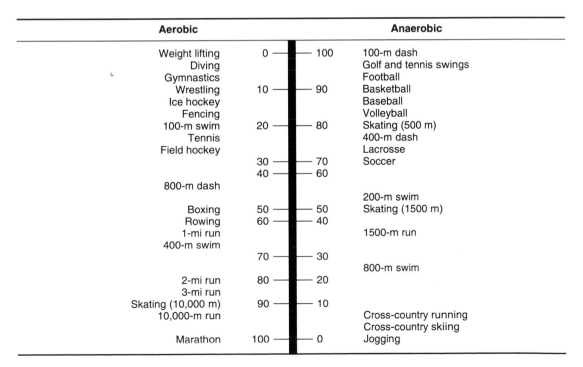

Aerobic			Anaerobic
Weight lifting	0	100	100-m dash
Diving			Golf and tennis swings
Gymnastics			Football
Wrestling	10	90	Basketball
Ice hockey			Baseball
Fencing			Volleyball
100-m swim	20	80	Skating (500 m)
Tennis			400-m dash
Field hockey			Lacrosse
	30	70	Soccer
	40	60	
800-m dash			
			200-m swim
Boxing	50	50	Skating (1500 m)
Rowing	60	40	
1-mi run			1500-m run
400-m swim			
	70	30	
			800-m swim
2-mi run	80	20	
3-mi run			
Skating (10,000 m)	90	10	
10,000-m run			Cross-country running
			Cross-country skiing
Marathon	100	0	Jogging

FIGURE 1. Relative Contributions of Aerobic and Anaerobic Energy Systems to Various Sports Activities (Adapted from Fox EL: Training of youth for sport. In Kelley VC (ed): *Practice of Pediatrics,* vol 10. Philadelphia, J.B. Lippincott, 1984; with permission.)

TABLE 4.   **Classification of Sports**

| | | Noncontact | | |
Contact Collision	Limited Contact Impact	Strenuous	Moderately Strenuous	Nonstrenuous
Boxing	Baseball	Aerobic	Badminton	Archery
Field hockey	Basketball	dance	Curling	Golf
Football	Bicycling	Crew	Table tennis	Riflery
Ice hockey	Diving	Fencing		
Lacrosse	Field events	Field events		
Martial arts	High jump	Discus		
Rodeo	Pole vault	Javelin		
Soccer	Gymnastics	Shot put		
Wrestling	Handball	Running		
	Horseback	Swimming		
	Ice skating	Tennis		
	Rollerskating	Weight-lifting		
	Skiing			
	Cross-country			
	Downhill			
	Water			
	Softball			
	Squash			
	Volleyball			

Reprinted from the American Academy of Pediatrics Committee on Sports Medicine: Recommendations forparticipating in competitive sports. *Pediatrics* 81:737–739, 1988; with permission.

Using an established form ensures that the major issues are addressed and brings some consistency to the process. Many forms have been advocated, Table 5 provides an example of one that includes appropriate historical questions.

Frequency

The preparticipation physical examination should be performed prior to initial athlete participation and prior to any new level of competition.

For the prepubescent, the initial examination should probably be performed in the office on an individual basis. The first sports physical is important because it may represent a healthy child's first interaction with the health care system. Many children have not been seen by a physician since their second set of immunizations at age 5 years.

For the pubescent or postpubescent athlete, the preparticipation examination can also be done when grade levels change (e.g., grade school, junior high school, high school, and college) and is often performed in the station technique. Between levels, an "intercurrent" review can be performed to determine if any *new* medical problems or injuries have occurred since the previous examina-

tion. Additional historical questions regarding new medications or new concerns can help the physician to identify potential problem areas. Such an intercurrent examination should include measurement of vital signs, such as height, weight, blood pressure, heart rate, and visual screening. An example of the intercurrent form is given in Table 6.

For the adult, the preparticipation examination should be part of a comprehensive physical examination unless a comprehensive examination has been done recently. Special considerations should be made for older individuals, especially if they have risk factors for coronary artery disease (hypertension, diabetes, hypercholesterolemia, smoking history, previous cardiac disease, strong family history, obesity, or sedentary lifestyle). A useful algorithm for the office-based method in adults is given in Figure 2.

Timing

Timing of the preparticipation examination should consider two points:
1. The examination should occur before a particular sport season has begun and should allow enough time for adequate rehabilitation of any problems that may be identified.

TABLE 5.　Preparticipation Physical Examination of Michigan State University

This is a screening evaluation and is not meant to, nor should it, take the place of a standard complete physical examination.

Name _____ Date _____ Date of birth _____ Sex _____
Address _____ Phone _____ Sport _____
Parent/guardian _____ Phone _____
Address _____ Emergency # _____
Family doctor _____ Address _____
Doctor's phone _____ Date of last exam _____

The following questions are to be answered *yes* or *no*.
Please check the appropriate box. Comment on all *yes* answers.

Have you ever:	Y	N	Comments
Been hospitalized or had surgery?	( )	( )	_____
Broken a bone or had a muscle injury?	( )	( )	_____
Had an injury to a joint?	( )	( )	_____

Please check appropriate box(es)
Knee ( )　　Shoulder ( )　　Ankle ( )　　Elbow ( )　　Wrist ( )　　Other ( )

Has anyone in your immediate family ever had:	Y	N	Comments
Diabetes (high blood sugar)?	( )	( )	_____
Sudden death (age <50)?	( )	( )	_____
High blood pressure?	( )	( )	_____
Heart attack (age < 50)?	( )	( )	_____
Asthma?	( )	( )	_____
High cholesterol?	( )	( )	_____

Have you ever had or do you now have:			
Chest pain with or after exercise?	( )	( )	_____
Dizziness with or after exercise?	( )	( )	_____
High blood pressure?	( )	( )	_____
Racing of the heart/irregular rhythm?	( )	( )	_____

Have you ever had or do you now have:			
Wheezing/cough with exercise or asthma?	( )	( )	_____
Weakness, fatigue, or anemia?	( )	( )	_____

Have you ever had:			
Loss of consciousness?	( )	( )	_____
Concussion?	( )	( )	_____
Convulsions (seizures) or epilepsy?	( )	( )	_____
Neck injury?	( )	( )	_____
"Stinger," "burner," or "pinched nerve"?	( )	( )	_____

Have you had or do you now have:			
Hearing loss or perforated eardrum?	( )	( )	_____
Headaches or migraines?	( )	( )	_____
Dental plate or orthodontic work?	( )	( )	_____
Impaired vision, wear glasses/contacts?	( )	( )	_____

Have you ever had:			
Heat exhaustion or intolerance?	( )	( )	_____

Additional comments or concerns _____

Have you had or do you now have:		
Hernia?	( )	( )
Loss of function or absence of testicle (boys)?	( )	( )
Weight problem (underweight or overweight)?	( )	( )
Menstrual problems (girls)?	( )	( )

Age of first period? _____ Last menstrual period _____

Have you in the past or do you currently use:		
Cigarettes, chewing tobacco, or marijuana?	( )	( )
Alcohol?	( )	( )
Recreational drugs?	( )	( )
Steroids?	( )	( )
Vitamins or supplements?	( )	( )
Weight-loss medications, laxatives, self-induced vomiting?	( )	( )

List any current medications (include over-the-counter and birth-control pills, vitamins, supplements) _____
List any allergies _____
Last tetanus shot _____
Any medical problem or injury since your last exam? _____

TABLE 5.   **Preparticipation Physical Examination of Michigan State Universty** *(Continued)*

PHYSICAL EXAMINATION *(to be completed by physician)*

Blood Pressure _____ Pulse _____ Height _____ Weight _____
Vision R 20/_____ L 20/_____ corrected Y / N

	Nml	Abnml	Comments
HEENT	( )	( )	_____
Thyroid	( )	( )	_____
Lymphatics	( )	( )	_____
Cardiac	( )	( )	_____
Lungs	( )	( )	_____
Skin	( )	( )	_____
Abdominal	( )	( )	_____
Genitalia	( )	( )	_____
Tanner stage (circle)			1 2 3 4 5
Musculoskeletal:			
Neck	( )	( )	_____
Shoulder	( )	( )	_____
Elbow	( )	( )	_____
Wrist, hand	( )	( )	_____
Back	( )	( )	_____
Knee	( )	( )	_____
Ankle, foot	( )	( )	_____

Other: _____

I certify that I have reviewed the history and examined the above student and recommend sports activity:

  clearance with no limitations _____
  clearance pending further evaluation or testing _____
  referral to _____ prior to clearance
  clearance with limitations _____
  disqualified from competition _____

Signature of examining physician _____ Date _____

2. It should not be performed so far ahead of a season that new problems are likely to develop in the interim. Conducting the examination roughly 4 to 6 weeks before the season is a reasonable and appropriate approach.

History

A specific, thorough history is the cornerstone of all medical evaluations, and the preparticipation examination is no exception. In the study by Goldberg et al.[22] of 701 athletes, 78% of those disqualified from sports participation had abnormalities detected through the history. The history should be focused to cover the cardiovascular, musculoskeletal, and neurologic systems, but it should also include questions that pertain to additional sports-related concerns, such as eating disorders, exercise-related bronchospasm, menstrual dysfunction, social and ergogenic drug use, and thermoregulatory dysfunction.

Cardiovascular System

In terms of the cardiovascular system, the important historical questions relate to the occurrence of **sudden cardiac death.** Roughly 5 in 100,000 young athletes have a condition that makes them vulnerable, and 10% of these, or 1 in 200,000 athletes, will experience sudden cardiac death.[15] Studies show that exercise increases the risk.[42] Thompson estimated that in athletes older than 40 years, there is 1 death for every 396,000 jogging hours.[52] In young athletes sudden cardiac death is rare, but always tragic and devastating for everyone involved. Every attempt should be made to detect abnormalities that may put the young athlete at risk for sudden cardiac death. In athletes less than 30 years old, the causes are most often related to structural cardiovascular abnormalities.[39] Maron's study of sudden cardiac death described structural cardiovascular abnormalities such as hypertrophic cardiomyopathy, anomalous origin of the left coronary artery, atherosclerotic disease, and ruptured aorta.[37] The causes of sudden cardiac death in a recent

TABLE 6. **Intercurrent Preparticipation Examination**

Master problem list	Date identified	Date resolved
1.		
2.		
3.		
4.		

Date of entrance physical examination _____

Past medical history: Since your initial preparticipation physical examination have you had any of the following (If yes, please explain what, where, and when):

	Y	N	Comments
1. Presently taking medication (include over-the-counter and birth-control pills)?	( )	( )	_____
2. Allergic to medicine, foods, bee stings?	( )	( )	_____
3. Wearing any *new* appliances—glasses, contacts, dentures, hearing aids?	( )	( )	_____
4. *New* medical problem requiring treatment or medication?	( )	( )	_____
5. Surgical operations or accidents?	( )	( )	_____
6. Injuries related to sports participation?	( )	( )	_____
7. Fainting or dizziness with exercise?	( )	( )	_____
8. Head injury or loss of consciousness?	( )	( )	_____
9. Date of last menstrual period (females)	( )	( )	_____

Review of Systems

Please check if you have developed any *new* problems to the following areas of your body since your last examination.

_____ Skin	_____ Neck	_____ Genital (include menstrual
_____ Head	_____ Lungs	for women
_____ Eyes	_____ Heart	_____ Knees
_____ Mouth/throat	_____ Abdomen	_____ Shoulders, arms, hands
_____ Nutrition/weight control	_____ Urination/bowel	_____ Hip, ankle, foot
_____ Blood	_____ Emotional	_____ Muscle strength

I would like to meet with the team physician _____

I certify that the above information is correct to the best of my knowledge.

Student/parent signature _____ Date _____

Physical Examination (to be completed by physician)

Vital Signs _____
Height _____ Weight _____
Blood pressure _____ Heart rate _____
Visual acuity R 20/_____ L20/_____ Corrected Y / N
Other testing _____ _____

Review by medical staff
   clearance with no limitations _____
   clearance pending further evaluation or testing _____
   referral to _____ prior to clearance
   clearance with limitations _____
   disqualified from competition _____

Signature of examining physician _____ Date _____

---

review[6] are summarized in Table 7. The predominant cause in older athletes is coronary artery disease.

Hypertrophic cardiomyopathy or idiopathic hypertrophic subaortic stenosis leads to symptoms and sudden death from hypertrophy associated with a decrease in heart chamber size and subsequent impairment of diastolic filling. The hypertrophy of the subaortic septum as well as anterior motion of the mitral valve during systole leads to obstruction of the outflow tract.[33] The ultimate etiology of sudden death is believed to be a malignant arrhythmia.

It is extremely important to attempt to identify these patients during the preparticipation examination because their presentation is often sudden cardiac death. Maron[35] found in his series of 78 patients that 40% were involved in exercise prior to their death. Symptoms, when present, included fatigue, syncope, palpitations, or severe dyspnea, es-

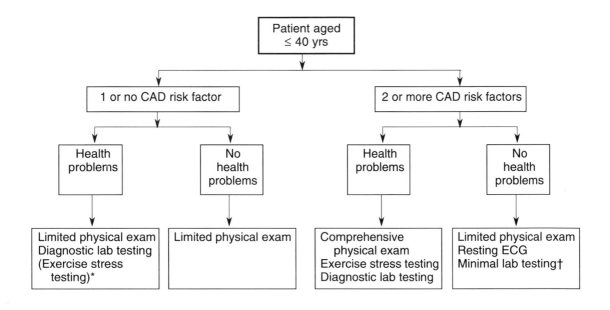

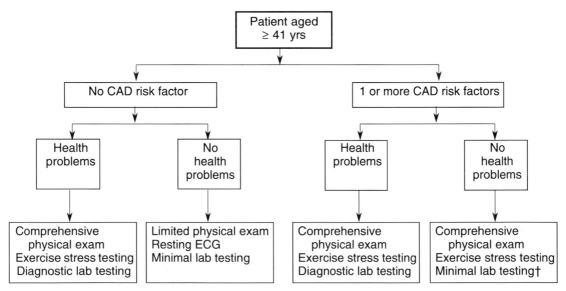

FIGURE 2. Recommended algorithm for the office-based preparticipation physical examination. *Risk factors* forcoronary artery disease (CAD) include hypertension, smoking, diabetes, hypercholesterolemia, previous coronaryartery disease, strong family history, and obesity or sedentary lifestyle. *Health problems* include cardiopulmonarydisease, neurologic disease, endocrinopathy, musculoskeletal disorder, psychiatric disorder, renal or hepatic disease,anemia, current drug use, and other chronic or acute diseases.

*Exercise stress testing is recommended if the patient has cardiopulmonary disease.

†Diagnostic laboratory testing is indicated if coronary heart disease risk factors include hyperlipidemia, hyperglycemia, or hyperuricemia.

Diagnostic laboratory testing can include fasting chemical survey, complete blood count, urinalysis, and lipid profile. Minimal laboratory testing can include chemical survey. (Adapted from Taylor RB: Pre-exercise evaluation: Which procedures are really needed? *Consultant* (Apr) 94–101, 1983; with permission.)

TABLE 7. **Causes of Sudden Death in Athletes**

Condition	Incidence (%)
Age 30 Years or Younger	
Anomalous coronary arteries	20.9
Hypertrophic cardiomyopathy	19.6
Coronary artery disease	9.0
Myocarditis	5.7
Conduction system abnormalities	4.4
Heatstroke	7.0
Sickle cell trait	3.8
Concentric left ventricular hypertrophy	3.2
Mitral valve prolapse	1.9
Aortic stenosis	1.3
Myocardial infarction without coronary artery disease	0.6
Other causes	10.1
Unknown	9.5
Age 40 Years or Older	
Coronary artery disease	88.7
Anomalous coronary arteries	4.2
Myocardial infarction without coronary artery disease	—
Hypertrophic cardiomyopathy	—
Myocarditis	7.1
Mitral valve prolapse	—
Mitral stenosis with left ventricular hypertrophy	—

pecially if associated with exertion. Because hypertrophic cardiomyopathy is an autosomal-dominant disorder, family history is extremely important. Maron found that 25% of patients with sudden cardiac death and hypertrophic cardiomypathy had a history of a sudden nontraumatic death of at least one parent or sibling <50 years of age.[36]

Numerous **coronary artery abnormalities** have been found to play a causative role in sudden cardiac death in young athletes. The most common abnormality is anomalous origin of the left coronary artery from the right sinus of Valsalva or from the right coronary artery itself. "Pistol Pete" Maravich, the 40-year-old former professional basketball player, died suddenly during a pick-up basketball game. At autopsy, he was found to have a single coronary artery and marked cardiac hypertrophy. The symptoms of aberrant coronary circulation are due to an inability of the coronary arteries to meet the increased cardiac demands of exercise (i.e., myocardial ischemia). The demands of exercise often lead to concentric hypertrophy of the myocardium, which further increases myocardial oxygen demand and can exacerbate the ischemia of aberrant circulation. Patients typically complain of exertional chest pain and syncope.

The other major cause of sudden cardiac death in young individuals is **cystic medial necrosis** of the aorta, which can result in aor-

TABLE 8. **Major Features of Marfan's Syndrome**

Family history
Cardiovascular abnormalities
  Cystic medial necrosis
  Aortic dilatation
  Aortic aneurysm
  Aortic dissection
  Aortic insufficiency
  Mitral valve prolapse
  Mitral regurgitation
Musculoskeletal abnormalities
  Kyphoscoliosis
  Anterior thorax deformities
    Pectus excavatum, pectus carinatum
  Tall, with limb length > trunk length
  Arachnodactyly
  Spina bifida
  Spondylolisthesis
Ocular disorders
  Ectopia lentis
  Myopia
  Iridodonesis

tic rupture. This condition is most prevalent in persons with **Marfan's syndrome,** an autosomal-dominant disorder characterized by generalized degeneration of connective tissue. Two of the four major features of Marfan's syndrome (Table 3) are needed to make the diagnosis:

1. Family history of Marfan's syndrome,
2. Cardiovascular abnormalities,
3. Musculoskeletal abnormalities, and
4. Ocular abnormalities.

A family history is present in 85% of patients.[42] Musculoskeletal abnormalities occur in virtually all patients and often provide the initial clue to the diagnosis. Arachnodactyly is present in 88% of patients and ocular disorders in 79%. The cardiac manifestations, which are the ultimate cause of sudden cardiac death, are present in virtually all patients by the third or fourth decade of life. The classic lesion is cystic medial necrosis that leads to a dilated aortic root. The three abnormalities that together account for 90% of deaths in patients with Marfan's syndrome are ruptured aortic aneurysm, aortic dissection, and severe aortic insufficiency. Patients with Marfan's syndrome may present with arrhythmias or with complaints of chest pain or syncope, either at rest or with exertion.

Atherosclerotic coronary artery disease rarely causes sudden cardiac death in the young athlete but accounts for almost 90% of cases in athletes over 30 years of age. In a study of 95 college football players, risk factors for coronary artery disease were assessed along with lipid profile, percent body fat, blood pressure, and aerobic capacity. Offensive linemen were found to have an overall increased risk for coronary heart disease.[41] It is important to consider the risk factors for coronary artery disease in prospective athletes and to review potential symptoms (Table 9). Symptoms of myocardial ischemia may be classic, such as chest pain or tightness with exertion, but often they are more vague, such as nausea and malaise with exercise, shoulder pain with exertion, syncope or near-syncope with exertion, or fatigue out of proportion to exercise. In diabetics, these symptoms may be masked, and "silent" ischemia may occur. If indicated by the history, further laboratory or diagnostic testing may be indicated.

TABLE 9. Risk Factors for Coronary Artery Disease

Hypertension
Diabetes mellitus
Previous coronary artery disease
Family history of premature coronary
  artery disease (<50 yrs)
Smoking history
Increased age
Male gender
Obesity
Sedentary lifestyle

Neurologic System

The second crucial part of the history involves the neurologic system. Although it is relatively easy to determine if previous neurologic injury has occurred, the natural history of neurologic injury in sports has yet to be fully elucidated. Many of the guidelines used in the past are based on anecdotal and commonsense practices, with little objective data to support them. Nonetheless, it is important to determine and to quantitate prior neurologic injury in the athlete. Gerberich[21] found that after a player sustains a first concussion, the chance of incurring a second concussion is more than four times greater than in a player who has never sustained a concussion. The "second impact syndrome," reported by Saunders and Harbaugh,[50] involves a second head trauma before full recovery from a previous one. This syndrome can lead to edema of the brain and possible death. Questions in the preparticipation examination need to address previous neurologic injury, including concussions, neck injuries, brachial plexus injuries ("burners" or "stingers"), and seizure disorders and their control, as well as any ongoing neurologic symptoms or postconcussive sequelae.

Musculoskeletal System

The last section of the preparticipation examination that needs to be discussed is the musculoskeletal system. It is important to consider any history of previous injury, surgery, fractures, or stress injury. If the older individual gives a history of significant morning stiffness, joint pain, or other rheumatologic symptoms, further testing may be indicated.

Other important historical issues include prior and current medical conditions, medication and drug use, missing organs, allergies, special devices or appliances used, and most recent tetanus booster.

Physical Examination

The physical examination should be short and should focus on the cardiovascular and musculoskeletal examination. Because of the low prevalence of disqualifying conditions among young athletes and the frequent lack of significant physical findings for such conditions, sensitivity is very low.[49] The conditions

TABLE 10. Review of Previous Studies of Conditions Causing Disqualification
of the Young Athlete

Study	No. of Subjects	No. Who Failed and Conditions Cited
Goldberg et al.[22]	701	9 (1.3%) 5 Knee instability 1 Recurrent concussions 1 Syncope with exercise, significant murmur 1 Recent femur fracture 1 Scoliosis
Thompson et al.[53]	2,382	31 (1.2%) 7 Significant heart murmurs 3 Undescended testicle 2 Patellofemoral syndrome 2 Postinjury spinal pain 2 Acute ankle instability 15 "other"
Magnes et al.[32]	10,540	47 (0.4%) 19 High blood pressure 6 Ophthalmic (blindness in one eye, retinal surgery) 5 Genitourinary (absent testicle, testicle mass) 4 Neurologic (concussion, intracranial bleeding) 2 Recent mononucleosis with splenomegaly 1 Morbid obesity 2 Musculoskeletal (unstable knee, unstable shoulder) 1 Congenital heart abnormality 1 Skin infection 1 Gynecologic (pregnancy) 1 Pulmonary (asthma) 1 Endocrinologic (abnormal glucose) 6 Irretrievable data

that may result in disqualification from participation are summarized in Table 10.

The physical examination should include measurements of height, weight, blood pressure, and heart rate. An assessment of visual acuity is important, and any pupil irregularity or asymmetry should be noted. It is important to recognize that the preparticipation physical examination can and should be sport- specific. Therefore, the otoscopic examination may be more important in a swimmer than in a tennis player. Likewise, a skin abnormality, such as herpes gladiotorum, is more important to recognize in a wrestler than in a golfer.

Cardiac screening often results in the detection of innocent flow murmurs. A systolic murmur accentuated by maneuvers that *decrease* left ventricular volume should raise concern, because it occurs in both hypertrophic cardiomyopathy (or idiopathic hypertrophic subaortic stenosis) and mitral regurgitation. A helpful screening maneuver is to listen to the murmur while the patient moves from a standing to a squatting position. This maneuver reduces the outflow obstruction and causes the pathological murmur to diminish, whereas innocent murmurs become louder.

All diastolic murmurs and a second heart sound that does not split should also be considered abnormal. A holosystolic murmur should raise the possibility of a ventricular septal defect. Some of the abnormalities of the cardiovascular examination in Marfan's syndrome and hypertrophic cardiomyopathy (or IHSS) are summarized in Table 11.

The musculoskeletal examination should focus on range of motion, strength of major muscle groups, and joint stability. A useful screen for musculoskeletal abnormalities is outlined in Table 12. The musculoskeletal examination should again be sport-specific and attempt to identify areas of weakness that may predispose an athlete to injury in a particular sport. If there are muscle imbalances, inflexibility, or strength deficits, a specific program can be initiated prior to participation. An assessment of the neurologic system with documentation of any preexisting abnormalities should be part of the examination.

Finally, in young athletes, Tanner staging should also be performed, with evaluation of secondary sexual characteristics (Table 13). Prospective studies by McKeag[40] have indicated that inappropriate maturational match-

TABLE 11. **Cardiovascular Abnormalities on Physical Examination in Conditions Causing Sudden Cardiac Death**

Idiopathic hypertrophic subaortic stenosis or Hypertrophic obstructive cardiomyopathy	Jugular venous pulse with prominent α wave
	Carotid pulse; short duration, brisk upstroke, often bifid (67%)
	Systolic ejection murmur at left lower sternal border (classic) murmur *increases* with standing, expiration, second and third phases of the Valsalva maneuver, *decreases* with squatting, inspiration
	Fourth heart sound at apex
Marfan's syndrome	Early ejection sound
	Aortic regurgitant murmur at right upper sternal border
	?Mitral valve prolapse with mitral regurgitant murmur
Aortic stenosis	Large α wave with severe aortic stenosis
	Narrow pulse pressure
	Systolic thrill at base of heart
	Apex beat displaced inferiorly and laterally (left ventricular hypertrophy)
	Early systolic ejection murmur
	Paradoxic splitting S2 (severe aortic stenosis)
	Fourth heart sound
Anomalous coronary artery	Mitral regurgitation sometimes present secondary to papillary muscle ischemia or infarction
	Examination often normal

TABLE 12. **Musculoskeletal Physical Examination**

Athletic Activity (Instructions)	Observations
1. Stand facing examiner	Acromioclavicular joints; general habitus
2. Look at ceiling, floor, over both shoulders, touch ears to shoulder	Cervical spine motion
3. Shrug shoulders (against resistance)	Trapezius strength
4. Abduct shoulders 90° (examiner resists at 90°)	Deltoid strength
5. Full external rotation of arms	Shoulder motion
6. Flex and extend elbows	Elbow motion
7. Arms at sides, elbows at 90° flexed; pronate and supinate	Elbow and wrist motion
8. Spread fingers; make fist	Hand and finger motion and deformities
9. Tighten (contract) quadriceps; relax quadriceps	Symmetry and knee effusion, ankle effusion
10. "Duck walk" 4 steps	Hip, knee and ankle motion
11. Back to examiner	Shoulder symmetry, scoliosis
12. Knees straight, touch toes	Scoliosis, hip motion, hamstring tightness
13. Raise up on toes, heels	Calf symmetry, leg strength

ing of athletes during high-school competition constitutes a major risk factor for subsequent injury in youth sports.

THE "ATHLETE'S HEART"

As early as 1899, Henschen "with the aid of only chest percussion demonstrated that the hearts of cross-country skiers were larger than those of sedentary individuals and that the athletes with the biggest hearts were those who won races."[56] The clinical and structural cardiac changes seen in the well-trained athlete depend, to some extent, on the kind of exercise performed. The two extremes are *dynamic exercise,* mostly isotonic, as in mara-

thon runners, and *static exercise,* mostly isometric, as in weight-lifters.

On physical examination, athletes who participate in dynamic exercise characteristically have bradycardia, increased stroke volume, and left ventricular hypertrophy. The second heart sound is often high-pitched and widely split. Because of augmentation of diastolic filling, and third heart sound is common. In 20 to 50% of athletes, a fourth heart sound is present, although this is more common in athletes participating in static exercise. A fourth heart sound is a cause for concern, because it can be heard in patients with hypertrophic cardiomyopathy or hypertension, both of which represent a stiff, noncompliant ventricle. The corresponding radiographic changes in the athlete's heart include an in-

TABLE 13.   Maturity Staging Guidelines for Boys and Girls

Boys Stage	Pubic Hair	Penis	Testis
1	Preadolescent (none)	——	——
2	Slight, long, slight pigmentation	Enlargement	Enlarged scrotum, pink, some ruga
3	Darker, starts to curl, small amount	Longer	Larger
4	Coarse, curly, adult type, small amount	Increase in size of glans, breadth of penis	Larger, scrotum darker
5	Adult, spread to inner thighs	Adult	

Girls Stage	Pubic Hair	Breasts
1	Preadolescent (none)	Preadolescent (no germinal button)
2	Sparse, lightly pigmented, straight medial border of labia	Breast and papilla elevated as small mound; areolar diameter increased
3	Darker, beginning to curl, increased	Breast and areola enlarged; no contour separation
4	Course, curly, abundant but less than adult	Areola papilla form secondary mound
5	Adult female triangle and spread to inner thighs	Mature, nipple projects, areola part of general breast contour

Adapted from Tanner JM: *Growth at Adolescence,* 2nd ed. Oxford, Blackwell Scientific Publications, 1962, pp 28–39; with permission.

creased cardiac silhouette, often described as a globular shape, and a cardiothoracic index greater than 0.5.

The electrocardiogram (ECG) can demonstrate changes due to prolonged and intense training. As with radiography, the findings are not always specific. Sinus bradycardia, junctional rhythms, first- and type-I second-degree block have been seen more frequently in athletes than in sedentary individuals[26,55] Similarly, ST-segment and T-wave abnormalities have been seen in athletes.[5,57] Voltage changes are commonly found in athletes. Both left and right ventricular hypertrophy have been described (using the criterion of Sokolow and Lyon[23]). Increased P-wave amplitude and notching have also been noted.[54] The ECG abnormalities seen in athletes often disappear with exercise.

Echocardiography allows noninvasive detection of such conditions as hypertrophic cardiomyopathy (or idiopathic hypertrophic subaortic stenosis), mitral valve prolapse, aortic root dilatation, and valvular lesions. Pellicia et al.[45] performed echocardiography in 947 elite athletes from a variety of sports. The thickness of the left ventricular wall was found to be greater than 13 mm (consistent with the diagnosis of hypertrophic cardiomyopathy) in only 16 (1.7%) of the athletes, most of whom were training in rowing sports. The highest value was 16 mm. All of these athletes had a large ventricular cavity (greater than 54 mm).

The authors concluded that a left ventricular wall thickness greater than 16 mm and hypertrophy in the setting of a small ventricular cavity should be considered abnormal.

The ratio of the thickness of the interventricular septum to the thickness of the left ventricular posterior wall (normally 1.3:1) has been used to define pathologic conditions. This ratio can be increased in athletes. It has been suggested that a better criterion is the ratio of the width of the interventricular septum to the left ventricular end-systolic diameter, with a value of 0.48 or more suggesting abnormality.[26]

The hypertrophic cardiomyopathy that most physicians recognize as a cause of sudden cardiac death is usually asymmetric, but assymetry can no longer be used as an exclusive criterion to differentiate pathologic from physiologic conditions. Sudden cardiac death has been reported in idiopathic concentric hypertrophy, although it is relatively uncommon.[7,34]

In summary, physiologic changes that occur in the heart in response to exercise training can sometimes be difficult to differentiate from pathologic conditions. Because these conditions are among the major causes of sudden cardiac death in athletes, it is important to pay particular attention to the historical questions and examination findings that might merit further testing. It is important to be familiar with some of the ECG "abnormalities" that are commonly seen in athletes and represent physiologic rather than pathologic changes. In patients with hypertrophic cardiomyopathy, 90% have an abnormal ECG[35]; the most sensitive diagnostic tool in this condition, as well as many others, is the echocardiogram.

ADDITIONAL TESTING AND EVALUATION

In the absence of a specific indication for laboratory testing, routine blood or urine testing is of little benefit.[49] In children, proteinuria is benign in all but 0.08% of cases.[44] Because exercise routinely produces trace amounts of hematuria and proteinuria, a dipstick urinalysis is not generally helpful.[22] Additional testing should take into account the individual athlete in terms of age, gender, anticipated exercise activity, and goals. In particular, the historical section of the preparticipation examination can help to determine what, if any, additional testing is required. In the presence of a strong family history of hypertrophic cardiomyopathy or Marfan's syndrome, further evaluation with an ECG and echocardiogram may be warranted. In women with a history of menstrual dysfunction, further evaluation should be considered, and the additional health screen questionnaire can help to direct these studies. In young individuals with a strong family history of coronary artery disease or hypercholesterolemia, careful attention to blood pressure is important. Obtaining a lipid profile is often helpful in such cases. In the older individual, a lipid profile and exercise testing may be a routine part of the comprehensive examination (see Figure 2). If abnormalities are detected in the physical examination, further testing or consultation may be indicated. The decision to obtain further testing should be tailored to the individual and directed by the history and physical findings.

ASSESSMENT

The assessment made at the conclusion of the preparticipation examination should be specific to the individual. Five major categories of recommendations can be made:

1. Clearance without limitations;
2. Clearance pending further investigation;
3. Clearance pending consultation;
4. Clearance with limitations; and
5. Disqualification or contraindication to participate.

Some abnormalities can be clarified by further testing or consultation, and others require surgery or rehabilitation prior to reevaluation. In terms of cardiovascular abnormalities, the sixteenth Bethesda Conference in 1984 remains the "gold standard" for recommendations,[58] including recommendations for further testing and limitation to different types of activities in accordance with the results. Although these recommendations have been criticized because of their overall conservatism, without good information regarding the natural history of some of these abnormalities, they remain the standard of care. The recommendations must be individualized and are usually made in conjunction with a consulting cardiologist. As more and more success is obtained with the repair of congenital heart disease, the information regarding natural history will certainly grow, and new recommendations may allow safer participation.

Many abnormalities that are detected may not necessarily preclude sports participation. For example, the patient with a renal contusion may be at risk for losing a kidney if he or she sustains a blow to the damaged kidney, yet the probability of such a blow is rather small; moreover, even if it were to occur, the probability of losing the kidney would also be small. These probabilities are difficult to predict, because so few data are available. In this situation, the physician must present to the athlete, or if the athlete is a minor, to the athlete and his or her parent or guardian, the potential risks of participation as they are known, along with recommendations. The athlete can then decide whether to take the risk. Written documentation of the conversation, recommendations, and decision of the athlete (and parents), along with signatures of the involved parties, is important.

The conditions that constitute absolute or relative contraindications for specific sports activity tend to fall into six major categories: (1) neurologic, (2) defects in paired organ systems, (3) organ enlargement, (4) active infection, (5) vertebral/pelvic defect, and (6) cardiopulmonary disorder. The decisions and recommendations are difficult to make, especially when certain absolute risks can be potentially harmful. In general, physicians need to be familiar with the risks of specific sports and conditions to provide pertinent information to the athlete.

Copies of the preparticipation examination should be distributed to the school physician or nurse, the parents, the primary-care physician, the team physician, and the team trainer so that a record is available at all practices and competitions.

CONCLUSION

The preparticipation examination for potential athletes of any age represents a special physician–patient interaction in which many important factors need to be considered. The assessment should be tailored to meet the needs of the individual as well as the main objectives of the examination. It should detect significant abnormalities that put the individual at increased risk of injury or cardiac event. Finally, it should provide an opportunity to introduce the individual to the health care system and to provide education. If done in a thorough and objective manner, with these guidelines in mind, the assessment will allow successful athletic participation for almost all individuals.

REFERENCES

1. Anderson W, Albrecht R, McKeag DB, et al: A national survey of alcohol and drug use by college athletes. *Phys Sportsmed* 19(2):91–104, 1991.
2. American College of Sports Medicine Publications: The female athlete triad—A closer look. *Sports Med Bull* 27(4):4, 1992.
3. Barrow GW, Saha S: Menstrual irregularity and stress fractures in collegiate female distance runners. *Am J Sports Med* 16:209–216, 1988.
4. Bullen BA, Skrinar GS, Bertins IZ, et al: Induction of menstrual disorders by strenuous exercise in untrained women. *N Eng J Med* 312:1349–1353, 1983.
5. Caselli G, Piovano G, Vernando A: A follow-up study of abnormalities of ventricular repolarization in athletes. In Lubich T, Vernando A (eds): *Sports Cardiology*. Bologna, Aulo Gaggi, 1980, pp 477–99.
6. Chillag S, Bates M, Voltin R, Jones D: Sudden death: Myocardial infarction in a runner with normal coronary arteries. *Phys Sportsmed* 18(3):89–94, 1990.
7. Craven CM: Sudden death in a young athlete: A case report. *Am J Sports Med* 20:621–623, 1992.
8. De Souza MJ, Maguire MS, Rubin D, Maresh CM: Effects of menstrual phase and amenorrhea on exercise responses in runners. *Med Sci Sports Exerc* 22:575–580, 1990.
9. Dibrezzo R, Fort IL, Brown B: Relationships among strength, endurance, weight and body fat during three phases of the menstrual cycle. *J Sports Med Phys Fitness* 31(1):89–94, 1991.
10. Drinkwater BL, Bremmer B, Chestnut CH III: Menstrual history as a determinant of current bone density in young athletes. *JAMA* 263:545–548, 1990.
11. Drinkwater BL, Nilson K, Chestnut CH III, et al: Bone mineral content of amenorrheic and eumenorrheic athletes. *N Eng J Med* 311:277–281, 1984.
12. Drinkwater BL, Nilson K, et al: Bone mineral density after resumption of menses in amenorrheic athletes. *JAMA* 256:380–382, 1986.
13. Dummer GM, Rosen LW, Heusner WW, et al: Pathogenic weight-control behaviors of young competitive swimmers. *Phys Sportsmed* 15(5):75–84, 1987.
14. Dyment PG: Another look at the sports preparticipation examination of the adolescent athlete. *J Adolesc Health Care.* 7(suppl 16):130s–132s, 1986.
15. Epstein SE, Maron BJ: Sudden death and the competitive athlete: Perspectives on preparticipation screening studies. *J Am Coll Cardiol* 7:220–230, 1986.
16. Fiatarone MA, Marks EC, Ryan DT, et al: High-intensity strength training in nonagenarians; Effects on skeletal muscle. *JAMA* 263:3029–3034, 1990.
17. Fields KB, Delaney M: Focusing the preparticipation sports examination. *J Fam Pract* 30:304–312, 1990.
18. Frisch RE, Gotz-Welbergen AV, McArthur JW: Delayed menarche and amenorrhea of college athletes in relation to age of onset of training. *JAMA* 246:1559–1563, 1981.
19. Gadpaille WJ, Sanborn CF, Wagner WW: Athletic amenorrhea, major affective disorders, and eating disorders. *Am J Psychiatry* 144:939–942, 1987.
20. Garrick JG, Smith NJ: Preparticipation sports assessment. *Pediatrics* 66:803–806, 1980.
21. Gerberich SG, Priest JD, Boen JR, et al: Concussion incidence and severity in secondary school varsity football players. *Am J Public Health* 73:1370–1375, 1983.
22. Goldberg B, Saraniti A, Witman P, et al: Preparticipation sports assessment: An objective evaluation. *Pediatrics* 66:736–745, 1980.
23. Hanne-Paparo N, Drory Y, Schoenfeld Y, et al: Common ECG changes in athletes. *Cardiology* 61:267–278, 1976.
24. Henschen K, Griffin L: Quoated in "Parent egos take the fun out of little league." *Psychol Today*, 1977, pp 18–22.
25. Hough DO, McKeag DM: Preparticipation examination results. Michigan State University (unpublished data), 1982.
26. Huston TP, Puffer JC, Rodney WM: The athletic heart syndrome. *N Eng J Med* 313(1):24–32, 1985.
27. Johnson MD: Tailoring the preparticipation exam to female athletes. *Phys Sportsmed* 20(7):61–72, 1992.
28. Kadel NJ, Teitz CC, Kronmal RA: Stress fractures in ballet dancers. *Am J Sports Med* 20:445–449, 1992.
29. Licata AA: Stress fractures in young athletic women: Case reports of unsuspected cortisol-induced osteoporosis. *Med Sci Sports Exerc* 24:955–957, 1992.
30. Linder CW, DuRant RH, Seklecki RM, et al: Preparticipation health screening of young athletes: Results of 1268 examinations. *Am J Sports Med* 9:187–193, 1981.
31. Lombardo JA: Preparticipation physical examination. *Prim Care Clin* 11:3–21, 1984.
32. Magnes SA, Henderson JM, Hunter SC: What conditions limit sports participation? Experience with 10,540 athletes. *Phys Sportsmed* 20(5):143–160, 1992.

33. Maron BJ, Bonow RO, Cannon RO, et al: Hypertrophic cardiomyopathy: Interrelations of clinical manifestations, pathophysiology, and therapy. *N Eng J Med* 316:780–789, 1987.
34. Maron BJ, Epstein SE, Roberts WC: Causes of sudden death in competitive athletes. *J Am Coll Cardiol* 7:204–214, 1986.
35. Maron BJ, Roberts WC, Epstein SE: Sudden death in hypertrophic cardiomyopathy: A profile of 78 patients. *Circulation* 65:1388–1394, 1982.
36. Maron BJ, Roberts WWC, Edwards JE, et al: Sudden death in patients with hypertrophic cardiomyopathy: Characterization of 26 patients with functional limitation. *Am J Cardiol* 41:532–538, 1978.
37. Maron BJ, Roberts WC, McAllister HA, et al: Sudden death in young athletes. *Circulation* 62:218–229, 1980.
38. Martens R: The uniqueness of the young athlete: Psychological considerations. *Am J Sports Med* 8:382–385, 1980.
39. McCaffrey FM, Braden DS, Strong WB: Sudden cardiac death in young athletes. *Am J Dis Child* 145:177–183, 1991.
40. McKeag DB: Preseason physical examination for the prevention of sports injuries. *Sports Med* 2:413–431, 1985.
41. Millard-Stafford M, Rosskoph LB, Sparling PB: Coronary heart disease: Risk profiles of college football players. *Phys Sportsmed* 17(9):151–163, 1989.
42. Missri JC, Swett DD: Marfan's syndrome: A review. *Cardiovas Rev Rep* 3:1645–1653, 1982.
43. Myburgh KH, Hutchins J, Fataar AB, et al: Low bone density is an etiologic factor for stress fractures in athletes. *Ann Intern Med* 113:754–759, 1990.
44. Peggs JF, Reinhardt RW, O'Brien JM: Proteinuria in adolescent sports physical examination. *J Fam Pract* 22:80–81, 1986.
45. Pelliccia A, Maron BJ, Spataro A, et al: The upper limit of physiologic cardiac hypertrophy in highly trained elite athletes. *N Eng J Med* 324:295–301, 1991.
46. Risser WL, Hoffman HM, Bellah GG Jr, et al: A cost-benefit analysis of preparticipation sports examinations of adolescent athletes. *J School Health* 55:270–273, 1985.
47. Risser WL, Hoffman HM, Bellah GG Jr: Frequency of preparticipation sports examination in secondary school athletes: Are the university interscholastic league guidelines appropriate? *Texas Med* 81:35–39, 1985.
48. Rosen LW, McKeag DB, Hough DO, Curley V: Pathogenic weight-control behavior in female athletes. *Phys Sportsmed* 15:79–86, 1986.
49. Runyan DK: The preparticipation examination of young athletes: Defining the essentials. *Clin Pediatr* 22:674–679, 1983.
50. Saunders RL, Harbaugh RE: The second impact in catastrophic contact-sports head trauma. *JAMA* 252:538–539, 1984.
51. Tennant FS Jr., Sorenson K, Day CM: Benefits of preparticipation sports examinations. *J Fam Pract* 13:287–288, 1981.
52. Thompson PD, Funk EJ, Carleton RA, et al: Incidence of death during jogging in Rhode Island from 1975 through 1980. *JAMA* 247:2535–2538, 1982.
53. Thompson TR, Andrish JT, Bergfeld JA: A prospective study of preparticipation sports examinations of 2670 young athletes: Methods and results. *Cleve Clin Q* 49:225–233, 1982.
54. Venerando A, Rulli V: Frequency, morphology, and meaning of the electrocardiographic anomalies found in olympic marathon runners and walkers. *J Sports Med* 3:135–141, 1964.
55. Zehender M, Meinertz T, Keul J, Just H: ECG variants and cardiac arrhythmias in athletes: Clinical relevance and prognostic importance. *Am Heart J* 119:1378–1391, 1990.
56. Zeppelli P: The athlete's heart: Differentiation of training effects from organic heart disease. *Prac Cardiol* 14(8):61–84, 1988.
57. Zeppilli P, Pirrami MM, Sassara M, Fenici R: Ventricular repolarization disturbances in athetes: Standardization of terminology, ethiopathogenetic spectrum and pathophysiologic mechanisms. *J Sports Med Phys Fitness* 21:322–335, 1981.
58. 16th Bethesda Conference: Cardiovascular abnormalities in the athlete. Recommendations regarding eligibility for competition. *J Am Coll Cardiol* 6:1186–1232, 1985.

Chapter 2

TISSUE INJURY AND HEALING: Using Medications, Modalities, and Exercise to Maximize Recovery

Susan L. Hubbell, MD, and Ralph M. Buschbacher, MD

An injury is "an act that damages or hurts."[25] Inflammation is "a local response to cellular injury marked by capillary dilation, leukocyte infiltration, redness, heat, and pain that serves as a mechanism initiating the elimination of noxious agents and of damaged tissue."[25] Thus, the initial phase of the inflammatory response is helpful in tissue repair as removal of damaged tissue is started. However, the later phases of swelling, pain, and decreased mobility are detrimental to full recovery. Our goals in the treatment of injury are to allow the initial phase of the inflammatory response to occur and to control the later phases.

TYPES OF MUSCULOSKELETAL INJURIES

Tissue damage can be classified by etiology as due to either macrotrauma or repetitive microtrauma. **Macrotrauma** is acute damage due to some strong force. The patient is usually aware of the incident that caused the damage and has an abrupt onset of pain as a result. The pain can be due to either direct trauma to the area in question or indirect transmission of force to that area.

Overuse of tissue from repetitive motion, stress, or stretching can cause **microtrauma**. If,

instead of being allowed to heal, the tissues are stressed or reinjured, the healing process becomes pathologic with chronic inflammation, weakness, stress fractures, and abnormal calcification resulting. At the microscopic level, failure of collagen fiber occurs. If left untreated, repetitive microtrauma may weaken body tissues to such an extent that microtraumatic injury is likely, if not inevitable.

TISSUE HEALING

Repair of soft-tissue injury involves replacement of damaged or lost cells and extracellular matrices. Replacement can occur either by regeneration of tissue that is structurally and functionally identical to normal tissue or by development of scar tissue.[21]

The healing process has several phases,[5,22] each of which lasts a varying amount of time. The first, the acute vascular inflammatory stage, lasts from 1 to 7 days. The release of vasoactive chemical mediators such as histamine, bradykinin, and prostaglandins promotes vasodilation and increased vascular permeability. Chemotactic agents cause increased cell mobility and direct cell movements to the inflamed area. Degradative enzymes catalyze the tissue components.

The second phase, occurring on days 7 to 21, is marked by collagen proliferation. Initially, the collagen is arranged in a random pattern. Stressing of the tissue promotes alignment of the fibrils in an organized pat-

Portions of this chapter were adapted with permission from Buschbacher RM (ed): *Musculoskeletal Disorders: A Practical Guide for Diagnosis and Rehabilitation.* Stoneham, MA, Butterworth-Heinemann, 1994.

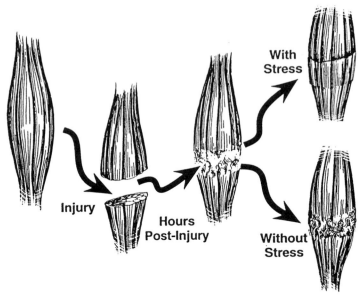

Injury

Hours
Post-Injury

With
Stress

Without
Stress

FIGURE 1.   Stress applied to a healing tendon promotes proper collagen orientation. (From Buschbacher RM (ed): *Musculoskeletal Disorders: A Practical Guide for Diagnosis and Rehabilitation.* Stoneham, MA, Butterworth-Heinemann, 1994; with permission.)

tern (Fig. 1) and also stimulates a proliferation of elastin fibrils, which limits scar formation and improves tensile strength.

The third phase involves remodeling and maturation of the new tissue and may last several months to several years. Ligaments and tendons may require 15 to 18 weeks to regain strength after immobilization is discontinued.[21]

All of the above phases are influenced by age, vascularity, nutrition, genetics, hormonal changes, innervation, and activity level.

SPECIFIC STRUCTURAL INJURY CONSIDERATIONS

Tendon and Ligament Injury

Tendons and ligaments are composed mostly of parallel collagen fibers. If they are not mobilized soon after injury (or surgery), they develop adhesions to the surrounding tissues. The loose connective tissue that ordinarily allows the tendons and ligaments to move freely turns to dense fibers that bind to the tendons and ligaments, limiting their function. Without stress from active movement, the collagen fibers remain disorganized and strength is reduced. Some ligaments, such as those in the back, must stretch to

allow proper body motion and thus contain elastin fibers. If these ligaments are immobilized and not put through an adequate range of motion, they lose their elastin. Loss of elastin decreases their strength and predisposes them to reinjury.

Ligamentous sprains are often graded as I, II, or III. Grade I injury is a microscopic tearing of the ligaments that causes pain. Joint stability is normal, but ligamentous testing causes pain. Grade II sprains involve tearing of some of the ligamentous fibers. Stability testing reveals laxity, with increased abnormal joint motion but a firm endpoint. Grade III sprains are complete disruptions of the ligaments.

Muscle Injury

A strain occurs when collagen fibers within muscles are torn. Such injuries usually heal well with little residual dysfunction. Muscles may also become contused or develop hematomas. Contusion and hematoma involve a crushing of muscle cells along with local bleeding. During healing, the injury may progress to the development of hard organized masses or even abnormally placed bone islands within the muscles. If a contused muscle is stressed too soon after injury, swelling may be aggravated and the condition worsened.

Such traumatically injured muscle should be rested until pain and acute inflammation are largely resolved. Compression and ice are useful acutely to prevent worsening of the damage.

Cartilage Injury

Cartilage may be fractured along with bone in a macrotraumatic injury. When this occurs in a joint, surgical fixation is often required. Because the normal hyaline cartilage cannot repair itself, a fibrocartilagenous scar is formed within the joint cartilage. This fibrocartilage is not as suited as a hyaline cartilage to function in a joint; therefore, future pain and degeneration may occur.

Bone Injury

Bone, like all other connective tissue, can be injured by macrotrauma or repetitive microtrauma. When macrotrauma causes a fracture, the osteoblasts within the periosteum lay down new bone in what is called a *callus*. The callus is formed and remodeled to provide complete healing of the bone.

Bone normally responds to a greater-than-average weight-bearing stress by slight resorption or weakening, followed by build-up to a level stronger than before. Thus, regular weight-bearing exercise increases bone density and creates a stronger bone. When the stressors are excessive and repeated, however, the initial slight resorption is not given enough time to heal; thus, the bone weakens and develops fracture lines, so-called *stress fractures.*

Stress fractures, like other fractures, cause the periosteum to react in an attempt to heal the defect. The fracture will heal if rested adequately, but if excessive stress is continued, the fracture will worsen. Stress fractures are common, for example, in runners who have recently increased their mileage or changed their footwear or running terrain.

INTERVENTIONS

Medications

The role of medications includes control of both pain and the inflammatory process.

Corticosteroids

Corticosteroids have a powerful anti- inflammatory effect that may disrupt the initial phases of the healing process. Corticosteroids should be avoided in the first few days after injury because their use may alter the regenerative pathways enough to impair normal healing.[10,14,24] In the later proliferative phases, corticosteroids may help to control edema and decrease a prolonged inflammatory response.[22] Local injection into a tendon sheath, bursa, or joint may be very helpful, although infiltration of the tendon itself should be avoided because it weakens the tendon, predisposing to rupture.[13] Topical corticosteroids have been administered with ultrasound (phonophoresis), with some reports claiming significant penetration of the medication in soft tissue.[9] Tables 1 and 2 list some of the most commonly used steroid preparations. Table 3 lists their associated side effects.

Nonsteroidal Antiinflammatory Drugs

Nonsteroidal antiinflammatory drugs (NSAIDs) block the production and release of prostaglandins.[12] NSAIDs have been shown to decrease pain and inflammation in the treatment of ankle sprains when given in the first 7 days after injury.[1,19] Unlike corticosteroids, NSAIDs have not been shown to delay the healing process. They are believed to be beneficial in the early days after acute injury, during rehabilitation, and in chronic overuse syndromes.[22] Patients using NSAIDs should be carefully monitored for side effects, especially gastrointestinal irritation. Topical anti-

TABLE 1. Oral Steroid Preparations Commonly Used in Musculoskeletal Disorders

Generic Name	Trade Name
Short-acting	
Cortisone	Cortone Acetate
Hydrocortisone	Cortef, Hydrocortone
Intermediate-acting	
Methylprednisolone	Medrol
Prednisolone	Delta-Cortef, Prelone
Prednisone	Deltasone, Orasone
Triamcinolone	Aristacort, Kenacort
Long-acting	
Betamethasone	Celestone
Dexamethasone	Decadron, Dexone, Hexadrol

TABLE 2.   Commonly Used Parenteral Steroid Preparations

Generic Name	Trade Name	Parenteral Administration*	
		Systemic	Local
Betamethasone			
Sodium phosphate	Celestone phosphate	IM, IV	IA, IL, ST
Acetate/sodium phosphate	Celestone Soluspan	IM	IA, IL, IS, ST
Dexamethasone			
Acetate	Decadron-LA	IM	IA, IL, ST
Sodium phosphate	Decadrol, Decadron phosphate	IM, IV	IA, IL, IS, ST
Hydrocortisone			
Sterile suspension	—	IM	
Acetate	Hydrocortone acetate		IA, IB, IL, IS, ST
Sodium phosphate	Hydrocortone phosphate	IM, IV, SC	
Sodium succinate	Solu-Cortef, A-HydroCort	IM, IV	
Methylprednisolone			
Acetate	Depo-Medrol	IM	IA, IL, ST
Sodium succinate	Solu-Medrol, A-MethaPred	IM, IV	
Prednisolone			
Acetate	Articulose-50, Predicort	IM	
Acetate/sodium phosphate	—	IM	IA, IB, IS, ST
Sodium phosphate	Hydeltrasol, Predicort RP	IM, IV	IA, IL, ST
Tebutate	Hydeltra TBA		IA, IL, ST
Triamcinolone			
Acetonide	Kenalog	IM	IA, IB, IL
Diacetate	Aristocort Forte, Triam-Forte	IM	IA,IL,IS,ST
Hexacetonide	Aristospan Intra-articular		IA, IL

*IM = intramuscular, IV = intravenous, SC = subcutaneous, IA = intraarticular, IB = intrabursal, IL = intralesional, IS= intrasynovial, ST = soft tissue

inflammatory gels have been shown to decrease pain and swelling in acute ankle sprains without systemic side effects.[6,16] Table 4 lists the commonly prescribed NSAIDs; Table 5 describes oral doses and cost; and Table 6 lists the most common side effects.

Acetylsalicylate (aspirin) should be avoided during the early phases of injury because of its antiplatelet activity, which can predispose to bleeding. This effect persists for the life of the platelet; in contrast, the antiplatelet effects of the other NSAIDs are temporary and dose-related.[8] Aspirin may be helpful in the later stages of healing for control of pain and edema.[12]

Analgesics

In acute pain due to injury, the first line of treatment is often pain control. Excessive pain leads to reflex muscle splinting and even more pain. To provide comfort, analgesics are often used along with ice and proper positioning and elevation of the injured area.

Acetaminophen is roughly equivalent to aspirin as an analgesic, but it has only weak anti-inflammatory properties. It interrupts prostaglandin-mediated pain stimuli in the central nervous system and is generally useful for treating mild- to-moderate pain. Because acetaminophen potentiates the pain-relieving properties of narcotic medications, it is available in various combinations with narcotics.

Narcotics activate or stimulate the body's own pain-control mechanisms within the central nervous system. They do not diminish awareness of pain but decrease the subjective distress of pain. The prototypical narcotic is morphine, and like morphine, the other narcotics generally have addictive qualities. The risk of addiction is small when narcotic medications are prescribed for acute pain and for short periods of time. Table 7 lists the frequently prescribed aspirin- and acetamino-

TABLE 3. Side Effects Associated with Steroid Use

Endocrine/metabolic
  Glucose intolerance
  HPA axis suppression
  Altered lipid metabolism
  Negative nitrogen balance
  Hypokalemia
  Hypercalciuria
Cardiovascular
  Hypertension
  Sodium and water retention
Central nervous system
  Euphoria
  Disorientation, confusion
  Hallucinations
  Paranoia
Musculoskeletal system
  Osteoporosis
  Growth suppression
  Aseptic necrosis of femoral head
  Myopathy
Gastrointestinal
  Nausea/vomiting
  Peptic ulcer disease(?)
  Increased appetite
Hematologic
  Leukocytosis
Immunologic
  ↓ Function of leukocytes
  ↑ Risk of infections
  May mask infections
Dermatologic
  Acne
  Striae
  Imparied wound healing
  Hypertrichosis
Ophthalmologic
  Cataracts
Allergic reactions
  Anaphylaxis
  Facial flushing
  Seizures

HPA = hypothalamo-pituitary-adrenocortical.

TABLE 4. Commonly Used Nonsteroidal Antiinflammatory Drugs

Chemical Class and Generic Name	Trade Name
Acetylated salicylates	
Aspirin	Multiple products
Nonacetylated salicylates	
Choline salicylate	Arthropan
Magnesium and choline salicylate	Trilisate
Magnesium salicylate	Magan, Mobidin, Doan's Caplets
Sodium salicylate	Multiple products
Salsalate	Disalcid
Diflunisal	Dolobid
Propionic acid derivatives	
Ibuprofen	Motrin, Rufen, Advil, more
Fenoprofen	Nalfon
Naproxen	Naprosyn, Anaprox
Ketoprofen	Orudis
Flurbiprofen	Ansaid
Ketorolac	Toradol
Pyrroleacetic acid derivatives	
Sulindac	Clinoril
Tolmetin	Tolectin
Indoleacetic acid derivatives	
Indomethacin	Indocin
Etodolac	Lodine
Anthranilic acid derivatives (fenamates)	
Mefanamic acid	Ponstel
Meclofenamate	Meclomen
Phenylacetic acid derivatives	
Diclofenac	Voltaren
Oxicams	
Piroxicam	Feldene
Pyrazolone derivatives	
Phenylbutazone	Butazolidin, Azolid

phen-narcotic products; Table 8 lists some of the most common side effects.

Oral Streptokinase-Streptodornase

Oral streptokinase-streptodornase has been tried in the early treatment of ankle sprains. Initial studies have demonstrated a decrease in pain, edema, hematoma, and analgesic intake.[3] Further studies are in progress.

Muscle Relaxants

Centrally acting muscle relaxants affect the activity of neurotransmitters in the central nervous system that help to regulate muscle tone. In general, their overall action is sedation rather than direct relaxation of muscle.[12] Nevertheless, they are often useful in treating musculoskeletal pain.

Physical Agents

Cryotherapy

Acute musculoskeletal trauma is one of the major indications for the use of cryotherapy.[5] Cold decreases blood flow, metabolic activity, and muscle tone. Cold therapy decreases edema and hemorrhage and provides analgesia. Nerve conductivity is decreased, and stretch reflexes are inhibited with deep cool-

TABLE 5. Usual Dosages and Cost of Commonly Used Oral NSAIDs

NSAID	Daily Analgesic Dose (mg)	Anti-Inflammatory Daily Dose	Daily Cost ($)
Acetylated salicylates			
Aspirin	650–975 every 4h	2.4–3.9* g	0.20
Nonacetylated salicylates			
Choline salicylate	435–870 every 4h	4.8–7.2* g	2.20
Magnesium and choline			
salicylate	2–3 g salicylate in 2–3 divided doses	1.5–4.5* g salicylate in 2–3 divided doses	3.31
Magnesium salicylate	300–600 every 4h	1.09–4.8* g	3.03
Sodium salicylate	325–650 every 4h	3.9–5.2* g	0.31
Salsalate	3000 in 2–3 divided doses	3 g in 2–3 divided doses*	0.62
Diflunisal	1000 load then 500 every 8–12h	250–500* mg twice daily	1.38
Propionic acid derivatives			
Ibuprofen	200–400 every 4–6h	1.2–3.2* g in 3–4 divided doses	1.39
Fenoprofen	200 every 4–6h	300–600* mg three or four times daily	2.85
Naproxen	500 load then 250 every 6–8h	250–500* mg twice daily	2.12
Ketoprofen	50 every 6–8h	150–300* mg in 3–4 divided doses	3.89
Flurbiprofen	50 four times daily	200–300* mg in 2–4 divided doses	3.30
Pyrroleacetic acid derivatives			
Sulindac	150–200 twice daily	150–200* mg twice daily	2.12
Tolmetin	—	600 mg–1.8* g in 3–4 divided doses	3.17
Indoleacetic acid derivatives			
Indomethacin	25–50 two to four times daily	25–50* mg two to four times daily	3.16
Etodolac	400 load then 200–400 every 6–8h	400 mg 2–3 times daily or 300 mg 3–4 times daily*	3.85
Anthranilic acid derivatives			
Mefenamic Acid	500 load then 250 every 6h*	—	3.22
Meclofenamate	50 every 4–6h	200–400* mg in 3–4 divided doses	3.61
Phenylacetic acid derivatives			
Diclofenac	—	150–200* mg in 2–4 divided doses	3.34
Oxicams			
Piroxicam	—	10 mg twice daily or 20* mg once daily	2.20
Pyrazolone derivatives			
Phenylbutazone	—	Initial: 300–600 mg in 3–4 divided doses. Maint: 100 mg 1–4 times daily*	0.62

*Dosage used to calculate cost based on average wholesale price. Source: *Redbook Drug Topics.* Oradell, NJ, Medical Economics, Inc. 1992.

TABLE 6. Common Side Effects of NSAIDs

Side Effect*	Diclofenac	Diflunisal	Fenoprofen	Flurbiprofen	Ibuprofen	Indomethacin	Etodolac	Ketoprofen	Meclofenamate	Mefenamic Acid	Naproxen	Phenylbutazone	Piroxicam	Sulindac	Tolmetin
Gastrointestinal															
Gastritis	—	1	1	1	1	—	1	1	—	—	—	1	—	1	2
Diarrhea	3	3	2	3	2	2	3	3	4	3	2	1	2	3	3
Nausea	3	3	3	3	3	3	3	3	4	3	3	3	3	3	4
Vomiting	1	2	3	2	2	2	2	2	—	—	1	1	1	2	3
CNS effects															
Headache	3	3	3	3	2	4	3	3	3	—	3	1	2	3	3
Mood changes	1	1	1	2	1	2	—	2	1	—	1	1	1	1	2
Drowsiness	1	2	3	2	1	1	2	2	—	—	3	1	2	1	2
Hepatic effects															
Hepatitis	1	1	1	1	1	1	—	1	—	1	1	1	1	1	1
↑ Liver function tests†	2	1	1	—	1	1	—	2	1	1	1	1	1	1	1
Dermatological															
Rash	2	3	3	1	3	1	1	2	3	—	3	2	2	3	2
Hives	1	1	2	1	1	1	1	1	2	—	1	1	1	—	1
Itching	2	1	3	1	2	1	1	1	2	—	3	1	2	2	2
Renal effects															
Fluid retention	3	1	2	—	2	2	—	3	2	—	3	3	2	2	3
Renal impairment	1	1	1	1	1	1	—	1	1	1	1	1	1	1	1
Cardiovascular‡															
Hypertension	1	—	—	1	1	1	—	1	—	—	—	1	1	1	3
Chest pain	1	1	—	1	—	1	—	—	—	—	—	—	—	—	2
↑ Congestive heart failure	1	—	—	1	1	1	—	1	—	—	1	1	1	1	1
Heartbeat change	1	1	3	1	1	1	1	1	1	1	2	—	1	1	—
Hematologic															
Leukopenia	1	—	—	1	1	1	1	—	1	1	1	1	2	1	—
Anemia	1	—	—	1	1	1	—	1	1	2	—	1	2	—	2
↓ Platelets	1	1	1	1	1	1	—	1	1	1	1	1	1	1	1
Ocular/otic															
Blurred vision	1	1	2	1	1	1	—	2	1	—	2	1	1	1	2
Ringing in ears	2	2	2	2	2	2	1	2	2	—	3	1	2	2	2
Hypersensitivity															
Anaphylaxis	1	1	1	1	1	1	1	1	—	—	1	1	1	1	1

*Incidence rates 4 = >10%, 3 = 3–9%, 2 = 1–3%, 1 = <1%, — = unknown.
†Greater than 3 times the upper limit of normal.
‡Cardiovascular effects may be secondary to NSAID-induced renal impairment.

TABLE 7. Frequently Used Narcotic-Analgesic Products

Trade Name	Amount of Analgesic* (mg)	Narcotic and Other Components
Aspirin/narcotic combinations		
Empirin 2	325	15 mg codeine
Empirin 3	325	30 mg codeine
Empirin 4	325	60 mg codeine
Synalgos-DC	356.4	16 mg dihydrocodeine bitartrate (30 mg caffeine)
Azdone	500	5 mg hydrocodone bitartrate
Percodan	325	4.5 mg oxycodone hydrochloride 0.38 mg oxycodone terephthalate
Talwin compound	325	12.5 mg pentazocine
Darvon with aspirin	325	65 mg propoxyphene
Darvon compound	389	32 mg propoxyphene (32.4 mg caffeine)
Darvon-N with aspirin	325	100 mg propoxyphene napsylate
Fiorinal	325	50 mg butalbital (40 mg caffeine)
Acetaminophen/narcotic combinations		
Tylenol No. 1	300	7.5 mg codeine
Tylenol No. 2	300	15 mg codeine
Tylenol No. 3	300	30 mg codeine
Tylenol No. 4	300	60 mg codeine
Lortab 5/500	500	5 mg hydrocodone bitartrate
Vicodin	500	5 mg hydrocodone bitartrate
Vicodin ES	500	7.5 mg hydrocodone bitartrate
Hydrogesic	500	5 mg hydrocodone bitartrate
Demerol-APAP	300	50 mg meperidine
Percocet	325	5 mg oxycodone
Tylox	500	5 mg oxycodone
Talacen	650	25 mg pentazocine
Darvocet-N 50	325	50 mg propoxyphene napsylate
Darvocet-N 100	650	100 mg propoxyphene napsylate
Fioricet	325	50 mg butalbital (40 mg caffeine)

*Aspirin or acetaminophen, respectively.

TABLE 8. Most Common Side Effects Associated with Narcotic Use

Gastrointestinal
  Constipation
  Nausea/vomiting
Central nervous system
  Dizziness
  Drowsiness
  Confusion
  Seizures (rare)
  Blurred or double vision
  False sense of well-being
Cardiovascular
  Hypotension
Respiratory
  Respiratory depression (with high doses)
Allergic (due to histamine release)
  Hypotension
  Flushing
  Wheezing
  Tachycardia

TABLE 9. Effects of Cryotherapy

Decreased pain
Decreased spasticity
Decreased blood flow
Decreased edema
Increased joint stiffness
Improved function in multiple sclerosis (cool pool or cold room)
Reduced damage from burns (if applied immediately)
Decreased joint inflammation
Decreased metabolic activity
Decreased nerve conduction velocity

Adapted from Kottke FJ, Lehmann JF: *Krusen's Handbook of Physical Medicine and Rehabilitation,* 4th ed. Philadelphia, W. B. Saunders, 1990.

ing. Sensory transmissions are blocked, and painful muscle splinting is decreased. Cold therapy is indicated for at least the first 48 hours after injury and should be continued after that time if persistent edema is noted and skin temperature is increased.[21] Ice should be applied in 12- to 15-minute time blocks followed by a rest period.[7,22] Cold whirlpool baths may also be prescribed. Prolonged use of cold should be avoided because of the potential for cold-induced vasodilation (hyperemia).[18]

If muscle splinting inhibits flexibility in the later stages of treatment, ice may be helpful when applied prior to stretching exercises. Table 9 lists the major effects of cryotherapy, and Table 10 the major contraindications.

Figure 2 illustrates the mechanism of action of both heat and cold therapies.

Heat

Heat treatments are contraindicated in the presence of acute inflammation, trauma, hemorrhage, edema, or ischemia.[5] Thus, heat modalities are not appropriate in the early stages of the healing process. In later stages, heat can be used to improve analgesia, promote blood flow, and decrease muscle tone.[5] (Fig. 2) Table 11 describes the more commonly used heating modalities, Tables 12 and 13 list effects and contraindications, respectively.

Ultrasound, a form of deep heating, can increase tissue damage if used too soon after injury.[5] It is indicated in the later phases of healing to enhance local circulation and to increase soft-tissue extensibility.[7,22] Ultrasound is also useful in the treatment of subacute tendinitis and bursitis and of joint and soft-tissue contractures. It has been shown to increase muscle blood flow and joint temperature.[17]

Superficial heating modalities such as hot packs, paraffin bath, fluidotherapy, and whirlpool may be used for treatment of injuries to the extremities after the acute phase.

Hydrotherapy

Hydrotherapy in a therapeutic swimming pool is helpful in the early stages of rehabilitation.[5] The buoyancy of the water allows the

TABLE 11. Common Heating Modalities

Conduction	Hot water bottle Heating pad Hydrocollator pack Paraffin bath	Superficial
Convection	Whirlpool Hubbard tank	
Conversion	Infrared lamp Ultrasound	Deep

TABLE 12. Effects of Therapeutic Heat

Increased collagen extensibility
Decreased joint stiffness
Increased inflammation
Reduced sensation of pain
General relaxation and sedation
Increased local blood flow
Mild consensual increase in blood flow
   (to the opposite limb)
Reduced spasticity
Increased core body temperature
Decreased gastrointestinal peristalsis and
   gastric acid production
Increased menstrual flow (deep heat)
Reduced menstrual cramping

Adapted from Kottke FJ, Lehmann JF: *Krusen's Handbook of Physical Medicine and Rehabilitation,* 4th ed.Philadelphia, W. B. Saunders, 1990.

TABLE 10. Contraindications to Cryotherapy

Anesthetic areas
Obtunded or unresponsive patient
Cold allergy
Cryoglobulinemia
Raynaud's phenomenon
Paroxysmal cold hemoglobinuria
Prolonged use over superficial nerves
Paramyotonia congenita
Delayed application after burns

Adapted from Kottke FJ, Lehmann JF: *Krusen's Handbook of Physical Medicine and Rehabilitation,* 4th ed.Philadelphia, W. B. Saunders, 1990.

FIGURE 2. The effects of heat and cold on decreasing muscle tension.
A, Heating certain afferent muscle spindle fibers causes them to have a decreased rate of firing, thus relaxing tonic muscle activity.
B, Cooling the skin facilitates the alpha-motor neurons, thus increasing spasticity and muscle stretch reflexes.
C, Cooling, the afferent muscle spindle fibers (deep cooling) causes a direct effect by inhibiting their firing, thus relaxing muscle spasticity.
D, Heating the Golgi tendon organ increases its firing which inhibits the alpha-motor neuron and decreases spasticity.
E, Direct effect of heat increases collagen extensibility.
(From Buschbacher RM (ed): Musculoskeletal Disorders: A Practical Guide for Diagnosis and Rehabilitation. Stoneham, MA, Butterworth-Heinemann, 1994, with permission.)

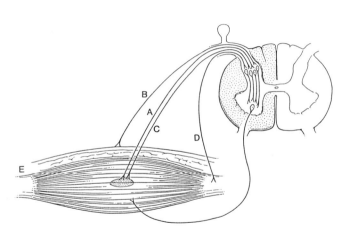

TABLE 13. Contraindications to the Use of Heat

Anesthetic area
Obtunded or uncommunicative patient
Impaired vascular flow to the limb
Acute injury
Acutely inflamed joints
Hemorrhagic conditions
Over the pregnant uterus
Over the testes
Over metallic implants (shortwave and microwave)
Over cemented metallic implants (ultrasound)
Over cancers
When used for multiple sessions over a child's
    ephiphyseal growth plate
Over the eyes
Over the spinal column after laminectomy (deep heat)
Over the heart (deep heat)
Over sites of infection (except over some superficial skin
    infections)

Adapted from Kottke FJ, Lehmann JF: *Krusen's Handbook of Physical Medicine and Rehabilitation,* 4th ed. Philadelphia, W. B. Saunders, 1990.

athlete to maintain and increase strength, range of motion, and endurance even before full weight-bearing is allowed.

Contrast Baths

Contrast baths (alternating heat and cold) may be helpful in decreasing edema and in the treatment of reflex sympathetic dystrophy.[5] They typically cause a vigorous hyperemia.

Transcutaneous Electrical Nerve Stimulation

Transcutaneous electrical nerve stimulation (TENS) units are useful for pain control following injury. They may help the athlete to participate in a strengthening and rehabilitation program.[7,22]

Pulsed High-Voltage Galvanic Stimulation

Pulsed high-voltage galvanic stimulation (PHVGS) has many effects, including decreases in pain, edema, muscle guarding, and disuse atrophy, as well as increases in local blood flow and tissue healing.[21] In treating athletes, PHVGS may help to decrease edema and to control pain in the early phases. It also may help to decrease muscle guarding, thus allowing better range of motion in later phases. Electrical stimulation may help to pre-

vent atrophy in a muscle that the patient cannot contract voluntarily.[15]

Biofeedback

Biofeedback may be helpful in muscle relaxation, reedeucation, and strengthening.[23]

Massage

Massage has several positive effects, including increased blood flow in muscles, increased lymph flow, relaxation of muscles, and decreased blood pressure. Massage also can help to loosen adherent scar tissue and to prevent the formation of adhesions and fibrous tissue. In addition, it has a relaxing sedative effect on the central nervous system.[7]

Rest and Exercise

Relative rest is important in the early stages of healing. Relative rest means avoiding exacerbating movements and allowing other motions to occur. This approach helps to decrease swelling, pain, and the complications of immobility. The familiar RICE protocol consists of *R*est, *I*ce, *C*ompression, and *E*levation.

Immobilization may be required after certain fractures as well as acutely inflamed joint conditions, ligament sprains, and tendinitis. Immobilization should be limited to a few days (if at all) for tendinitis and sprains but may be necessary for periods of up to 2 weeks for inflamed joints.

Although rest is initially protective of the damaged organ, prolonged rest results in progressive loss of functional capacity (including the muscular, skeletal, cardiovascular, respiratory, urogenital, digestive, integumentary, and nervous systems).[14] Total inactivity of muscle results in a loss of up to 5% of muscle strength per day.[20] Young healthy subjects on bedrest lose an average of 1.0 to 1.5% per day of initial strength.[20] Loss of 1.3 to 5.5% per day was observed during immobilization in a plaster case.[20] Immobilization also results in loss of muscle mass, decreased cross-sectional area of both type I and type II fibers, and decrease in activities of mitochondrial enzymes.[2] Joint contractures also occur after prolonged immobilization. Intraarticular and ligamentous adhesions are two contributing factors.[11] In some conditions, loss of motion occurs after only a few days of immobilization because of the formation of dense connective tissue to replace the normal, loose areolar tissue.[14] Ligamentous contraction due to contractile proteins in ligament fibroblasts has also been proposed as a possible cause of joint contracture due to immobilization.[4] Decreased endurance, decreased coordination, and osteoporosis occur as well.[15]

Early protected motion is recommended after injury, followed by a gradual progression of physical activity.[15] Exhaustive physical activity should be avoided early in the recovery process because it may cause a drop in functional capacity.[15] The rate of recovery of muscular strength with exercise is slower than the rate of loss during immobilization. One can expect only a 10% increase in strength per week with a daily program of maximal exercise.[15] Endurance improves at a similar rate.[15] The tensile and maximal static strength of tendons improves with physical training.[21] During range-of-motion exercises, prolonged steady stretch has been shown to be more effective than intermittent or short-term stretching.[15]

Proprioceptive exercises must be included in the rehabilitation program because loss of sense of position occurs with ligament disruption and is an important factor in reinjury.

Isometric strengthening exercises can be performed even while joint motion is limited. In most cases, it is recommended that range of motion of the joint be 75% of normal before advancing to an isotonic strengthening program.[22] Progressive resistive exercise and endurance programs then follow.

REHABILITATION PROGRESSION

It is sometimes helpful to divide the rehabilitation of musculoskeletal disorders into four overlapping phases.

Phase I is the initial period when inflammation and pain must be controlled for both macrotraumatic injury and overuse conditions. The RICE protocol is commonly used after sports injury. In addition, NSAIDs may reduce inflammation, especially in overuse conditions such as tendinitis or bursitis. Ice is a helpful adjunct to treatment that relieves pain and reduces edema, especially in the acute postinjury period (or until swelling subsides). Ice is also useful for overuse conditions both before and after exercise to avoid aggravating inflammation. Heat is generally used in the subacute period (after 1 to 2 days). It is also helpful in overuse syndromes. Phase I usually lasts for 1 to 2 weeks. It is important not to lose fitness of the rest of the body while the affected body part is rested.

Phase II, the mobilization phase, is the most important phase of rehabilitation. When a part of the body hurts, it is natural to try not to move it. Such self-splinting is helpful for a while, but when done for too long, it results in contracture, decreased strength and function, and ultimately more pain. As soon as inflammation is controlled, the patient must work on restoring and maintaining normal range of motion. Obviously, when joints are unstable or after supporting structures have been torn—for example, after ankle sprain or shoulder dislocation—flexibility exercises are not encouraged in the damaged structures. Slightly less flexibility in the defective area compared with the normal side is sometimes allowable as long as flexibility in other planes is maintained.

Superficial or deep heating is often useful while working on flexibility. It is most effective if applied during stretching because warm collagen is more easily deformed.[15] Late in phase II isometric exercises may be started.

Phase III is the strengthening phase. When starting this phase of rehabilitation, it is important first not to lose the gains made in phases I and II. Isometrics are continued, and isotonic and isokinetic strengthening exercises are added. As a general guideline, one should start with relatively low-weight and moderate-to-high repetitions and progress to higher-weight, low-repetition exercises as tolerated.

Phase IV—functional restoration—is the part of rehabilitation that is often neglected. It is not enough to achieve good flexibility and strength in the therapy department alone. Functional tasks similar to those that are to be resumed must be practiced before return to activity. This allows the athlete to return to the previous level of function with less likelihood of reinjury.

REFERENCES

1. Bahamonde LA, Saavedra H: Comparison of the analgesic and antiinflammatory effects of diclofenac potassium versus piroxicam versus placebo in ankle sprain patients. *J Int Med Res* 18(2):104–111, 1990.

2. Booth FW, Gollnick PD: Effects of disuse on the structure and function of skeletal muscle. *Med Sci Sports Exerc* 15:415–420, 1983.

3. Calandre EP, Ruiz-Morales M, Lopez-Gollonet JM, et al. Efficacy of oral streptokinase-streptodornase in the treatement of ankle sprains. *Clin Orthop Rel Res* 263:210–214, 1991.

4. Dahners LE, Banes AJ, Burridge KWT: The relationship of actin to ligament contraction. *Clin Orthop* 210:246–252, 1986.

5. DeLisa JA: *Rehabilitation of Medicine: Principles and Practice.* Philadelphia, J.B. Lippincott, 1988.

6. Diebschlag W, Nocker W, Bullingham R: A double-blind study of the efficacy of topical ketorolac tromethamine gel in the treatment of ankle sprain, in comparison to placebo and etofenamate. *J Clin Pharmacol* 30 (1):92–99, 1990.

7. Duncombe A, Hopp JF: Modalities of physical treatment. *Phys Med Rehabil State Art Rev* 5(3):493–519, 1991.

8. Goodman AG, Gilman LS, Gilman A: *The Pharmacological Basis of Therapeutics,* 8th ed. New York, Pergamon Press, 1990.

9. Griffin JE, Touchstone JC, Liu A: Ultrasonic movement of cortisol into pig tissue: II. Movement into paravertebral nerve. *Am J Phys Med* 44:20–25, 1965.

10. Halpern AA, Horowitz BG, Nagel DA: Tendon ruptures associated with corticosteroid therapy. *West J Med* 127:378–432, 1977.

11. Jhee WH: Exercise and rest. In Schwab CD (ed): Musculoskeletal Pain. *Phys Med Rehabil State Art Rev* 5(3):527–536, 1991.

12. Kawahara NE, Spunt AL: Pharmacologic agents in musculoskeletal pain. In Schwab CD (ed): Musculoskeletal Pain. *Phys Med Rehabil State Art Rev* 5(3):479–492, 1991.

13. Kennedy JC, Baxter-Willis R: The effects of local steroid injections on tendons: A biochemical and microscopic correlative study. *Am J Sports Med* 4:11–18, 1976.

14. Kottke FJ: The effects of limitation of activity on the human body. *JAMA* 196:825–830, 1966.

15. Kottke FJ, Lehmann JF: *Krusen's Handbook of Physical Medicine and Rehabilitation,* 4th ed. Philadelphia, W.B. Saunders, 1990.

16. Lee EH, Lee PY, Ngai AT, Chiu EH: Treatment of acute soft tissue trauma with a topical non-steroidal antiinflammatory drug. *Singapore Med J* 32:238–241, 1991.

17. Lehmann JF: *Therapeutic Heat and Cold,* 3rd ed. Baltimore, Williams & Wilkins, 1982.

18. McMaster WC, Liddle S: Cryotherapy influence on post traumatic limb edema. *Clin Orthop* 150:283–287, 1980.

19. Moran M: An observer-blind comparison of diclofenac potassium, piroxicam and placebo in the treatment of ankle sprains. *Curr Med Res Opin* 12(4):268–274, 1990.

20. Muller EA: Influence of training and of inactivity on muscle strength. *Arch Phys Med Rehabil* 51:449–462, 1970.

21. Renstrom PAFH, Leadbetter WB: Tendinitis I: Basic Concepts. *Clin Sports Med* 11:505–519, 533–572, 1992.

22. Saal JA: General principles and guidelines for rehabilitation of the injured athlete. In: Saal JA (ed): Rehabilitation of sports injuries. *Phys Med Rehabil State Art Rev* 1(4):523–535, 1987.

23. Schwab CD (ed): Musculoskeletal Pain. *Phys Med State Art Rev* 5(3):447–652, 1991.

24. Sweetham R: Corticosteroids arthropathy and tendon rupture. *J Bone Joint Surg* 518A:397–398, 1969.

25. *Webster's Ninth New Collegiate Dictionary.* Springfield, MA, Merriam-Webster, 1991.

Chapter 3

STRENGTH TRAINING AND FLEXIBILITY

Michael F. Dillingham, MD, and Joel S. Saal, MD

The combination of strength training and flexibility into a single review facilitates the important integration of this knowledge in training and rehabilitation.

Despite an abundance of data on basic and applied aspects of strength training, we lack scientific agreement on its application, particularly in post-injury rehabilitation. Adding to this dilemma are notable problems in various study designs: (1) limited sample size; (2) limited duration, often fitting the arbitrary confines of a school semester or quarter (this duration is too short to evaluate a serious athletic training response beyond initial neural adaptations and so misses meaningful changes of muscle mass); (3) poor statistical analysis; (4) use of untrained subjects, which may alter test results because of their skill, motivation, and/or tolerance of pain; and (5) lack of control of variables such as general nutrition or health and protocol compliance.

Testing of isolated muscle preparations does not correlate well with muscle behavior in vivo. The distribution and metabolic parameters of animal muscle fiber vary somewhat from those of human muscle. Especially in the smaller animals used for studies, contraction velocities tend to be greater than in humans, and the tendency to have muscles of the single-fiber-type is much higher.

The importance of flexibility training in injury prevention and performance enhancement remains a strong empirical observation that has not been well supported in the available clinical literature. Nonetheless, there is adequate basis for the continued use of specific stretching programs in a conditioning and athletic training protocol. The nature of flexibility is complex, with an interplay of connective tissue, the biophysics and neurophysiology of motor control, and human joint kinematics.

Currently available information about strength and flexibility is not only helpful, but even required for medical personnel who deal in sports or who prescribe exercise programs. This chapter is intended to help in formulating a conceptual framework for the practical application of strength and flexibility training.

PHYSIOLOGIC ASPECTS OF STRENGTH

Muscle Fiber Types

Various schemes have been used to classify muscles, including color (red, white), metabolic activity (oxidative, glycolytic), time to peak tension (fast, slow), and histochemical schemes (type I, type II). In animal studies, the fast-slow classification is commonly used with metabolic modifiers (e.g., fast fatigue resistance, fast oxidative) whereas in humans the histochemical scheme predominates. In this scheme, the myofibrillar adenosine triphosphatase (ATPase) stain identifies three myosin isoforms:

  type I, correlating with slow twitch;
  type IIa, correlating with fast oxidative–glycolytic, fatigue-resistant; and
  type IIb, correlating with fast glycolytic–oxidative, fatigue-sensitive.

Note: This chapter is an update on two previous articles published in 1987 in *Physical Medicine and Rehabilitation: State of the Art Reviews*.

A fourth category, type IIc, contains different fibers in differing schemes. In one scheme, it describes a purely glycolytic fast fiber; in other schemes, a fiber that is intermediate between type I and type II. As the naming scheme implies, type I slow fibers are primarily oxidative (aerobic), using mitochondrially based oxidative reactions (respiration) to produce large amounts of ATP, whereas type II fast fibers combine oxidative and nonoxidative (anaerobic) glycolytic pathways.

Fiber type is a function of the alpha-motor neuron supplying the muscle and results directly from neural influence. Under normal circumstances, the proportion of fiber type varies from person to person. This variance is genetically determined. Experimentally, fiber types can be changed with reinnervation and with chronic electric stimulation. Endurance training can induce a change from type IIb to the more aerobic type IIa and even changes a few type IIa fibers to type I. There is no evidence of conversion of type I fibers to type II fibers. Although most human muscle is a mosaic of approximately one-half type I and one-half type II fibers, highly trained athletes may have extreme fiber distributions based on the combination of genetics and prolonged training. The situation in humans contrasts with the findings in animals, especially smaller animals, which may have unmixed muscles.

The different isoforms of myosin vary in the speed at which they split ATP (from 300 to 600 times/s). This is the key factor yielding variation in the velocity of shortening; i.e., the cycling of cross-bridges. The maximal velocity of shortening of the type II fiber is about 6 fiber lengths/s; of a type I fiber, about 2 fiber lengths/s. The speed of contraction is 40 to 90 ms for type II and 90 to 140 ms for type I fiber.

The power of the fast-twitch fiber is greater than that of the slow-twitch fiber at all velocities of shortening. Its peak power is 4 times that of the slow-twitch fiber because of its greater velocity. Even in evenly mixed muscle at low velocity, the fast fibers still provide 2.5 times the contribution of the slow fibers to total power. In animal models, a mixed muscle has only 55% of the peak power of a similar-sized pure fast muscle. Only at very low velocities can slow and fast fibers make near-equal contributions to power. At moderate velocity, slow fibers make only a slight contribution. For practical purposes, at high velocities, power is a function of fast fibers only. In dynamic contraction, fast type II fibers dominate. The type IIa fast oxidative fiber can sustain moderate power even better than a slow fiber. The greatest difference between fiber types, however, may be anaerobic (glycolytic) capacity, which can vary as much as 600% between fast and slow fibers. Most fast fibers have only 30% to 40% of the aerobic (oxidative) enzymes of a slow fiber.

For burst-type activities requiring peak power, the fast twitch fiber must be trained. The slow fibers are important as an endurance background or base in the setting of strength training. They are also important to provide a depot for the metabolism of byproducts of anaerobic glycolytic metabolism (i.e., the oxidation of lactate in the mitochondrial oxidative system). An individual's genetic make-up determines the distribution of muscle fiber type and probably potential muscle size.

Metabolism

At rest, muscle consumes only 20% of the body's normal oxygen consumption (i.e., 20% of 300 mL/min); at $VO_{2 max}$ it consumes 2000 to 2200 mL/min in women and 3000 to 3500 mL/min in men. These values may be twice as high in world-class endurance athletes in whom muscle consumes 90% of the O_2 at $VO_{2 max}$. Oxygen is not stored, and therefore, the rate-limiting factor for muscle oxidative metabolism (respiration) is cardiovascular. Oxidative metabolism converts 50% of its chemical energy to heat and 50% to energy. The overall efficiency of muscular activity in converting chemical energy to mechanical work is between 30% and 35%. As glycogen and free fatty acids are stored, the rate-limiting factor in their use is the active membrane transport system.

As Brooks and Fahey[2] observe:

The design of the training regimen to improve performance in any physical activity should begin with an evaluation of which energy system or systems are involved.

Energy sources are described with various terms, e.g., immediate, ultra-short-term, short-term, and endurance. Basically, however, such terms are meant to describe the time duration through which an energy source is utilized. An abrupt switch from aerobic to anaerobic metabolism does not occur.

The first energy sources to be considered are

most frequently described as *immediate:* adenosine triphosphate (ATP) and creatine phosphate (CP) (Fig. 1), which are sometimes referred to as phosphagen. The ATP in muscle is sufficient to allow approximately 1 to 2 s of activity or 1 to 3 maximal contractions against a heavy load. A combination of stored ATP and creatine phosphate allows approximately 6 to 8 seconds of acute burst activity or short sprint activity. During this time, a reaction of creatine phosphate plus adenosine diphosphate (ADP) replinishes the ATP supply. After depletion, the normally large levels of creatine phosphate can be reestablished in a matter of minutes. The enzymes of this energy system (and those of glycolysis) are water- soluble and exist in the sarcoplasm near the contractile proteins to facilitate rapid muscle activation and recovery. Because creatine phosphate is a small diffusible molecule, it is an easy, convenient way to move energy to different sites and acts as an energy buffer. It is probable, however, that up to 20% of immediate energy needs are met by glycolysis, which clearly is not the critical pathway at this time.

The immediate period has also been referred to as *alactic.* In a teleologic sense, it allows time for glycolytic metabolism, which begins in the first second of activity, to ramp up. By 10 s into an intense activity, the original ATP and creatine phosphate have been utilized. Glycolysis is working at a near-maximal rate. In a sprint, the rate of glycolytic activity is 1000 times baseline and this increased rate accounts for the inefficiency of the glycolytic anaerobic system. Glycolysis produces pyruvate, which is converted to lactate (if not picked up by mitochondria) plus 3 ATP per glycogen split (2 per glucose utilized). In contrast, 39 ATPs are produced from each glucose split from glycogen during complete oxidative metabolism, which yields ATP, H_2O, CO_2, and heat.

Lactate is cleared slowly from the cells, but its clearance is rate-limited. It can be reconverted rapidly to pyruvate for uptake to the mitochondria, but this process is also rate-limited. Therefore, at maximal activity, oxidative metabolism is able to use about 10% of the pyruvate produced. A large accumulation of lactate occurs in muscle, despite the fact that by 40 to 50s of activity, oxidative systems have been activated and 50% of energy production is oxidative. This process of oxidative metabolism, which consumes lactate produced within the fiber or by adjacent fibers, requires increases in muscle circulation, cardiac output, and pulmonary ventilation. If these factors are sufficient, maximal mitochondrial activity is possible.

The final rate-limiting factor in prolonged aerobic activity is substrate transport of glucose and free fatty acids to the muscle. This transport limits oxidative capacity to approximately 50% of VO_{2max} once the intracellular substrate stores are utilized. Subsarcolemmal mitochondria energize the active transport process involved in oxidative metabolism. During the ultra-short-term activity period of less than 1 minute, anaerobic metabolism is maximal, providing energy to replenish the stores of ATP and creatine phosphate. In addition, anaerobic oxidative metabolism has the opportunity to initiate and ramp up. During this period, 60% of the energy produced is anaerobic.

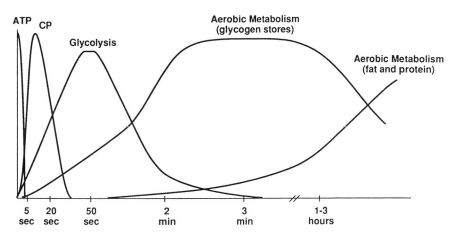

FIGURE 1. Energy systems used during immediate (< 10 s), ultra-short-term (10–50 s), short-term (50 s–??), and endurance (duration?) periods of exercise. CP = creatine phosphate.

If dynamic exercise is carried out at maximal capacity, blood lactate levels reach their maximal value within 40 to 45 s. It takes hours, however, to equilibrate high levels of plasma and intracellular lactate levels. If the levels of lactate within muscle are too high, glycolysis is actually inhibited. Strength training at 60% to 70% of maximum for multiple sets may actually deplete glycogen stores in a minority of muscle fibers. Once depleted, it takes approximately 1 day to reestablish normal storage levels of glycogen in muscle.

In prolonged exercise, such as a 1-hour run, muscle activity is primarily of the endurance type. Most of the energy is provided from aerobic metabolism using stored glycogen and free fatty acids within the cell as well as circulating glucose and free fatty acids.

The effects of training on muscle metabolism and metabolic capacity vary. The concentration of creatine phosphate is changed little by weight or endurance training. Glycolysis improves somewhat if the training is of the high-intensity or interval type. However, the oxidative metabolic machinery can be most affected by training. With adequate training, mitochondrial volume can increase to double the baseline. Endurance training results in greater use of fat as an energy source, thus sparing the glycogen stores and increasing endurance. Clearance and tolerance of lactate are also improved. There is an increased sensitivity to insulin and increased concentration of lipase to allow more efficient use of energy sources.

Intracellular glycogen stores can increase up to 50% as part of the adaptive process, although lipid stores are not changed. Increased myoglobin concentration allows better oxygen transport to the muscle. Endurance training leads to increased numbers and volume of capillaries as well as increased cardiac output and oxidative metabolism. Heavy-load, low-repetition training (Olympic lifting) has no effect on oxidative pathways or enzymes. Heavy-load, high-repetition training (bodybuilding style) has some effect on oxidative enzymes and capillary numbers but not on capillary density. Only endurance training brings about the full effect of the adaptations described above.

Muscle Activity

At this point, it is appropriate to consider how muscle fibers contract. Broadly speaking,

the two categories of contraction are *static* and *dynamic*. Static contraction is described as isometric, whereas dynamic contractions are either concentric (shortening) or eccentric (lengthening). Muscles almost never work in an isolated type of contraction, nor is activity constant in its force (isotonic) or velocity (isokinetic).

Isometric contraction implies that both ends of the muscle are fixed and that no motion results from the contraction. Thus, no mechanical work is performed, and energy is dissipated as heat. Maximal isometric tension can be produced at 1.2 times the resting length of muscle. The resting length of muscle is the length that the muscle assumes when lying free (detached from its ends). Isometric tension falls to zero at the point of maximal shortening; it is also zero at twice the resting length because at this length actin and myosin do not overlap. A maximal isometric contraction can be held for only a few seconds; a 50% contraction can be held for approximately 1 minute; and a 10% to 15% contraction can be held virtually indefinitely as an aerobic activity.

Isometrics, however, result in little endurance training. They provide strength training only at the joint angle being used. They do not improve a muscle's ability to exert force rapidly (rate of force development). They also provide little stimulus for muscle hypertrophy or endurance. Though heavily studied because of ease of laboratory preparation, isometric exercise has little use in strength training. In rehabilitation, it is used as a fall-back position if pain or limited range of motion prohibits other forms of training.

Dynamic muscle contractions are the general focus of strength training. Shortening, concentric contractions are also described as positive contractions. External work is done and is a function of how far a given weight is moved. Mechanical efficiency (the ratio of external work performed to extra energy produced) of this kind of contraction is generally 20% to 25%, with the rest of the energy dissipated as heat. Mechanical efficiency decreases with increased shortening velocities and increases to as much as 45% by use of the stretch-shortening cycle (e.g., a brief, short squat before jumping). The contribution of the stretch-shortening cycle (also known as plyometric exercises) to efficiency increases with increasing prestretch load. This effect is partly due to a "recapture" of elastic strain energy in the muscle-tendon complex, which is released on shortening, and to release of energy stores in tendon (up to 15% of the total force generated). It is also due to reflex potentiation of muscle activity by muscle spindle activity. The elastic component of muscle and tendon, which works in series, allows higher force because the muscle itself can work at increased length and lower velocity of contraction.

Most physiologic strength activity involves a stretch-shortening cycle with wide variation in the length, duration, and amount of stretch. This variation results from normal occurrence of impact and gravity on body segments. In addition to the benefits mentioned above, the stretch-shortening cycle with its increased muscle stiffness also improves deceleration and impact absorption by the stretched muscle; it should be viewed as a category of motor activity separate from concentric or eccentric exercise. Long stretch-shortening cycles involve large angular displacements over a time course of greater than 250 ms, whereas short cycles have small angular displacements at 100 to 250 ms.

Lengthening eccentric contractions are also described as negative contractions. Under some circumstances, mechanical efficiency can be as high as 60%. It is increased by increased stretch velocity.

Under normal circumstances the muscle is under slight tension. The usual range of shortening or lengthening falls between 0.7 and 1.2 times the normal resting length. Thus, maximal tension can be achieved at physiologic ranges. The tension decreases with shortening and increases with lengthening. With passive stretching, elastic tension can increase up to twice that of equilibrium, which is described as the length obtained by an unattached muscle.

The highest force is generated by a fast eccentric contraction and the lowest by a fast concentric contraction. Eccentric contractions can generate greater force and power maximums than concentric contractions at any given velocity of stretch. In fact, an integrated electromyogram (EMG) shows less activity for the same force level in eccentric contraction than in concentric contraction. In addition, there is less oxygen consumption, and greater mechanical energy is produced than for similar concentric contraction.

The greatest power can be generated at 25% to 30% of maximal contraction velocity. In activity of very short duration (e.g., 1 lift; known as a tetanic contraction), maximal strength (i.e., maximal force at a given velocity) is essentially the same as maximal power (i.e., work per unit time). In longer events, power becomes a function of both strength and the metabolic capacity to generate ATP. Power also increases with a better rate of force development. Unfortunately, in athletic training, the terms *strength* and *power* are not always used according to their strict definitions. Strength is used to express an ability to exert a high force, whereas power may be used to describe an explosive movement. In reviewing the potential strength of muscle, certain principles need to be kept in mind: Power equals force times the velocity of shortening. Potential power is proportional to the number of active sarcomeres in parallel. The number of sarcomeres in a cross-section determines the potential maximal force generated by muscle. Thus, the total mass of the muscle determines its power. Velocity is proportional to the number of active sarcomeres in a series; thus, fiber length determines the potential maximal velocity of contraction.

Viewed in another way, longer muscles can contract more quickly because there are more sarcomeres with greater shortening per unit time. The maximal tension in muscle is a function of cross-sectional area. Maximal tension is believed to be 23 to 45 N/cm^2. Because pennation of fibers increases the effect of cross-section, pennated muscles tend to be specialized for strength, whereas long muscles with a fusiform organization of sarcomeres tend to be specialized for speed and power.

In vivo muscle does not act like muscle in an in vitro isolated pattern. Full resting length is indeed the position of greatest possible tension, but other in vivo factors exist that modify the effect of muscle contraction (e.g., the lever arm, the angle of pull, the insertion or origin of the muscle, and various external forces). In addition, fiber type, recruitment pattern, coordination and speed of cycling pattern, and agonist and antagonist contractions all affect what we measure as strength. In a variety of subjects, muscle strength can vary 10% to 20% in a given day when measured with the same activity.

It is apparent that muscle length determines speed of contraction and that cross-sectional area determines the potential maximal force. The highest power is generated at approximately one-forth of the maximal velocity of contraction. These factors should be taken into consideration with training. Movements in strength training should be full-range and controlled. "Cheating" by using momentum to move heavier weights than might otherwise be lifted should generally be avoided, except for the last few repetitions at fatigue level. The controlled motion of concentric and eccentric contraction is the best way to provide muscle stimulus.

Recruitment

As mentioned earlier, muscle size, cross-section, and velocity are not the only factors that determine power output and strength. Coordination of neural factors is also critical.

The force generated in a motor unit from two nerve stimuli is greater than that generated from one stimulus. This process is described as summation. During high frequencies of stimulation, muscle is tetanic and cannot relax. This phenomenon is known as a *fusion of contraction.*

Motor units contain from as few as half a dozen muscle fibers to as many as several thousand. The larger motor neurons innervate the faster fibers, which occur in the larger units. The range of stimulation for slow fibers is 5 to 30 Hz with fusion at 20 Hz; for fast fibers it is usually 30 to 60 Hz with fusion at 50 Hz. The rate of stimulation is proportional to excitation of the central nervous system. Because force production is a function of the rate of fiber stimulation, maximal force requires that all units fire at a high rate, a goal achieved only with training. When more motor units are called on to contract, the process is known as *muscle recruitment.* Thus strength is achieved through both rate coding (summation) and recruitment.

Certain facts have been learned from integrated EMG. Voluntary isometric contraction reveals a linear relationship of EMG activity relative to tension. Voluntary concentric contraction shows activity proportional to tension, but the slope is less with an eccentric contraction; i.e., an eccentric contraction requires less excitation to achieve a given tension. A relaxed muscle has no integrated EMG activity. With any type of maximal contraction, all motor units fire.

We also know that small, slow, fatigue- resistant type I fibers of low threshold and low force output are recruited first, followed by the larger, faster type II fibers of high threshold and high force output. This so-called *size principle* predicts the typical pattern of central excitation most of the time. Because of the nature of fast-twitch fibers, a high frequency of stimulation is needed to produce tetany. Maximal force requires complete recruitment of both slow- and fast-twitch fibers, and rate coding allows synchronous fusion tetany in each motor unit.

Practically speaking, slow-contracting muscle units are recruited first in activities of low force-demand. Firing frequency is low. As more strength is demanded, firing rate increases. The previously involved motor units thereby create a greater contraction force. Lastly, new larger motor units are recruited. Exceptions to the size principle do occur with certain ballistic movements in which larger units are first recruited.

Neural training is important in the early stages of strength training. Integrated EMG activity rises in the first 3 to 4 weeks of training. Stretch may inhibit the agonist in the untrained, but it facilitates the agonist in the trained individual (the stretch-shortening cycle). The agonist is also reflexly potentiated. The bilateral deficit (i.e., the sum of forces in a bilateral simultaneous move is less than the sum of the limbs working alone) is eliminated in the trained individual.

In addition to increased firing rate and recruitment, the rate of force development increases when training is velocity-specific. Ballistic training leads to a premovement silence in the stretch-shortening cycle; thus, there are no refractory fibers. It also can produce increased firing rates of up to 120 Hz. Recruitment of subgroup motor units also occurs with repetitive specific-movement training related to joint angle; as a result, fibers are activated with mechanical advantage. Training also facilitates agonist co-contraction, which decelerates, stabilizes, and protects the joint with a counterbalancing force and therefore allows precision of movement. Synchronization of motor units occurs most effectively during brief maximal contractions. The recruiting order of motor units is fixed for specific moves and varies with different positions and velocity of movement. It is reasonable to train a muscle in more than one position with more than one type of motion and with near-maximal contraction.

The neural coordination provided by such strength training is additive to the effects of hypertrophy and training of energy systems. Together, they facilitate the purpose of strength training, which is to accelerate a given mass more rapidly. Neural coordination, which is important to strength, implies the need for specificity. It also implies the need for proper technique so that learned patterning is appropriate to the activity desired. Neural coordination is additive to the effects of hypertrophy, which increases cross-section and mass of muscle, and to the effects of metabolic training, which increases the energy systems necessary for strength activity.

Fatigue

The layman's definition of fatigue is failure to maintain power output. Fatigue is a normal occurrence and is, in a sense, protective, preventing overwork, muscle overload, and excessive damage.

Psychological factors, especially the individual's ability to tolerate discomfort, are involved with the perception of fatigue. Muscle discomfort is generally associated primarily with an aerobic state and accumulation of lactate and hydrogen ions. Blood flow increases with muscle contraction but starts to decrease at a voluntary contraction of about 30% of maximal. As one approaches maximal voluntary contraction, blood flow may be severely reduced, thereby requiring anaerobic metabolism. With practice and mental conditioning, the central nervous system can maintain full activation during the anaerobic state.

It is unlikely that neural activation plays a critical role in fatigue during normal exercise activity. Therefore, the loss of strength or power due to fatigue results from changes in the muscle contractile system at maximal effort. The same is true of repetitive submaximal effort. Integrated EMG activity falls with fatigue, but a feedback mechanism seems to allow enough motor-unit firing to elicit the maximal possible effort, regardless of the level of fatigue. The motor-unit firing rate remains at the minimum necessary for maximal stimulation of the muscle performing the task.

Fatigue occurs when phosphagen (ATP and creatine phosphate) is exhausted. Glycolysis begins in the first second of maximal exercise, and within a few seconds it contributes significantly to the energy generated. Performance at submaximal but relatively high-cycle workloads depends on muscle glycogen stores, although free fatty acids contribute energy substrate as well. Fatigue in prolonged exercises results from glycogen depletion in type I (slow/oxidative) and type IIa (fast/oxidative) fibers. In intense exercise, fatigue probably results from glycogen depletion in type IIb fibers. Type II fibers have fewer cross-bridges than type I at any given time; consequently, they need more ATP per unit force.

At the cellular level, two significant processes probably contribute to muscle contractile failure. The myosin-actin cross-bridges are stimulated by the release of calcium from the sarcoplasmic reticulum and by coupling to the tropomyosin molecule. (The calcium pump uses about 30% of a muscle's ATP.) The increased concentration of hydrogen ions associated with lactate accumulation interferes with these activities. In addition, the breakage of the cross-bridges between actin and myosin requires energy from ATP. Generation of ATP is reduced because of reduced myosin-kinase activity at low pH and low ATP/ADP ratios. In addition to reducing speed of cross-bridge cycling, the increased concentrations of hydrogen ions and phosphate also reduce the total number of cross-bridges and the force generated by the cross-bridges. The net result is a reduction in the maximal force and the maximal velocity of muscle contraction.

One of the significant effects of strength training is to teach the athlete to tolerate fatigue and discomfort with vigorous exercise. Once this goal is achieved with time and practice, "true muscular failure" becomes a function solely dependent on the muscle contractile elements rather than on voluntary activation of the central nervous system.

Sex Differences

Beginning in childhood, males are stronger than females, generating a greater tension per volume of muscle. This strength difference is magnified by different socially established patterns of use, especially in the upper limbs. If activities are similar, however, there is little real difference in strength between prepubertal males and females. With the onset of puberty, the male will develop up to 10 times the androgenic hormone level of a child or female. Though muscle mass increases in females, it increases up to 40% more in males who may be as much as 50% stronger. The fast fibers have a greater cross-sectional area in males than in females.

Muscle glycogen synthesis and fat oxidative capacity probably do not respond to training as quickly in females as in males, although there is little difference in male and female fiber mix, blood lactate levels, fat metabolism, or muscle glycogen. Adult males have more muscle cell nuclei than adult females and thus a greater potential for hypertrophy. Strengthening in the adult male occurs both by muscle hypertrophy and by recruitment. The muscle hypertrophy involves increased contractile protein mass. Children, females, and older males increase strength primarily by recruitment and do not have the same capacity for muscle hypertrophy as younger adult males. The difference between males and females is greatest in strength training that is oriented toward power rather than endurance, because power training is specific to the type II fibers, which are most susceptible to hypertrophy. Though females may increase the cross-section by 15%, males can increase cross-section and volume of type II fibers by up to 40% with training.

Age Differences

During puberty, strength and muscle mass are highly influenced by training, especially in males. Strength is generally maximal between 20 and 30 years of age. Muscle mass relative to total body mass starts to fall in the fifth decade, with an accelerated loss beginning in the seventh decade. Approximately 30% of muscle mass is lost between ages 30 and 70 years. Women, however, lose less strength with aging because they are not as dependent on anabolic hormones and muscle hypertrophy as a source of strength. Although the elderly can increase strength through training, gains are limited. They are unable to achieve significant muscle hypertrophy. With age, motor units, especially the type II units that are necessary for strength and power, are lost. In addition, the remaining muscle also suffers a decrease in enzyme activity (glycolytic more than oxidative) and mitochondrial mass; thus, it is able to generate less ATP per volume of muscle. Age is also associated with an increased threshold of activation of motor units and a longer recovery time. Myosin, ATP, and creatine phosphate also decrease in concentration. The decline in strength varies among arms, trunk, and legs, partially depending on the habitual activity patterns of the individual.

In a trained individual, however, strength at age 65 can be approximately 80% of the lifetime maximum. The routine loss of strength measured in a normal western population is probably due equally to lifestyle as well as biologic factors. Additional factors, including decreased flexibility and arthritis, play a role in loss of strength associated with increasing age.

PRINCIPLES OF STRENGTH TRAINING

The three principles of strength training are overload, variability, and specificity.

Overload.   The neuromuscular unit is capable of adapting to appropriate stimuli. The greater the overload, the greater the adaptation. In addition, the greater the overload, the greater the recovery time after exercise.

Four basic factors are involved in overload training: intensity, volume, duration, and rest. The applied stimulus should be gradual and progressive but cycled discontinuously. This will allow neural adaptation, muscle hypertrophy, and development of the stressed metabolic systems. Overload increases immediate energy systems not through increased concentration of enzyme per unit volume, but through increasing muscle volume by hypertrophy. It increases potential strength by increasing the cross-sectional area and mass of muscle through hypertrophy. Overload increases endurance capacity by increasing mitochondrial volume and by various other changes in the oxidative metabolic pathway.

Variability.   A variety of exercise helps to prevent psychological burn-out and physical maladaptation. Repetitive, unvaried, heavy weight-training programs lead to a plateau in results, and occasionally to loss of strength and overtraining injuries. Variation avoids such problems and allows subunits of the training cycle that are specific to subset needs of the athlete or patient. For instance, reasonably varied training may include a period of high-volume, moderately heavy lifts for hypertrophy; a period of high-volume, heavy lifts for strength; a period of emphasis on power with lighter weights for velocity training and more plyometrics to train the stretch-shortening cycle; and a period of low-volume, light-weight exercise to prepare for maximal lift or competition. Within these large units (which may cover weeks or months), rest periods and underload are provided. Carefully planned variability is the basis of periodization with macro- and microcycles that allow rest and narrowly defined specificity training.

Specificity.   Specificity of exercise is a critical factor in neuromuscular training. Whereas overload encourages development of metabolic systems and muscle size, specificity encourages metabolic systems and, most importantly, neural coordination. As mentioned earlier, variability protects the athlete during training and allows the breakdown of training into subunits that optimize the goal of specificity. Strength can be increased by activation of prime movers, better co-contraction of synergists, and increased inhibition of antagonists. Untrained persons cannot fully activate muscles, especially in the high- threshold muscle motor units. Recruitment patterns of muscle are relatively passive. Specificity applies to velocity of contraction, to joint position during the contraction, and to the type of contraction carried out. An established pattern of recruitment can be modified by sensory input. Muscular strength gains in a particular activity can be achieved by training.

In strength training, it is important to practice technique. As stated before, practice should be properly performed to develop appropriate neural patterning and habits. Both of the force generators—overload and velocity—need to be trained. Velocity is improved by selecting loads that allow training at different speeds (i.e., the force velocity principle). Maximal velocity varies as a function of the maximal cycling rate of cross-bridges, not as a result of neurologic factors.

Muscle Growth

Muscle growth occurs primarily by enlarging the number and size of myofibrils and the associated sarcoplasm. Fiber-splitting (hyperplasia), which for some time was thought to be a source of muscle enlargement, probably does not occur, although myofibril split is part of the hypertrophic process. Heavy resistance training increases the cross-section of both type I and type II fibers; however, the increase is more marked in type II fibers, because they are involved in the adaptive response to heavy resistance training. Initially muscle fiber girth is increased at the expense of extracellular space. Later, the cross-section enlarges, with fibril-splitting and the increase of myofibrils as actin and myosin filament are added. Since the half-life of contractile proteins is short (7 to 15 days) and the half-life of sarcoplasmic proteins is even shorter, adaptation is facilitated. Because of higher rate of protein syn-

thesis, type II fibers hypertrophy more readily than type I. Heavy strength training involves a general decrease in the concentration of mitochondria because type II fibers are trained more specifically than type I; however, the total volume of mitochondria does increase. The sarcoplasm:myofibril ratio may decrease slightly. There is no change in capillary: fiber ratio in heavy strength training (in endurance training, the ratio increases; in body builders, the density also increases somewhat). Oxidative enzymes increase with most training. These factors increase the fatigue resistance of the muscle. The number of muscle fibers is unchanged.

In most athletes, increases in connective tissue are proportional to the hypertrophy achieved. However, athletes taking steroids have less contractile tissue per cross-section than athletes who do not take steroids. The amounts of muscle glycogen, creatine phosphate, and ATP increase with strength training. The increase in creatine phosphate and ATP allows more repetitions near the 1- repetition maximal lift. It is important to note, however, that the change in strength is not directly proportional to the increase in muscle cross-section, because neural adaptations as well as changes in isoform of cross- bridging proteins, changes in the force of cross-bridges, and changes in the percentage of activated cross-bridges all play a role.

Several theories have been advanced to define the critical stimulus for muscle growth. According to one theory, the amount of tension involved causes an increase in protein synthesis and metabolic change. The more likely mechanism, however, is damage caused by forced contraction, especially eccentric contraction. This damage results in a temporary decrease in strength and power. Hypertrophy is a repair response to the damage, hence, to the practical and theorically based observation that the greatest gains in strength come from heavy resistance activity carried out every 3 to 4 days. Daily lifting leads to decreased strength. The stimulus to gene expression and muscle size is probably mechanical via strength and/or force generation or their sequelae.

Muscle Soreness

There are two types of muscle soreness: *immediate* and *delayed*. The delayed reaction occurs 24 to 48 hours after activity and probably represents an overuse injury. Eccentric contractions are noted to cause more soreness than concentric contractions, probably because of the greater microtrauma involved in eccentric activity.

Types of Exercise

Isometrics are used to maintain tone, to train or maintain a pattern of contraction, or to strengthen a particular weak point in the range of motion. Though useful in a painful joint, they are rarely used in late rehabilitation or strength training.

Most advanced strength training is done with *dynamic* contraction (concentric and/or eccentric), using the constant resistance of free weights or sectorized machines. Variable cams are occasionally used on sectorized or plate-loaded machines, ostensibly to allow more constant load throughout the entire range of motion, but they have not been proved to be superior to free weights. The stretch-shortening cycle (plyometrics) is also felt to be an important part of training, especially for explosive movements (e.g., jumping, discus).

The goal of strength training is hypertrophy and enhanced neural coordination. In addition to the basic principles already covered, adequate rest is necessary between sets and between workouts. Most strength-training athletes do 3 or more sets of 4 to 8 repetitions. Rest between sets allows full tension to be obtained with the next set. Large muscles are worked no more than twice a week. Rest plus periodicity avoids overstressing the musculoskeletal system, reduces injury, and allows rapid biologic adaptation and maintenance of interest.

In a typical strength-training program, the initial phase, often referred to as setting a "base," is reminiscent of the 3-times-per-week pattern of physical therapy practice. It involves highly repetitious exercise with endurance and muscle-toning as goals (e.g., 3 to 4 sets of 10 to 12 repetitions). Of importance, it also develops the flexibility necessary to undergo true strength training. The true strength building phase follows with workouts that are heavier and less frequent. The first part of any workout is warm-up and stretch, easily done with 1 to 2 sets of very light weights through a full range of motion. The actual strategies for strengthening vary greatly. The technique appropriate to the athlete desiring

a warm-up, some endurance work, and some strength work (i.e., athletes cross-training or lifting for general health reasons) is known as pyramiding. The exercise is begun with lower weights and higher repetitions (12 to 15) for stretch, endurance, and warm-up and progresses through several more sets, each with higher weights and fewer repetitions (e.g., 8 to 10 and finally 4 to 6).

For free weights, dumbbells can be used in lieu of a routine Olympic bar or weight machines; they allow better isolation of muscles and the development of symmetric strength and coordination. Modification of the type of weight used permits higher degrees of interest and motivation. The use of machines offers variety and is safer when partners are not available to "spot" particular exercises. Most frequently, workouts are organized by body parts or regions to increase concentrations and to allow adequate rest on a 3- to 4-day cycle. Typical bodybuilding or cross-training workouts may include the back and chest on one day, arms and shoulders on another day, and legs on still another day. Major compound moves, such as the clean and jerk (*see* Chapter 12 on bodybuilding), that train more than one body part are also cycled in 3 to 4-day intervals. Maximal efforts are frequently reserved for alternate workouts, with an effort level of approximately 85% on the lighter workout.

In strength training, there are two basic types of lifting: compound and isolation exercise. Compound exercise involves synergistic muscles; for example, for lower limb strengthening, squats or leg presses can be performed, as they involve the use of the hamstrings, quadriceps, and gluteals, among other muscles. Isolation exercise is generally added to the compound exercise.

In the lower limbs, knee extensions work the lower part of the quadriceps, and, depending on the angle, the whole quadriceps upward to the hip. Exercises for some muscles should be done in different positions. For example, the biceps and triceps work somewhat differently at different angles. Working with the arm at the side or out in front stresses the biceps in a different manner. In addition, because of the way biceps works, it is susceptible to variations in hand position on the bar or on the dumbbell. The triceps can be worked at the side, straight ahead, or overhead, depending on the desired training effect or for variety in the training routine.

There is no set way to carry out strengthening activity, but the principles of overload and specificity have to be kept in mind. Muscle must be stressed adequately to cause breakdown so that hypertrophy can occur. Muscles also should be worked with their synergists so that better neural patterning and recruitment can occur. Muscles exercised in different positions train neural patterning. Finally, strengthening activities that mimic the motions or activities necessary in a particular sport should be included. This obviously requires a knowledge of the muscles used and the kinesiology involved in any particular sport activity or maneuver. For example, athletes can strengthen the muscles used in jumping by doing cleans. Throwers require isolated strengthening of various muscles in the shoulder girdle, including those that control the scapula, as well as patterned activities that strengthen the pattern of throwing. Free weights, exercise machines, pulleys, or elastic resistance exercises, such as rubber tubing, are helpful in this regard. A key element is knowledge of sport-activity dynamics. Much of the art or the sport of strengthening assumes that the participant has a sense of feedback from his or her own body. One must learn when the body has been overworked and when modification of the training scheme is necessary. This knowledge comes only with time and experimentation.

Mention should be made of circuit training, which is generally performed on machines that require little or no setup, so that it can be done quickly. The participants move rapidly from one machine to the next. Some manufacturers have made exaggerated claims about the aerobic benefits and strength gains possible on the circuit with brief, intense exercise of multiple body parts. In fact, aerobic benefit is limited. Strength and endurance may be maintained, but little hypertrophy or strength gains beyond neural patterning are achieved.

Weight Training for Athletes

In general, programs designed for athletes by strength coaches at all levels involve a combination of the specificity of the bodybuilder's activities and the speed and coordination typical of Olympic lifters. This strategy is a mix of compound and isolation exercises. The exercises done by recreation athletes and post-therapy patients generally borrow heavily from bodybuilding techniques.

The critical underlying concepts that apply to any strength-training technique for the general population or for subspecialized populations are overload and specificity. Strength gains and hypertrophy occur with strength overload. Endurance overload promotes endurance rather then strength. In addition, the speed of activity may be improved as a function of velocity of the lift.

Persons outside the competitive arena rarely train only for speed, endurance, or strength but rather have some combination in mind. They prioritize the type of training to achieve the gains necessary for their particular goal. As a practical matter, strength training cannot be isolated from endurance and speed in most activities. For example, putting the shot is a power event, but it requires particular coordination and speed, as do other power events (e.g., the discus and hammer throw). A football player may train for strength, but he also needs elements of aerobic endurance to function at the highest level throughout a game. Strength training, therefore, should rarely be done in isolation; certain aspects of muscular endurance have to be considered. In summary, understanding the physiologic basis of strength training allows a rational rehabilitation program to be designed.

FLEXIBILITY

Flexibility implies an ease of attaining a certain range of motion against resistance from the physical properties of tissue. Dynamic flexibility describes the ability of a body part to move quickly, whereas passive flexibility describes the amplitude of a range of movement.

Biophysical Aspects of Flexibility

The muscle-tendon unit is the key structure in flexibility. Because it must withstand forces greater than body weight delivered over a small area, injury is usually due to inadequate dynamic flexibility and overuse syndromes. The relative contribution of various individual tissues to stretch elongation has not been established, but in the most widely accepted view, the major role is played by muscle, followed by loose areolar connective tissue and then dense connective tissue (ligament and tendon).

The mechanical behavior of a muscle is due, in part, to its connective tissue components. Each muscle has a significant amount of connective tissue within separate compartments. The layers of connective tissue are the epimysium, perimysium, and endomysium. These sheaths determine the viscoelastic properties of muscle and are the mechanism of transmission of muscle forces to tendon and therefore eventually to bone.

Connective tissues respond to stretch in a viscoelastic manner. This property of connective tissue and the contract/relax properties of muscle determine response to stretching. Muscle fibers and connective tissue (tendons and connective tissue surrounding muscle) are aligned in series along the axis of applied stretch, whereas muscle itself is composed of contractile and elastic elements arranged in parallel.

Tendon Factors in Stretch

In the laboratory, when tendon is subjected to a tensile force, its response is depicted graphically by a stress/strain curve, with stress defined as force per unit area and strain as the ratio of percent link change to original length. As shown in Figure 2, this function is not linear. A greater deformation at low loads is followed by a rapid increase in stress until rapid deformation occurs (rupture). The initial change is related to the gradual elongation of elastic fibers, along with a straightening of the wavy arrangements of collagen fibers. This is followed by rupture of small collagen fibers with disruption of cross-links. The shape of the curve can be altered by prestretching the tendon.

The flexibility of the tendon varies inversely with its length; a tendon of greater length shows greater flexibility. Within the initial part of the stress/strain curve, the deformation is time-dependent, a feature known as *creep* (percentage length change/time at constant applied force). A low load applied for a prolonged time produces a greater length change than a large force applied rapidly.

Isometric warm-up allows stretching at physiologic levels to elongate the muscle tendon unit more effectively. Furthermore, additional force is required to cause connective tissue failure in warmed-up muscle. The amount of force required to cause damage is also influenced by temperature, local blood flow, and nutritional state. A stretching program, therefore, should include the regular application of forces in a gradual and prolonged manner with adequate tissue temperature.

Muscle Factors in Stretch

Whole muscle is a heterogeneous structure, with components of varying flexibility. From external to internal organization, each muscle contains an outer connective tissue sheath (epimysium), an inner connective tissue sheath surrounding fiber groups (perimysium), a layer surrounding the individual fibers (endomysium), and the sarcolemma (membrane that delineates individual fibers).

The main force-generating muscle cells, known as extrafusal fibers, are innervated by alpha-motor neurons. These are the contractile elements and determine the power of the muscle. In parallel with extrafusal fibers are the intrafusal fibers (muscle spindles), which

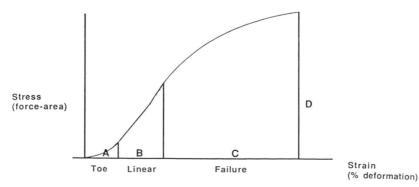

FIGURE 2. Representative stress/strain deformation curve for tendon. *A* = toe, *B* = linear deformation, *C* = failure (individual fibrils), *D* = rupture. (Adapted from Stromberg D, Wiekerhielm C: Viscoelastic description of a collagenous tissue in simple elongation. *J Appl Physiol* 26:857–862, 1969.)

are innervated by gamma-motor neurons. Although given a contractile function, they primarily serve the purpose of length/tension control for the muscle as a whole. Their length and tension are determined by the input of the gamma-motor neuron, the activity of which, in turn, is influenced by numerous factors, including suprasegmental input via descending cerebellar and cortical tracts and segmental input through direct sources (muscle tension and force development via the segmental innervation by alpha-motor neuron) as well as indirect sources (central overlap of cutaneous afferents and receptors of multiple types). In this manner, there can be multiple simultaneous inputs to the determination of muscle length and tension at a given time.

In addition, receptors in the musculotendinous unit (Golgi-tendon organ) operate in a fail-safe manner (all or none) at the point of critical stresses to the structure, delivering inhibitory input, preventing further muscle contraction and thereby allowing lengthening and facilitating relaxation. When the muscle spindle is stretched, it sends impulses to the spinal cord, which reflexively causes the muscle to contract. If the stretch is maintained (> 6 s), the Golgi tendon organ fires, causing relaxation. This process has direct implications for slow, prolonged stretching and for specific adaptations of stretching techniques. The resetting of the length/tension baseline in muscle may be achieved by the slow application of a stretch.

Neuromuscular Facilitation

The length- and tension-setting physiology is the basis for the techniques of proprioceptive neuromuscular facilitation.[13] First developed as a means of increasing strength in paralyzed limbs, these exercises gained popularity in treating spasticity and subsequently in application to normal limbs. As a result, we have been inundated with numerous stretching techniques with varying degrees of direct neurophysiologic rationale. Although these methods have been demonstrated to be effective in increasing flexibility, evidence regarding the specific basis for the observed effect is conflicting. In Moore and Hutton's[14] study of female gymnasts, EMG activity during stretch was greater and mobility gains were greater in the PNF group. A preceding muscle contraction causes a lingering afterdischarge that results in persistent muscle activation.

Importance of Flexibility

Although it has been demonstrated that the application of flexibility programs can prevent muscle injuries, it has been difficult to document the benefits of flexibility on other injury prevention.

The relationship between degree of flexibility and the occurrence of major knee injuries (ligament disruption, internal derangement) has received a great deal of attention in the literature. The results, however, are far from conclusive. Nicholas[15] demonstrated a correlation between five tests of laxity/flexibility and the occurrence of third-degree muscle strains and major knee injuries in a group of professional football players. Subsequent studies by other authors, however, have produced conflicting results.[12] The major predictive factor for joint injury is a previous joint injury or the presence of excessive joint laxity, and not necessarily inadequate flexibility.

Muscle Tears

A prospective study of flexibility programs in soccer players showed a correlation of improved range of motion and a decrease in the incidence of muscle tears.[12] In addition, this study revealed less flexibility in hip range of motion in soccer players than in age-matched controls. A more recent review of all studies of soccer injuries suggested an important role for flexibility in the prevention of injury, especially in older players. Muscle strain and tendinitis are more common in older and less flexible soccer players, and up to 11% of all injuries are related to poor flexibility.

In the setting of injury, flexibility takes on an even more crucial role in the function of the athlete. When strength has been lost or when pain limits force production, the resistance offered by soft tissues can lead to abnormal movement patterns. The abnormal joint excursion allows further maladaptive shortening of soft tissues as well as excessive forces on joints, establishing the possibility of further soft-tissue and joint compressive injury. Restoration of adequate flexibility on a regional basis, along with specific strength and movement training, is a cornerstone of physical rehabilitation.

In certain settings, however, withholding stretching is appropriate. For example, a hypermobile structure, such as an unstable joint, requires stabilization, not mobilization. This situation is common in spine and shoulder rehabilitation. In the presence of anterior instability of the shoulder, stretching of the posterior capsule while allowing adaptive shortening of the anterior capsule is the program of choice. Conversely, a frozen or severely hypomobile joint requires mobilization (for a capsular stretch) as well as stretching of extraarticular structures, with care to avoid undue joint compression. Following ankle injuries, it is important to restore the normal anterior ankle glide at the tibiotalar joint to avoid anterior joint compression. This is accomplished by a combination of mobilization in an anteroposterior plane as well as stretching in the Achilles tendon and medial joint structures. In general, these principles govern the major use of flexibility within rehabilitation of sports and other musculoskeletal injuries.

Less controversy surrounds the importance of inflexibility of soft tissue (i.e., muscle and tendon) in the pathogenesis of tendinitis than in the etiology of major joint injury. Inflexibility is considered by many researchers to play a causative role in Achilles tendinitis. The exact mechanism, however, is not clear. Although biomechanic properties of tendons have been shown to involve a change in fiber pattern after application of stretching force in vitro, it is not known whether this also occurs in vivo. The sites of tendinitis have been demonstrated to coincide with areas of relatively lower blood flow than neighboring portions of tendon. No data prove that flexibility training alters that blood flow per se.

As previously mentioned, the relative change in length with an applied stretching force is much smaller for tendon than for muscle. Although common stretching maneuvers may deliver some force to the tendon itself, the majority of deformation probably occurs in the muscle bellies. Therefore, the symptomatic improvements noted with flexibility programs in the treatment of tendinitis may be largely due to a change in muscle function, probably the eccentric shock and stress-absorbing function, rather than simply to change in the biomechanic profile of the tendon substance. Despite the mechanical uncertainties, flexibility training appears to be valuable in the treatment and prevention of many sites of tendinitis.

METHODS OF STRETCHING

Stretching techniques have evolved over recent years to include numerous options for improving flexibility.[11,16] Although each method has its share of faithful supporters, the distinct superiority of one method has not been demonstrated.

There are indications for the relative superiority of a given method in individual clinical situations. Prevention of injury (as in general warm-up), treatment of specific joint injury, flexibility needs in the presence of pain, and muscle spasm require modification of the basic method. The objectives of a flexibility program must be established in relation to the specific needs of the athlete; to obtain and maintain a level of flexibility is the general goal. Progressive daily gains in range of motion are unnecessary once an adequate level has been achieved. The postures utilized are designed to optimize stretch on the target tissue while minimizing stress on vulnerable surrounding structures (most notably the spine and knees).

The stretching options available can be divided into four categories: ballistic, static, passive, and neuromuscular facilitation. In addition, each of these methods can be combined with various therapeutic modalities.

Ballistic stretching employs the rapid application of force in a repeated manner in a bouncing, throwing, or jerking maneuver. This method was in standard use a few decades ago but is no longer recommended. The rapid increase in force can cause injury and is less efficient than other available methods. It causes a reflex muscle contraction and may actually impair stretching activity.

Passive stretching is performed with a partner applying a stretch to a relaxed extremity. This method has limited usefulness because of the increased risk of injury. There must be excellent communication between the partners, with slow and sensitive application of force. Gymnasts, dancers, football kickers, and soccer players have used this method for hamstring and hip adductor stretching. This method is commonly employed in the training room and physical therapy department and is safest in these contexts.

Static stretching, the easiest and probably the safest method of increasing flexibility, is recommended for preparticipation exercise in combination with warm-up. A position that applies a gradual stretch to the body part is held with steady force for a period of 15 to 60 seconds.

The duration of the applied stretch has recently been suggested to be equally effective at 15 compared with 45 to 60 seconds. This is the basis of yoga-type stretching and was advocated by deVries.[11] The added advantage of decreased muscular soreness after exercise supports the use of static stretching methods. Yoga-type stretching can be highly effective, although specific cautions are necessary. These methods have been tested over the centuries, but they carry a definite risk of injury if performed incorrectly or in the presence of certain injuries (specific joint instabilities or degenerative disc disease, especially cervical).

Neuromuscular facilitation techniques have been demonstrated in numerous studies to be effective methods for stretching. Most of these methods require an experienced partner (usually a physical therapist or trainer). Hold-relax and contract-relax (with or without agonist contraction) are the activities most frequently employed. In the experienced and attentive athlete, the contract-relax technique with added agonist contraction can be a highly effective and safe method. For hamstring stretch, the hamstrings are isometrically contracted for 5 s, while a gentle submaximal hip flexor contraction is maintained. We recommend this method for quadriceps, hamstring, and the gastrocnemius/soleus/Achilles complex.[9] A cross-training effect on contralateral hip flexibility has been demonstrated with proprioceptive neuromuscular facilitation techniques. This effect has a direct implication for flexibility training in the contralateral immobilized leg in the injured athlete.

In addition to manipulation of the neuromuscular system to enhance flexibility, the thermal characteristics of connective tissue can be exploited in certain circumstances. Warm-up exercises or conduction heating methods prior to stretching take advantage of the viscoelastic nature or collagen with increased temperature within the physiologic range. Warm-up prior to stretch or instead of stretch has failed to increase the level of flexibility (except in ankle dorsiflexion). Ease of stretch and prevention of injuries have not been studied, however, and this consideration is equally important. Therefore, we recommend 5 to 10 minutes of warm-up activity prior to stretching in the form of light jogging, fast walking, or stationary bike work.

Cold application has been used after flexibility training to take advantage of the thermal characteristics of connective tissue. Once plastic deformation has occurred, lowering the temperature can theoretically prolong the length changes. This strategy has not been proved to be effective, except in the setting of treatment of an injury. In this setting, muscle spasm and painful inhibition of joint and limb range of movement can be suppressed by cold application in the form of ice massage, cold immersion, or ice packs (time period for use varies with each method). The use of a vapocoolant spray has no significant benefit for flexibility gains in the absence of treatment of the injury. However, in the setting of injury in which muscle spasm is a factor, this modality can be highly effective (myofascial syndromes). Stimulation of cutaneous afferent nerves with the coolant spray can cause muscle relaxation on a physiologic basis similar to PNF techniques.

Although data suggest that ultrasound deep heating improves static or passive stretching, few data at this time support its routine use in the absence of an injury or fixed joint contracture.

The ideal flexibility program, therefore, should include a combination of stretching and mobilizing techniques (stretching across the long axis of the joint and mobilizing along the translational and rotational axes). A combination of passive, static, and proprioceptive neuromuscular facilitation techniques should be used, with specific target sites and motions for each sport.

Within each sport, needs will vary according to individual flexibility profiles. The program should be designed with these factors in mind and should be performed routinely: 3 times per week in off-season, and daily during the regular season. Gains in flexibility have been shown to be superior in athletes who stretch after activity. Therefore, a pre- and a post-competition routine should be established. The "after" routine can be more specific and abbreviated, focusing on muscle groups most stressfully involved in the athletic event. Since the short-term effects of stretching diminish significantly after 90 minutes, the program should be performed well within this time frame for at least 15 to 20 minutes, which appears to be the minimal time period for achieving adequate gains in temperature and extensibility. We recommend five repetitions for each motion, with each extremity. The duration of "hold" on static stretches should be 15 s with the initial stretch and should progress to 30 s on the last repetition. Stretches of longer duration have not been demonstrated to have increased effectiveness. Self-mobilization exercises at the segmental level of the thoracic and lumbar spine are recommended for most athletes who require upper body rotation and load bearing. Finally, stretching and mobilization techniques should be performed with careful attention to form to stay within the window of safety and effectiveness.

SELECTED READINGS

Physiology of Strength Training
1. Asterland, A, Rodahl, K: *Work Physiology: Physiologic Basis of Exercise.* New York, McGraw Hill, 1986.
2. Brooks, S, Fahey, J: *Exercise Physiology: Human Bioenergetics and Its Applications.* New York, John Wiley & Sons, 1984.
3. Dirix A, et al: *The Olympic Book of Sports Medicine,* vol 1. Oxford, Blackwell Scientific Publications, 1988.
4. Jones, SM, McCartney, N, McComas, AJ (eds): *Human Muscle Power.* Champagne, IL, Human Kinetic Publishers, 1986.
5. Komi PV: *Strength and Power in Sport.* Oxford, Blackwell Scientific Publications, 1992.

Practical Training Manuals
6. Pearl, W, Moran, MT: *Weight Training for Men and Women: Getting Stronger.* Bolinas, CA, Shelter Publications, 1986.
7. Schwarzenegger A: *Encyclopedia of Modern Bodybuilding.* New York, Simon & Schuster, 1985.

Periodicals
8. *Strength Training and Coaching.* Journal of the National Strength Coaches Association.

Flexibility
9. Agre J: Hamstring injuries: Proposed aetiological factors, prevention, and treatment. *Sports Med* 2:21–33, 1985.
10. Curwin S, Stanish W: *Tendinitis: Its Etiology and Treatment.* Lexington, MA, D. C. Heath, 1984.
11. de Vries H: Evaluation of static stretching procedures for improvement of flexibility. *Res Q* 33:222–229, 1962.
12. Ekstrand J, Gillquist J: The avoidability of soccer injuries. *Int J Sports Med* 4:124–128, 1983.
13. Knott M, Voss D: *Proprioceptive Neuromuscular Facilitation: Patterns and Techniques.* New York, Harper & Row, 1956. As cited in Basmajian J: *Therapeutic Exercise,* 3rd ed. Baltimore, Williams & Wilkins, 1978.
14. Moore M, Hutton R: Electromyographic investigation of muscle stretching techniques. *Med Sci Sports Exerc* 12:322–329, 1980.
15. Nicholas J: Injuries to knee ligaments: Relationship to looseness and tightness in football players. *JAMA* 212:2236–2239, 1970.
16. Wallin D, Ekblom B, Grahn R, Nordenborg T: Improvement of muscle flexibility: A comparison between two techniques. *Am J Sports Med* 13:263–268, 1985.

Chapter 4

REHABILITATION OF THROWING AND RACQUET SPORT INJURIES

James R. Andrews, MD, James A. Whiteside, MD, and Kevin E. Wilk, PT

The "overhead" athlete, such as the thrower or racquet sport athlete, presents a significant challenge to the clinician. This athlete must process a shoulder joint loose enough to accomplish the motion necessary to throw a baseball or to strike an overhead tennis serve, while exhibiting efficient muscular control to provide dynamic stability and to allow pain-free function. The key to sports performance is functional limb stability.

The overhead athlete places tremendous stress on the shoulder and elbow complex during sport activities. During throwing, the forces at the glenohumeral joint can exceed the body weight of the thrower. It is the function of the static (osseous and ligamentous structures) and dynamic (neuromuscular control) stabilizers to provide functional stability and to control these forces during overhead sport movements. The elbow complex, with its intimate joint congruency and thus excellent static stability, is less dependent on the dynamic stabilizers. This chapter reviews the anatomy and biomechanics of the shoulder and elbow complex during throwing and tennis activities. In addition, various rehabilitative techniques are discussed.

ANATOMY, KINEMATICS, AND BASIC INJURY MECHANISMS OF THE SHOULDER

Scapulothoracic Joint

The anatomic foundation of the shoulder girdle is the scapulothoracic articulation, which is formed by the ventral surface of the scapula and the posterior chest wall; it is the platform on which efficient shoulder motion depends. The scapula is moved superiorly by action of the superior fibers of the trapezius, levator scapula, and rhomboid muscles and inferiorly by the inferior trapezius fibers and pectoralis minor. Ventral motion is produced by the serratus anterior, pectoralis minor, and pectoralis major. Dorsal movement is caused by the posterior pull of the rhomboids and the middle and inferior trapezius. Rotation of the scapula is due to a combination of these movements. There is a 2:1 ratio of glenohumeral to scapulothoracic movement during arm flexion/extension and abduction/adduction. With repetitive forceful stress, the costal surface of the scapula may develop osteophyte formation at the inferior and superior medial borders. In addition, the soft-tissue supporting structures can become inflamed and may develop palpable tender areas.

Glenohumeral Joint

The glenohumeral joint is designed for motion with precarious stability restraints. The humeral head is held against the shallow glenoid concavity by capsular, tendinous, ligamentous, and muscular support. The relationship is analogous to a golf ball on a tee. If the support structure is inherently loose, stretched by overzealous activity or inflamed by repetitive overloading, the head of the humerus tends to be seated imperfectly within the glenoid fossa. It may even be driven over the labral rim by the power muscles (pectoralis major, deltoid, and latissimus dorsi) of the shoulder girdle.

The articular capsule of the glenohumeral joint is reinforced superiorly by the tendons of the supraspinatus; anteriorly by the subscapularis; posteriorly by the infraspinatus and teres minor; and inferiorly by the long head of the triceps. The coracohumeral ligament provides additional support to the superior part of the capsule as it blends with the supraspinatus tendon. Although at times difficult to individualize, three areas reinforce the anterior joint capsule: the superior, middle, and inferior glenohumeral ligaments. The inferior ligament is the most important and provides additional protection against joint subluxation. In addition, the overlying musculature adds to the integrity of the glenohumeral articulation.

The concavity of the glenoid fossa is deepened by the densely fibrous, triangular-shaped labrum that is attached to its circumference. The tendon of the long head of the biceps attaches directly to and is contiguous with the superior rim of the labrum and serves to depress the humeral head. In the overhead athlete, the long head of the biceps can be avulsed from the labrum by muscular activity in the follow-through phase of throwing.[1-3]

The shoulder joint is capable of essentially every definable motion. The humerus is flexed by the pectoralis major, anterior deltoid, coracorbrachialis, and (when the forearm is flexed) the biceps. It is extended by the latissimus dorsi, teres major, posterior deltoid, and (when the forearm is extended) the triceps. Abduction is produced by the deltoid and the supraspinatus. Adduction is the function of the subscapularis, pectoralis major, latissimus dorsi, and teres minor. The humerus is externally rotated by the infraspinatus and teres minor and internally rotated by the subscapularis, latissimus dorsi, teres major, pectoralis major, and anterior deltoid. The humerus is circumducted by a specific combination of these muscles.

In abducted shoulder motion, the subscapularis acts to stabilize and to roll the humeral head posteriorly in the glenoid fossa to counteract the tendency for anterior subluxation. The supraspinatus, which is in action with the deltoid throughout its entire range of motion, serves to maintain proper glenohumeral alignment. The infraspinatus and teres minor contribute a firm and steady counterforce to prevent anterior displacement of the humeral head; they also act to depress the humeral head. The latissimus dorsi pulls the humeral head posteriorly, extends the humerus, and depresses the shoulder. The lower fibers of the pectoralis major also depress the shoulder girdle.

Acromioclavicular Joint

The acromioclavicular joint is a diarthrodial articulation between the lateral end of the clavicle and the medial margin of the acromion of the scapula. The ligamentous support of the acromioclavicular joint is relatively lax and weak to allow the acromion and clavicle to glide and slide on one another in anterior/posterior and superior/inferior directions. It also allows some rotational motion of the clavicle. Acute ligamentous injuries occur with falls on the point of the shoulder, the top of the shoulder, the flexed elbow, or the outstretched hand. Such joint injuries or sprains are graded I through VI in respect to the separation of the clavicle from the acromion or the distance of the coracoid process from the clavicle.[24a]

The acromioclavicular joint may develop degenerative changes or bony resorption after acromioclavicular separation and mild repeated localized trauma. Osteolytic lesions of the lateral end of the clavicle may also occur without trauma in persons who train by weight lifting. Symptoms in osteolysis of the distal end of the clavicle are usually insidious in onset and mildly painful, but they can progress to cause significant shoulder disability. Disturbing symptoms of aching after exercise and localized pain when doing push-ups, chins, and dips or when throwing are often reported.

When degenerative changes occur in the acromioclavicular joint, decreased gliding and rotation may occur alone or in concert with pathology of the sternoclavicular joint. If glenohumeral motion is restricted, there may be a compensatory increase in laxity of the acromioclavicular joint to aid in shoulder motion.

Sternoclavicular Joint

The medial end of the clavicle articulates with and is firmly attached to the manubrium and the cartilage of the first rib. Joint integrity depends on its strong ligamentous support. Three planes of motion are allowed at the sternoclavicular joint: posterior/anterior, cephalad/caudad, and rotation. Violent medially directed forces to the lateral shoulder or direct trauma to the clavicle may cause an acute dislocation of the joint. As the arm is abducted and externally rotated in throwing or an overhead swing, posterior retraction of the shoulder results in anterior stretching of the sternoclavicular joint. On the follow-through of these motions, a rotational stress is developed medially in the sternoclavicular joint. Such repetitive motions may produce stress that develops into clinical sprains with minimal symptoms. If the ligamentous supports become sufficiently irritated by the repeated microtrauma of stretching, the sternoclavicular joint may become swollen and tender and may limit full shoulder motion. The sternoclavicular articulation may develop decreased range of motion from weight training and with advanced age. It may also develop increased motion as a compensatory mechanism for decreased glenohumeral and acromioclavicular mobility.

SHOULDER FUNCTION

For the shoulder to function with optimal proficiency in sports and in daily activity, there must be a harmonious and synchronous balance of muscular action. This balance must work through unimpeded and healthy articulations in a sound, well-conditioned body that is devoid of significant congenital or acquired abnormalities. Previous musculoskeletal injuries must have been ameliorated. Muscular strength and flexibility should be at preinjury levels, and educated, rational practice and performance plans should have been made, implemented, and instituted with proper supervision. Such an ideal situation is difficult to achieve and even more difficult to maintain.

To be proficient at a sport, practice is necessary. This necessitates repetitions of the same motion to perfect technique and to make the motion "second nature." With such use, the body can increase in strength and size due to muscle hypertrophy and bony enlargement. It can also develop problems such as irregular articular cartilage wear, ligamentous and tendinous microtrauma and inflammation, formation of scar tissue, and abnormal calcifi-

cation of soft tissue. With microscopic scarring, adjacent surfaces that previously moved on each other as smoothly as two pieces of silk become as rough as two pieces of thick corduroy. When actively moved, the affected area produces a rough, irregular excursion of opposing surfaces that is appreciated as crepitation. If the same activity is allowed to persist, the scarred tissues develop poor mechanical properties. As more activity is imposed on the traumatized area, further insults may result in pain, edema, hemorrhage, and fibrosis. This can lead to soft-tissue failure at load levels that previously were well tolerated.

ANATOMY, KINEMATICS, AND BASIC INJURY MECHANISMS OF THE ELBOW

The elbow is a hinged joint composed of the humerus, radius, and ulna, whose bony stability is produced by the olecranon, olecranon fossa complex, and the radial head/capitellum. The radioulnar portion of the joint allows the forearm to move in pronation/supination. Secondary soft-tissue stability is produced by flexor-pronator musculature. The primary soft-tissue stability of the elbow is the function of the ulnar (medial) collateral ligament, which serves to resist valgus and extension stresses in throwing and racquet sports. All three areas of restraint (osseous, muscular, and ligamentous) must function adequately to ensure stability and to counterbalance stress forces. Proximal-distal stability is provided by the articulation of the humerus and the ulna, which allows for 150° to 0° of flexion and extension of the elbow. The radioulnar portion of the joint allows 90° of supination and 70° of pronation of the forearm. The elbow normally has a slight valgus angulation, which is known as the carrying angle. The carrying angle (measured in full extension) is normally up to 10–15° in men and up to 20° in women. When the elbow is flexed, the angle reverts to 5–10° of varus position.

Humeroulnar Joint

The humeroulnar articulation consists of:
1. The trochlear notch in the humerus (for articulation with the trochlea of the ulna);
2. The olecranon process of the ulna (for

articulation with the olecranon fossa of the humerus); and

3. The coronoid process of the ulna (for articulation with its corresponding coronoid fossa in the humerus).

As the olecranon engages the olecranon fossa over the last 30° of extension, it creates great mediolateral elbow stability. Valgus stress in this position results in an abutment of the medial olecranon process against the medial olecranon fossa. In contrast, hyperextension stress causes straight posterior and posterolateral abutment of the olecranon in the olecranon fossa.

Radiocapitellar Joint

The humeral capitellum is convex. The radial head is concave and is free to rotate about the capitellum in pronation and supination. When the elbow is stressed in valgus, the radiocapitellar joint sustains compressive loads. It serves as a secondary stabilizer to such medial valgus forces and supplements the medial collateral ligament. Changes in articular cartilage can be caused both in the capitellum and in the radial head by compression and repetitive microtraumatic forces of pronation-supination.

Proximal Radioulnar Joint

The proximal radioulnar articulation is between the radial head and the radial notch of the ulna. It is estimated that approximately one-fifth of the radial head is in contact with the ulna at any given time. Stability of this joint depends on the integrity of the annular ligament, which communicates with the radial collateral ligament laterally and the ulna anteriorly. The radioulnar joint articulation is infrequently the site of athletic injury.

Ligamentous Structures

Radial (Lateral) Collateral Ligament

The radial collateral ligament originates from the lateral epicondyle and inserts primarily on the annular ligament that surrounds the head of the radius. A few of its fibers also attach to the radial notch of the

ulna. Since this ligament connects bone to soft tissue, it provides limited support. Additional lateral support against varus stress is assumed partially by the anconeus muscle, which originates on the lateral epicondyle and inserts into the radial border of the ulna.

Ulnar (Medial) Collateral Ligament

The ulnar (medial) collateral ligament is a ligamentous complex. The anterior oblique component originates from the medial epicondyle of the humerus and inserts just posterior to the coronoid process of the ulna. The posterior oblique component arises from the same point on the medial condyle and inserts on the ulna in the area of the mid-olecranon. The transverse portion of the ulnar collateral ligament is not primarily involved in medial stability. Portions of the anterior oblique band of the ulnar collateral ligament are taut both in flexion and in extension. The posterior oblique band of the ligament, however, is taut only in flexion and not in extension. As long as the anterior oblique band is intact, injury to the posterior band of the ligament does not result in elbow instability. The ulnar (medial) collateral ligament is known as the cornerstone of the throwing elbow; stabilization is its primary function.[4]

Musculotendinous Elbow Structures

The flexors of the elbow joint—the brachialis, biceps, and brachioradialis—function to decelerate elbow motion and are subject to repetitive, stressful overloading. The flexor-pronator muscle group originates from the medial epicondyle and consists of the flexor carpi radialis, flexor digitorum sublimis, pronator teres, palmaris longus, and flexor carpi ulnaris muscles. The flexor-pronator muscle mass serves as a dynamic secondary stabilizer of the elbow to resist valgus tensile forces.

The extensor forearm mass, the brachioradialis, extensor carpi radialis longus and brevis, and a portion of the common extensor tendons originates from the distal lateral humerus. In the throwing athlete, the major elbow decelerator for this group is the brachioradialis. The extensor carpi radialis brevis and longus are often involved in lateral epicondylitis.

INJURY MECHANISMS
IN ELBOW COMPARTMENTS

Anterior Compartment

A repetitious overhead throwing or hitting motion can produce anterior capsular sprains, flexor pronator muscle tears, bicipital muscle strains, and bicipital tendinitis. Repetitive, traumatic hyperextension of the elbow also produces anterior capsular stress. Such stress can be caused if hyperextension overload stress is superimposed on joint hyperelasticity, insufficient strength, or improper biomechanics. This clinical condition is sometimes confused with bicipital or brachial tendinitis or even osteochondritis of the trochlear groove. The history of a sudden, sharp pain and marked weakness in flexion is a tip-off of distal rupture of the biceps tendon at its insertion into the tuberosity of the radius. Mild pain, weakness, and tenderness of the anterior elbow associated with decreased flexion and supination support the diagnosis of bicipital or brachial tendinitis.

Lateral Compartment

Lateral elbow problems are usually caused by compressive forces between the humeral capitellum and the adjacent radial head. Such compression occurs in valgus stress and is associated with stretch injury to the radial joint. In the skeletally immature athlete, Panner coined the term "osteochondrosis" to describe an osteochondritis-like pathology of the capitellum. This osteochondrosis, which is not associated with loose body formation, tends to occur in the 7- to 10-year-old age group, whereas lateral osteochondritis dissecans typically occurs in the 11- to 15-year-old age group. Some investigators feel that osteochondrosis is an early stage of osteochondritis. If not treated, it may progress to the typical osteochondritis dissecans that exhibits loose body formation, bony rarefaction, craters, and flattening of the capitellum.

Lateral epicondylitis (tennis elbow) is caused by stress on the forearm and wrist extensors at the moment of extensor mass contraction. Repetitive overloading, which is the major cause of extensor tendinitis, primarily affects the extensor carpi radialis brevis muscle.

Posterior Compartment

Elbow problems of the posterior compartment are most often osseous in nature. With throwing and extension, the olecranon is wedged against the medial wall of the olecranon fossa. This can cause osteophyte and loose-bone body formation. Repeated hyperextension (valgus extension overload) is seen in the early acceleration phase of pitching or in the mid-phase of serving in racquet sports and produces abutment posteriorly.[5,6]

Apophysitis can be caused by forceful contraction of the triceps on the secondary ossification centers of the olecranon. In the adolescent, avulsion of the triceps at its insertion or a stress reaction at the recently fused olecranon apophysis can be noted. Inflammation of the olecranon bursa at the tip of the elbow can be produced by direct trauma or by chronic repetitive pressure on the elbow. Bleeding or a serous accumulation in the olecranon bursa may produce local discomfort and decreased range of motion. Fractures in the posterior elbow usually result from a direct blow along with a concomitant forceful contraction of the triceps.

Medial Compartment

Medial elbow pain most often ensues from medial epicondylitis, strain of the ulnar collateral ligament or flexor–pronator mass, ulnar nerve neuritis, and ulnar stress fractures. Medial elbow pain is reproduced by stress testing of the forearm valgus, which produces traction force to the medial soft tissues. Flexor tendinitis needs to be differentiated from ulnar (medial) collateral ligament sprain. In a sprain, tenderness is noted directly over the ulnar collateral ligament, and pain in enhanced by forced valgus stress. In flexor tendinitis tenderness is noted over the flexor muscles and medial epicondyle, and pain is caused by forced wrist flexion and forearm pronation.

The term "Little League elbow" refers to a traction-avulsion apophysitis of the medial humeral epicondyle. Repetitive, stressful tension forces across the physis are developed in the early acceleration phase of throwing, producing local tenderness and swelling, decreased joint extension, and pain on valgus stressing. Both the flexor pronator muscle group and the ulnar collateral ligament originate on the apophysis and may be involved in production of symptoms.

In the older athlete, medial epicondylitis can develop in the trailing elbow with batting. It can also be caused by hitting the forehand in tennis with the elbow forward of the racquet head. This motion results in a tensile stretch on the origins of the flexor–pronator muscle group. Medial muscle soreness may be compounded by ulnar neuritis, which can develop as a result of repetitive valgus traction.

PERIPHERAL NERVE PROBLEMS ABOUT THE SHOULDER AND ELBOW

Musculocutaneous Nerve

The musculocutaneous nerve can be injured in the shoulder by dislocation of the anterior shoulder, fracture of the coracoid process, severe shoulder contusions, or a muscle-splitting surgical approach to the anterior shoulder. Such nerve damage in the shoulder may produce weakness in elbow flexion and forearm supination, along with atrophy of the biceps and brachialis muscles and forearm dysesthesias. After innervating the elbow flexors, the musculocutaneous nerve passes into the forearm as the lateral antebrachial cutaneous nerve. It lies between the biceps aponeurosis and the fascia of the brachialis in the antecubital fossa of the anterior compartment. Trauma to this area or tendinitis of the bicipital tendon can produce sensory deficits of the forearm by compromising this nerve.

Radial Nerve

At the lateral elbow, the radial nerve divides into a posterior interosseous motor nerve and a superficial sensory branch. Compression of the motor nerve by the supinator muscle (arcade of Frohse) at the level of the humeroradial joint produces weakness of the forearm extensors and deep muscle aching. Symptoms are exacerbated by repeated activity of the supinator. Tenderness localized over the supinator muscle rather than the lateral epicondyle or conjoint tendon helps to differentiate this entity from lateral epicondylitis.

Median Nerve

At the elbow, the median nerve supplies motor innervation to the flexor-pronator muscles. Entrapment or contusion of the median nerve can occur just proximal to the medial elbow or anteriorly between the two heads of the pronator teres (pronator teres syndrome) or at the arch of flexor digitorum superficialis (anterior interosseous nerve syndrome). Aching of the volar forearm and pain exaggerated by flexor-pronator activity with the elbow in extension are typical of the pronator teres syndrome. Anterior interosseous nerve syndrome may cause proximal forearm pain and weakness of the flexor pollicis longus, pronator quadrators, and flexor digitorum profundus (of digits 2 and 3).

Ulnar Nerve

The ulnar nerve lies between the olecranon and the medial epicondyle in a superficial groove (ulnar sulcus). The ulnar nerve then enters the forearm between the ulna and the heads of the flexor carpi ulnaris muscle (cubital tunnel). A thickening of soft tissue at the cubital tunnel may cause ulnar entrapment neuritis. Repetitive overload throwing, however, tends to accentuate the normal stretching of the ulnar nerve, especially during the cocking and acceleration phases. Subluxations and, on rare occasions, dislocations of the ulnar nerve from the ulnar sulcus may occur. An athlete with ulnar neuropathy usually complains of posteromedial elbow discomfort and intermittent paresthesias in the fourth and fifth fingers. The symptoms are aggravated by throwing maneuvers and improved by rest.

Axillary Nerve

The axillary nerve is commonly injured in dislocations of the anterior shoulder, which lead to weakness in abduction and external rotation. There may be an area of decreased skin sensation over the lateral deltoid at the so-called axillary patch.

Suprascapular Nerve

The suprascapular nerve may be injured by traction stress during the deceleration phase of pitching. Such an injury may lead to infraspinatus weakness or combined supraspinatus/infraspinatus weakness. Abduction and/or external rotation of the shoulder may be impaired.

Thoracic Nerve

The serratus anterior muscle is innervated by the long thoracic nerve. This muscle functions as a powerful abductor, rotator, and stabilizer of the scapula. Damage to the long thoracic nerve can cause scapular winging and an inability to abduct or flex the arm fully. In some cases the nerve is only minimally involved in brachial plexus pathology, and in these cases an insidious weakness in shoulder stabilization may develop. This condition is often painless and, without observable scapular winging, is difficult to detect; it may cause decreased athletic prowess.

DISLOCATIONS OF THE ELBOW

Anterior/posterior stability of the elbow is the function of intact soft tissue, the medial and lateral collateral ligaments, and the integrity of the coronoid process/coronoid fossa. Elbow dislocations are generally the result of hyperextension, in which the olecranon is forced into the olecranon fossa and the trochlea is levered over the coronoid process. The ulnar (medial) collateral ligament is usually ruptured by this injury, and associated fractures may occur. Anterior dislocation of the elbow is much less common and much more severe.

VASCULAR PROBLEMS ABOUT THE SHOULDER AND ELBOW

Subclavian/axillary artery occlusion or thrombosis of the subclavian/axillary veins may produce both shoulder and elbow symptoms. Specifically, in the cocking phase of pitching in which a considerable amount of torque is produced, the middle-third of the axillary artery is subject to compression. This may cause symptoms of aching and early fatigue of the forearm muscles as well as coolness and paleness of the forearm and fingers. Symptoms are often referred to as "deep" and are often initially felt about the elbow.

BIOMECHANICS OF THROWING

Throwing is a highly stressful, violent, and skillful activity that requires flexibility, strength, power, endurance, coordination, and timing. The throwing action requires excessive motion, precisely coordinated movement, and a synchronized muscle-firing pattern, all of which must occur at a velocity faster than any other upper-extremity sport movement. To accomplish this difficult task, the shoulder must be capable of a tremendous amount of passive and dynamic motion. Although excessive motion is required for throwing, the shoulder complex and elbow must still maintain functional stability. This stability is accomplished through capsular and ligamentous restraints and by the contribution of the neuromuscular system. Minimal stability is afforded by osseous configuration. The throw can be broken down into five specific phases:

1. Wind-up,
2. Arm-cocking,
3. Arm acceleration,
4. Arm deceleration, and
5. Follow-through.

The wind-up phase exhibits the most variability from thrower to thrower. The goal of the wind-up is to establish an advantageous position from which to throw that also serves as a distraction to the hitter. During the wind-up the thrower must be balanced and establish good biomechanical alignment. Except for the potential energy of lifting of the lead leg, very little energy is generated in the wind-up phase of throwing.

Arm-cocking and acceleration are highly dynamic phases in the throwing motion. The thrower generates energy in different segments of the body and then quickly and systematically passes this energy to the ball. Proper timing and sequence of the motions are imperative to highly skilled throwing. Arm-cocking begins when the ball is taken out of the glove, and arm acceleration begins when maximal external rotation has occurred. During arm-cocking, the lead foot makes ground contact, and the hips, lead foot, and shoulders rotate to face the target. The angular velocity of the shoulder during the arm-cocking phase is approximately 1100 °/s.[12] At the extreme of the arm-cocking position the shoulder is abducted between 90° to 100°,[13] and the arm is externally rotated between 145° to 180°.[13] The elbow is flexed to approximately 90°. The internal rotators are eccentrically loaded and also elastically stretched. During the early cocking phase, the deltoid muscle exhibits a high level of activity; during mid-cocking, the supraspinatus, infraspinatus, and teres minor are highly active.[17,18] During the latter stages of arm- cocking, the subscapularis and latissimus dorsi exhibit a high level of activity, whereas the pectoralis major and serratus anterior exhibit a moderate level.[17,18] By the end of this stage, a tremendous amount of potential energy is available in the legs, trunks, and hips to be transferred to the throwing motion.

Once the arm reaches maximal external rotation, the elbow begins to extend, and the acceleration phase begins. While the arm extends at the elbow, internal rotation begins at the shoulder. During the acceleration phase, the angular velocity of the glenohumeral joint exceeds 7000°/s.[13] The angular velocity of elbow extension exceeds 2500°/s.[13] Regardless of what type of pitch is thrown or the style of the individual thrower, at ball release the throwing shoulder is abducted about 90° to 100°. The difference between an "overhand" and a "sidearm" baseball pitcher is not the abduction of the shoulder but rather the degree of lateral tilt of the trunk. Biomechanic analysis of throwing appears to indicate that approximately 90° of abduction is the strongest angle for the shoulder during the throw. During the acceleration phase, the rotator cuff and deltoid muscles exhibit a low level of activity, whereas the pectoralis major and latissimus dorsi muscles contract concentrically at a high level to accelerate the arm. The serratus anterior also exhibits a high level of muscular activity during this phase.

After ball release, the arm continues to extend at the elbow, rotates internally, and adducts horizontally at the shoulder. Because of the internal rotation, the hand appears to pronate. During this deceleration phase, the posterior shoulder muscles (posterior deltoid, infraspinatus, teres minor) contract eccentrically to decelerate the arm to prevent distraction of the glenohumeral joint.[12,17,18] The distractive forces at the glenohumeral joint are approximately equal to body weight.[8,11] The elbow joint must also decelerate before it reaches full extension. The elbow flexors contract to control the large extension moment. During this phase, the deltoid, rotator cuff, and serratus anterior muscles, exhibit a high level of activity.[8,17,18] The pectoralis major and latissimus dorsi exhibit a moderate level of muscular activity.[8,17,18]

The energy generated during the acceleration and deceleration phases of throwing must be dissipated after the ball is released. The key to a good follow-through is to allow the larger body parts to help in dissipating the energy in the throwing arm.[13] To reduce the required forces of deceleration, the throwing arm should exhibit a complete follow-through path, which allows the energy to be dissipated over a longer time. With a correct follow-through movement, the throwing hand should reach the opposite leg. A pitcher who ends up with his hand toward the target will most likely place excessive distraction loads on his shoulder.

BIOMECHANICS OF TENNIS

Most tennis arm movements require high-velocity dynamic muscular contractions during the serve and ground strokes. During the acceleration phase of the serve of highly skilled players, the maximal internal rotation velocity exceeds 2300°/s (Dillman CJ, unpublished data). The tennis serve can be divided into four specific phases: the wind-up, cocking, acceleration, and follow-through.

The wind-up phase is characterized by assuming a serving stance. The ball is tossed by the contralateral hand. The cocking phase begins following ball toss and terminates at the point of maximal external rotation of the shoulder. The maximal external rotation during the cocking phase is approximately 155°, with abduction between 80° and 85°.[10] The acceleration phase of the tennis serve begins at maximal external rotation and terminates at ball impact. During the phase, high muscular activity has been recorded in the pectoralis major, subscapularis, latissimus dorsi, and serratus anterior.[24,28] The arm and racket head are accelerating at a speed near 2500°/s, and peak muscular activity occurs just prior to ball impact. The final phase in the tennis serve is the follow-through. This phase is characterized by the deceleration of the arm through moderately high levels of muscle activity of the posterior rotator cuff, serratus anterior, biceps brachii, deltoid, and latissimus dorsi.[24]

The forehand and backhand ground strokes can be broken down into three phases: preparation, acceleration, and follow-through. During the preparation phase of either the forehand or backhand, muscular activity is relatively low. The acceleration phase exhibits very high muscular activity. During the forehand stroke, the subscapularis, biceps brachii, pectoralis major, and serratus anterior muscles exhibit significant activity.[24] Acceleration during the backhand stroke consists of high muscular activity of the middle deltoid, supraspinatus, infraspinatus, biceps brachii, and serratus anterior muscles.[24] During follow-through for the forehand ground stroke, moderately high muscular activity is seen in the serratus anterior, subscapularis, infraspinatus, and biceps brachii. Follow-through activity during the backhand is moderately high for the biceps, middle deltoid, supraspinatus, and infraspinatus muscles.

Biomechanic analysis of the angular velocities during the forehand ground stroke indicates a peak internal rotation angular velocity of 365° to 700°/s.[26] A common forehand stroke is the topspin ground stroke, which is advantageous to the player because it improves the velocity of the ball and control of the shot. The stroke path from low to high requires proper timing, positioning, and preparation. Improper biomechanics in the unskilled player results in a "rolling over" of the ball to achieve topspin. This improperly produced stroke, achieved by excessive internal rotation of the shoulder and pronation of the forearm, may eventually lead to overuse injuries, tissue breakdown of the rotator cuff, medial epicondylitis, or chronic tendinitis.

Peak angular velocities of external rotation during the backhand stroke in highly skilled players range between 328° to 1600°/s.[26] Improper biomechanic technique is commonly seen during the tennis backhand. The player should use legs and hips and provide angular acceleration velocity through torso rotation rather than with shoulder and arm motion. Improper technique is commonly noted in the unskilled player who stresses the elbow and forearm to strike a backhand. This type of incorrect stroke commonly leads to overuse tendinitis of the wrist extensors. Use of a two-hand backhand has been recommended for some players with upper-extremity injury, particularly "tennis elbow," because it allows bilateral upper-extremity force generation, load-sharing, and greater trunk rotation.

Most injuries to the shoulder complex in the thrower or racquet sport athlete develop as a result of repetitive microtraumatic forces that eventually can lead to acquired tissue failure. Usually these injuries can be effectively managed with appropriate and aggressive conservative treatment, but occasionally they require surgical intervention. The elbow complex exhibits a similar pathomechanic scenario. Most elbow injuries in the overhead athlete are due to repetitive, overload trauma. Often, as in the case of the thrower, microtraumatic forces can lead to subsequent tissue failure such as ulnar collateral ligament ruptures, osteochondritis, and abnormal osseous formation, all of which frequently require surgery to reestablish normal function.

REHABILITATION

Whether the treatment is conservative or surgical, rehabilitation plays a vital role in achieving a successful outcome. The rehabilitation process must be progressive with the ultimate goal of a rapid return to pain-free sport function. A functional, reliable rehabilitation program is based on six basic principles of rehabilitation:

1. Successful treatment is based on a team approach, with the physician, patient, and therapist/trainer working together toward a common goal.
2. The effects of immobilization must be minimized. Early motion and strengthening are preferred whenever possible.
3. Healing tissue should never be overstressed.
4. The patient must fulfill specific objective criteria to proceed from one stage to the next (Table 1).
5. The rehabilitation program must be based on sound, current clinical and scientific research.
6. The rehabilitation program must be adaptable to each patient to allow for individualization and specificity of sport activities.

Phase One:
Immediate Phase Rehabilitation

Shoulder

Immediately after shoulder injury or surgery, motion is allowed in a protected, minimally painful range of motion. Immediate motion minimizes the deleterious effects of immobilization, such as articular degeneration, muscular atrophy, and adverse collagen formation. The glenohumeral joint depends on the surrounding musculature for dynamic functional stability. Thus, strict immobilization results in inefficient dynamic stabilization through disuse atrophy, muscle substitution, and decreased neuromuscular control. Immediate motion exercises should be emphasized through the use of an L-bar (Breg Corporation, Vista, CA) to promote active assisted range-of-motion exercises. The motions emphasized include shoulder flexion and shoulder external and internal rotation. During shoulder flexion, the patient should be carefully instructed to lead with the thumb to

TABLE 1. Four Exercise Phases

Phase I—Immediate motion stage
   Immediate motion exercises
   Isometrics
   Stretching
   Weight-bearing contractions
Phase II—Intermediate stage
   Stretching
   Isotonics
   Manual resistance
   Neuromuscular control drills
Phase III—Advanced strengthening stage
   Isotonics—eccentric/concentric
   Plyometrics
   Isokinetics
   Neuromuscular control drills
Phase IV—Return to activity stage
   Continued strengthening program ("thrower's ten")
   Interval sport programs

create humeral external rotation and thus to clear the greater tuberosity from under the coracoacromial arch and to prevent supraspinatus impingement (Fig. 1). Exercises for external and internal rotation of the shoulder are usually initiated at 0° of shoulder abduction or in the plane of the scapula. Exercises are performed as tolerated, in 45° and lastly 90° of abduction (Fig. 2). Capsular stretches for the inferior, posterior, and anterior portions of the glenohumeral joint capsule are also initiated early in rehabilitation. Early motion exercises help to normalize the arthrokinematics of the joint and also to neuromodulate the patient's pain.

Immediately after a shoulder injury or surgery, it is common to observe a functional decrease in strength of the rotator cuff musculature secondary to pain, swelling, and trauma. The function of the rotator cuff is to stabilize dynamically and to steer the humeral head during arm movements. Therefore, it is critical to restore rotator cuff function as soon as possible. This can be achieved with the use of isometric contractions, which should be performed submaximally, at multiple angles, and in pain-free positions. The muscles to be emphasized include the external/internal rotators at 0° of abduction and in 0° and 30° of rotation (Fig. 3A), the abductors at 30° and 60° of elevation (Fig. 3B), the supraspinatus muscle in the

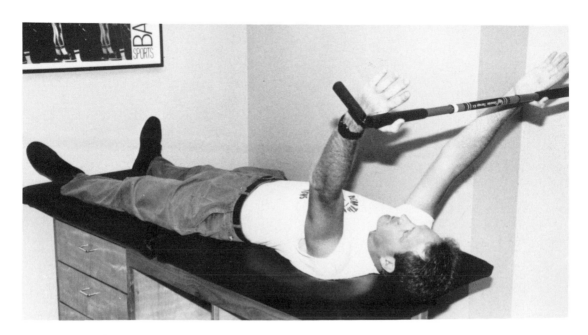

FIGURE 1. Active assisted shoulder flexion motion using an L-bar for motion stimulus.

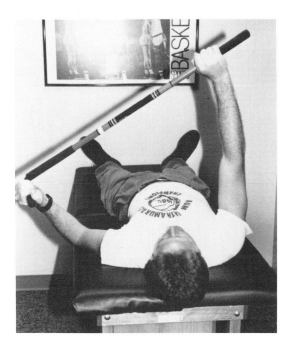

FIGURE 2. Active assisted shoulder external rotation motion using an L-bar with the shoulder at 45° of abduction.

empty-can position (scaption) at 30° and 60° of elevation (Fig. 3C), and the elbow flexors.

Isometric contractions serve to reestablish dynamic control of the humeral head and are vital to the successful outcome of the rehabilitation program. In addition, weight-bearing exercises are incorporated to elicit a co-contraction of the surrounding shoulder muscles. These drills are performed with the patient standing or kneeling. The patient places a constant force through the hands that is proportionate to body weight. Then the patient is instructed to shift weight from side to side, forward to back, and diagonally. As the patient improves, the drills can be progressed with manual resistance, hands on a large ball or small ball, and two hands to one hand. Additionally, a large Swiss ball may facilitate scapular and spinal extensors.

The goals of the exercises in phase one are

1. To reestablish normal motion of the shoulder complex,
2. To retard muscular atrophy,
3. To reestablish dynamic control of the humeral head, and

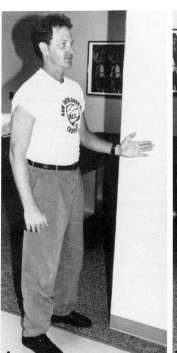
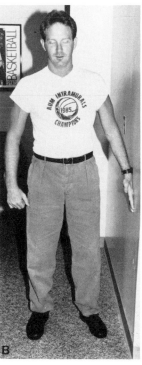
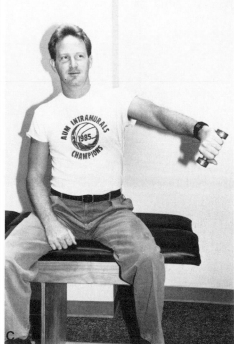

FIGURE 3. *A,* Isometric muscular contraction of shoulder's external rotators. *B,* Isometric muscular contraction of shoulder's abductors. *C,* The "empty-can" movement, shoulder "scaption" with internal rotation to isolate the supraspinatus muscle.

4. To decrease the patient's pain and inflammation.

Elbow

In contrast to the shoulder, the elbow joint complex is less dependent on the dynamic stabilizers. Most of its stability comes from joint congruency and osseous configuration. Because of this enhanced osseous stability, reestablishing elbow motion after injury or surgery is critical. When this goal is not successfully attained, an elbow flexion contraction is common. Many factors contribute to the development of elbow flexion contractures, including intimate congruency of the elbow joint complex (especially of the humeroulnar joint), tightness of the elbow capsule, and the tendency of the anterior capsule to scar and become adhesive. The anterior capsule is relatively thin and highly sensitive to injury. In addition, the brachialis muscle inserts into the capsule and crosses the anterior capsule as a muscle rather than as tendinous tissue. Thus, injury or immobilization of the elbow results in excessive scarring of the capsule and functional muscle splinting. To counteract these capsular restrictions, mobilizations are performed to both the humeroulnar and humeroradial joints. To regain elbow extension, a posterior glide of the ulna on the humerus is performed. Another extremely effective exercise in obtaining full extension is passive elbow extension with a hand-held weight to produce a passive overpressure extension stretch.[30] This stretch uses a long-duration/low-intensity application that appears to produce enhanced elongation of the collagen tissue.[22,29] Isometric strengthening drills are performed for the elbow, wrist, and forearm musculature to prevent muscular atrophy.

Phase Two Rehabilitation

Shoulder

Phase-two strengthening exercises are progressed from submaximal isometric muscular contractions to submaximal isotonic contractions. The goals of this phase are to improve muscular strength, endurance, and neuromuscular control of the shoulder complex. During this phase, scapulothoracic stabilization exercises are emphasized. Before a patient is allowed to perform phase-two exercises, specific criteria must be exhibited on clinical examination: (1) full, nonpainful range of motion, (2) minimal pain and tenderness, and (3) good strength (four-fifths on manual muscle testing) of the shoulder's internal/external rotators and flexor muscles. These criteria ensure proper rate of progression during the rehabilitation process.

The exercises performed in this phase are submaximal isotonic muscular contractions for the glenohumeral and scapulothoracic musculature. Low-weight submaximal contractions are used because most of the shoulder muscles are small and do not require large weights to achieve a maximal challenge. Slightly heavier weights are used to strengthen the "prime-mover" muscles of the shoulder complex—the pectoralis major, deltoid, latissimus dorsi, and teres major.

The rotator cuff exercises are expanded to include sidelying external rotation with a dumbbell to strengthen the external rotators (infraspinatus, teres minor). The internal rotators (subscapularis, pectoralis major, latissimus dorsi) are exercised in either sidelying or in standing. Early exercises for strengthening the internal and external rotators are performed in the zero position (0° abduction). As the patient improves, they are performed in 45° and later 90° of abduction. Several authors have suggested that rotator-strengthening exercises should be done in a position referred to as the scapular plane, which is 20° to 30° of shoulder flexion and 30° to 40° of abduction.[12,14,25] This position is advocated because it places minimal stress on the inferior capsule, may enhance supraspinatus microvascularity, and appears to be a more functional movement plane. Some clinicians believe that strengthening of the internal and external rotators should be performed in a continuum from an inherently stable position to a less stable position. In addition, it is believed that later strengthening exercises should be performed in more functional positions.

Isolated movements to strengthen the supraspinatus muscle have been the topic of several investigations. Jobe[5] reported highest electromyographic (EMG) activity of the supraspinatus muscle during the "scaption" or empty-can movement (Fig. 3C). Blackburn[7] reported increased muscular activity of the supraspinatus during horizontal arm abduction to 100° with external rotation, with the patient in the prone position.

Adequate strength of the scapulothoracic muscles is imperative for normal function of the glenohumeral joint. The scapulothoracic articulation must provide a stable base and proximal stability to allow distal mobility of the arm. The primary function of the scapula is to change positions dynamically and to provide stability, thus maintaining a consistent length-tension relationship of the rotator cuff muscles.[16]

Moseley has studied the scapulothoracic muscles with EMG during various exercises.[23] He reported that four exercises appeared to enhance the recruitment of the scapular muscles of the shoulder complex: scaption, rowing, press-up, and push-up. A four-part scapulothoracic exercise program has been established on the basis of these data: (1) prone horizontal abduction (neutral arm position) for strengthening of the rhomboideus minor/major muscles; (2) a push-up exercise for the serratus anterior and pectoralis muscles; (3) a prone rowing maneuver with an isometric hold to enhance muscular activity of the upper trapezius and levator scapulae muscles; and (4) an isometric press-up (Fig. 4) to create high muscular activity for the pectoralis major and minor and the latissimus dorsi muscles.

During this phase, it is extremely important to combine single-plane isotonic strengthening exercises with multiplane diagonal patterns using synergistic movement sequences, such as proprioceptive neuromuscular facilitation exercises.[21] A common diagonal pattern is the D_2 flexion/extension exercise pattern.[21] During flexion the patient is asked to elevate, abduct, and externally rotate the arm against manual resistance. To enhance stabilization of the rotator cuff, the clinician may ask the patient to hold at various points in the range as manual resistance is applied.[31] This technique, referred to as rhythmic stabilization, enhances the dynamic stability of the glenohumeral joint; the authors have found a significant benefit to the overhead athlete.[31]

Scapulothoracic muscular strength is important to the overhead athlete, but neuromuscular control is imperative to high performance. Exercises for neuromuscular control improve volitional motor control and movement of the scapula.[31,32] These exercises are performed with the patient side-lying on the contralateral side. The involved shoulder is free to move, and the hand is placed on the table with the arm abducted to 90° and internally rotated. The patient is asked to elevate

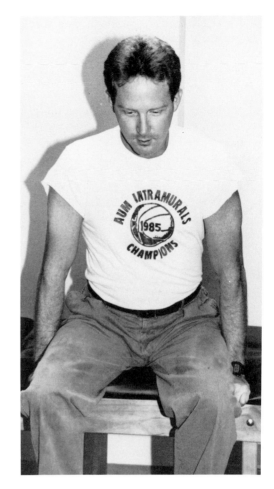

FIGURE 4. Shoulder press-up movement; can be performed with an isometric contraction or isotonic.

and depress, then protract and retract the scapula—with all movements performed slowly. The quality, not the quantity, of the movement is most important. The goal is to isolate nonsubstituted scapular movements. The drill begins with single-plane and progresses to multiplane movements, such as circles and diagonals.[31,32]

In addition, during this phase of exercises, it is extremely important to continue stretching to maintain shoulder motion. Most often these exercises include capsular self stretches and L-bar stretches.

Elbow

Elbow muscular stretches should be performed to ensure the maintenance and continued improvement of elbow motion, especially in extension. The athlete should progress to isotonic muscle-strengthening exercises with dumbbells or exercise tubing. The elbow flexors/extensors, pronators/supinators, and the wrist flexor/extensor muscles should be aggressively exercised. Endurance exercise should be emphasized particularly for the elbow flexors, wrist flexors, and pronators, which appear to play a significant role in dynamic stability of the humeroulnar joint.

Phase Three Rehabilitation

Shoulder

Phase-three exercises are considered dynamic strengthening exercises with the goals of improving muscular strength, power, and endurance. The emphasis of phase-three exercises for the overhead competitive athlete is a high-energy, eccentric contraction performed in a functional position. Because of stress to the musculotendinous unit and surrounding soft tissue, the patient must meet specific criteria before performing these drills. The patient must exhibit:

1. Full, nonpainful motion,
2. No pain or tenderness, and
3. Strength equal to 70% of the contralateral shoulder (documented objectively on isokinetic evaluation).

The exercises performed in this phase include isotonic dumbbell movements, exercise tubing movements for concentric/eccentric contractions, plyometrics, and neuromuscular control drills. The internal and external rotators are exercised with tubing in the 90° abducted/90° elbow-flexed position for the overhead athlete (Fig. 5). Exercise tubing is also used for biceps/triceps strengthening, rowing, and diagonal D_2 movement patterns. Again, diagonal movements can be performed with isometric holds at various points in the range of motion to strengthen the humeral head stabilizers.[32] Isotonic strengthening exercises with the dumbbell are continued for the deltoid, supraspinatus, forearm, and wrist musculature.

Plyometric drills, which are also initiated in this phase, are quick, powerful movements involving a prestretch of the muscle that activates its stretch-shortening activity. In turn, this stretch-shortening activates the muscle spindle and results in a facilitated concentric shortening contraction. Overhead sport

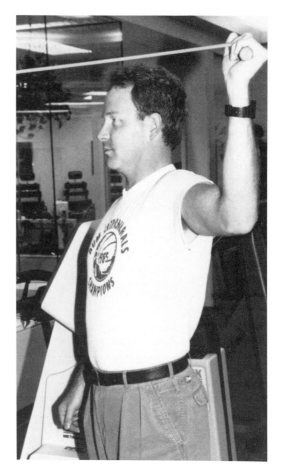

FIGURE 5. Strengthening exercises for internal and external rotators of the shoulder, performed in the 90/90° position.

movements such as throwing use a stretch-shortening type of contraction to accomplish explosive arm velocity.[8]

The plyometric exercise drill uses a three-phase movement. The first is the setting or eccentric phase, in which a rapid eccentric load is applied to the muscles. This stimulates the muscle's spindles, causing a muscle stretch reflex. The second phase is amortization, i.e., the amount of time between the initiation of the eccentric contraction and the beginning of the concentric contraction. Last is the response phase, which represents the resultant facilitated concentric contraction. Wilk[33] has described a plyometric exercise program for the throwing athlete (Table 2). The plyometric exercise drills provide the athlete with a functional progression from strengthening exercises to throwing movements and drills and prepare the shoulder muscles for the repetitive, microtraumatic

TABLE 2. **Plyometric Drills for the Upper Extremity**

Throwing Movements
Two-hand soccer throw
Two-hand chest pass
Two-hand side-to-side throw
Two-hand side throw
One-hand step and pass
One-hand baseball throw
Tubing plyometric exercise for internal and external rotation
Tubing diagonal plyometric exercises
Tubing biceps plyometric exercises
Plyometric push-ups

overload that will be applied during overhead sport activities. Plyometrics exercises can be performed for the musculature of both the shoulder and elbow joint.

Isokinetic exercise can be extremely beneficial in improving muscular strength, power, and endurance through high-speed training. Shoulder internal/external rotation is a commonly performed isokinetic movement. Clinicians have demonstrated significant variations in torque production, depending on the subject's test position. Soderberg and Blaschek[7] evaluated external and internal rotation in six different test positions and concluded that internal rotation exhibited increased torque production in the neutral position (0° to 20° of abduction) and that external rotation was increased in both the neutral position and the 90° abduction/90° elbow-flexion position. Greenfield[14] reported enhanced values of external rotation torque in the plane of the scapula versus the frontal plane. Ellenbecker[9] and later Hellwig[15], however, reported no significant differences in external rotation torque in the two test positions. Therefore, the clinician should be aware of potentially significant variations in torque productions when the arm position is changed. Wilk et al. have published descriptive data about the muscular performance value of the professional baseball pitcher.[34]

By considering these investigations, the pathophysiology of the rotator cuff, and the functional anatomy of the glenohumeral joint complex, a continuum of exercise positions for the internal and external rotators can be developed. The progression of this continuum is from 0° abduction (Fig. 6a) through the scapular phase (Fig. 6b) and finally to the 90°/90° position (Fig. 6c). By employing this continuum, the glenohumeral joint progresses from maximal to minimal static stability; therefore,

the demands on the rotator cuff muscles for dynamic stabilization also increase. Throughout the strengthening phase of the shoulder, verbal feedback from the patient is required. If shoulder symptoms develop at any stage, the activity is reduced to an asymptomatic level and readvanced only when adequate dynamic stability of the humeral head is attained. The authors believe that it is necessary for the competitive throwing or racquet sport athlete to exercise in functional positions, such as 90° of abduction.

Elbow

Isokinetic testing and exercise also can be performed for the elbow and wrist musculature. Elbow flexion/extension is a commonly used testing movement to document objectively the performance of the biceps and triceps muscles.

Phase Four: Activity Phase of Rehabilitation

The last phase of the rehabilitation program is the return to activity. The overhead athlete is encouraged to continue specific exercises to address strength deficits and to improve strength related to functional demands. A strengthening program for the overhead athlete addresses the appropriate musculotendinous units and challenges the muscles safely. This program is referred to as the "Thrower's Ten Program" (Table 3). The athlete must initiate a program of progressive and gradual functional rehabilitation to promote the safe return to unrestricted overhead sport activities. The specific criteria a patient must exhibit to enter this functional progression stage are:

1. Full, nonpainful motion,
2. No pain or tenderness,
3. Muscular strength that is satisfactory for functional demands, and
4. A satisfactory clinical examination.

Once these criteria are accomplished, an interval sport program may be initiated for the overhead athlete. The purpose of the interval sport program is to increase progressively and systematically the demands placed on the shoulder and elbow while performing the intended sporting activity. For the throwing athlete, the number, distance, intensity, and types of pitches are monitored and pro-

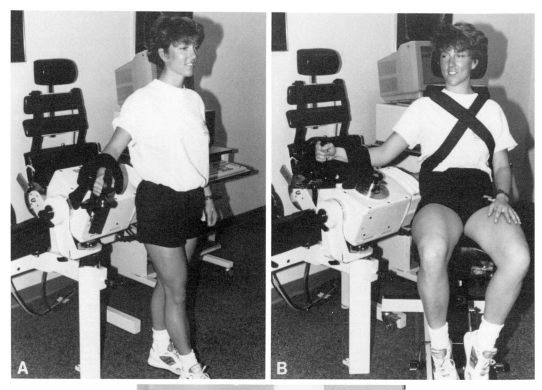

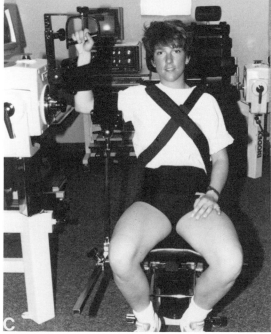

FIGURE 6.   Rotator cuff strengthening continuum. **A,** Moderate neutral position; **B,** Plane of the scapula; **C,** 90/90°
position.

TABLE 3. Thrower's Ten Program

1. Prone horizontal shoulder abduction
2. Seated rowing
3. Dumbbell deltoid
4. Dumbbell scaption
5. Tubing internal and external rotation 90/90
6. Tubing D$_2$ flexion/extension (holds)
7. Push-ups
8. Press-ups
9. Biceps/triceps curls
10. Wrist flexion/extension and pronation/supination
    Jogging
    Stretch
    Abdomen work
    Squat throws

gressed to facilitate a successful return to competition. Tables 4 and 5 illustrate the interval programs for the thrower. For the tennis player, the number, types, and intensity of strokes are progressed. Table 6 illustrates the functional interval tennis program.

For shoulder and elbow rehabilitation to be successful, the entire team must perform expertly and in concert. The athlete must be dedicated and diligent to continue the maintenance baseline exercises into the performance seasons and to report early any negative change in performance or significant discomfort.

TABLE 4. Interval Throwing Program—Phase I

45′ phase

Step 1:
a. Warm-up throwing
b. 45′ (25 throws)
c. Rest 15 minutes
d. Warm-up throwing
e. 45′ (25 throws)

Step 2:
a. Warm-up throwing
b. 45′ (25 throws)
c. Rest 10 minutes
d. Warm-up throwing
e. 45′ (25 throws)
f. Rest 10 minutes
g. Warm-up throwing
h. 45′ (25 throws)

60′ phase

Step 3:
a. Warm-up throwing
b. 60′ (25 throws)
c. Rest 15 minutes
d. Warm-up throwing
e. 60′ (25 throws)

Step 4:
a. Warm-up throwing
b. 60′ (25 throws)
c. Rest 10 minutes
d. Warm-up throwing
e. 60′ (25 throws)
f. Rest 10 minutes
g. Warm-up throwing
h. 60′ (25 throws)

90′ phase

Step 5:
a. Warm-up throwing
b. 90′ (25 throws)
c. Rest 15 minutes
d. Warm-up throwing
e. 90′ (25 throws)

Step 6:
a. Warm-up throwing
b. 90′ (25 throws)
c. Rest 10 minutes
d. Warm-up throwing
e. 90′ (25 throws)
f. Rest 10 minutes
g. Warm-up throwing
h. 90′ (25 throws)

120′ phase

Step 7:
a. Warm-up throwing
b. 120′ (25 throws)
c. Rest 15 minutes
d. Warm-up throwing
e. 120′ (25 throws)

Step 8:
a. Warm-up throwing
b. 120′ (25 throws)
c. Rest 10 minutes
d. Warm-up throwing
e. 120′ (25 throws)
f. Rest 10 minutes
g. Warm-up throwing
h. 120′ (25 throws)

150′ phase

Step 9:
a. Warm-up throwing
b. 150′ (25 throws)
c. Rest 15 minutes
d. Warm-up throwing
e. 150′ (25 throws)

Step 10:
a. Warm-up throwing
b. 150′ (25 throws)
c. Rest 10 minutes
d. Warm-up throwing
e. 150′ (25 throws)
f. Rest 10 minutes
g. Warm-up throwing
h. 150′ (25 throws)

180′ phase

Step 11:
a. Warm-up throwing
b. 180′ (25 throws)
c. Rest 15 minutes
d. Warm-up throwing
e. 180′ (25 throws)

Step 12:
a. Warm-up throwing
b. 180′ (25 throws)
c. Rest 10 minutes
d. Warm-up throwing
e. 180′ (25 throws)
f. Rest 10 minutes
g. Warm-up throwing
h. 180′ (25 throws)

Step 13:
a. Warm-up throwing
b. 180′ (25 throws)
c. Rest 10 minutes
d. Warm-up throwing
e. 180′ (25 throws)
f. Rest 10 minutes
g. Warm-up throwing
h. 180′ (25 throws)

Step 14:
Begin throwing off the mound or return to respective position

TABLE 5. **Interval Throwing Program—Phase II***

Stage one: fastball only	(Use interval throwing to 120' Phase as warm-up.)

Step 1:   Interval throwing
               15 throws off mound 50%
Step 2:   Interval throwing
               30 throws off mound 50%
Step 3:   Interval throwing
               45 throws off mound 50%
Step 4:   Interval throwing
               60 throws off mound 50%
Step 5:   Interval throwing   (Use speed gun to aid in effort control.)
               30 throws off mound 75%
Step 6:   30 throws off mound 75%
               45 throws off mound 50%
Step 7:   45 throws off mound 75%
               15 throws off mound 50%
Step 8:   60 throws off mound 75%

Stage two: fastball only
Step 9:   45 throws off mound 75%
               15 throws in batting practice
Step 10   45 throws off mound 75%
               30 throws in batting practice
Step 11:   45 throws off mound 75%
               45 throws in batting practice

Stage three
Step 12:   30 throws off mound 75% warm-up
               15 throws off mound 50% breaking balls
               45–60 throws in batting practice (fastball only)
Step 13:   30 throws off mound 75%
               30 breaking balls 75%
               30 throws in batting practice
Step 14:   30 throws off mound 75%
               60–90 throws in batting practice 25% breaking balls
Step 15:   Simulated game: progressing by 15 throws per workout

*All throwing off the mound should be done in the presence of a pitching coach to stress proper throwing mechanics.

TABLE 6. **Interval Tennis Program**

Day	1st Week	2nd Week	3rd Week	4th Week
Monday*	12 FH	25 FH	30 FH	30 FH
	8 BH	15 BH	25 BH	30 BH
	10-min rest	10-min rest	10 OH	10 OH
	13 FH	25 FH	10-min rest	10-min rest
	7 BH	15 BH	30 FH	Play 3 games
			25 BH	10 FH
			10 OH	10 BH
				5 OH
Wednesday*	15 FH	30 FH	30 FH	30 FH
	8 BH	20 BH	25 BH	30 BH
	10-min rest	10-min rest	15 OH	10 OH
	15 Fh	30 FH	10-min rest	10-min rest
	7 BH	20 BH	30 FH	Play set
			25 BH	10 FH
			15 OH	10 BH
				5 OH
Friday*	15 FH	30 FH	30 FH	30 FH
	10 BH	25 BH	30 BH	30 BH
	10-min rest	10-min rest	15 OH	10 OH
	15 Fh	30 FH	10-min rest	10-min rest
	10 BH	15 BH	30 FH	Play 1½ sets
		10 OH	15 OH	10 FH
			10-min rest	10 BH
			30 FH	3 OH
			30 BH	
			15 OH	

OH = overhead shots; FH = forehand ground stroke; BH = backhand ground strokes.
*Ice after each day of play.

REFERENCES

1. Andrews JR, Kupferman SP, Dillman CJ: Labral tears in throwing and racquet sports. *Clin Sports Med* 10:901–912, 1991.
2. Andrews JR, Carson WG: The arthroscopic treatment of glenoid labral tears in the throwing athlete. *Orthop Trans* 8:44–49, 1984.
3. Andrews JR, Carson WG, McLeod WD: Glenoid labrum tears related to the long head of the biceps. *Am J Sports Med* 13:337, 1985.
4. Andrews JR, Schemmel SP, Whiteside JA: Evaluation, treatment and prevention of elbow injuries in throwing athletes. In Nicholas JA, Hershman EB (eds): *The Upper Extremity in Sports Medicine.* Philadelphia, C. V. Mosby, 1990, pp 781–826.
5. Andrews JR: *Bony Injuries About the Elbow in the Throwing Athlete. Instructional course lectures no. 34.* St. Louis, C. V. Mosby, 1985.
6. Andrews JR, Miller RH: Arthroscopic surgery of the elbow. In Chapman MW (ed): *Operative Orthopaedics.* Philadelphia, Lippincott, 1988, pp 1571–1577.
7. Blackburn TA, McLeod WD, White B: EMG analysis of posterior rotator cuff exercises. *Athl Training* 25:40–45, 1990.
8. Dillman CJ: Proper mechanics of pitching. *Sports Med Update* 5:15, 1990.
9. Ellenbecker TS, Feiring DC, Dehart RL: Isokinetic shoulder strength: Coronal versus scapular plane testing in the upper extremity. *Phys Ther* 72(suppl):580, 1992.
10. Elliott B, Marsh T, Blanksby B: A three dimensional cinematographic analysis of the tennis serve. *Int J Sport Biomech* 2:260, 1986.
11. Feltner M, Dapena J: Dynamics of the shoulder and elbow joints of the throwing arm during the baseball pitch. *Int J Sport Biomech* 2:235, 1986.
12. Fleisig GS, Dillman CJ, Andrews JR: Proper mechanics for baseball pitching. *Clin Sports Med* 1:151, 1989.
13. Fleisig GS, Dillman CJ, Andrews JR: Biomechanics of the shoulder during throwing. In Andrews JR, Wilk KE (eds): *The Athlete's Shoulder.* New York, Churchill Livingstone, 1994.
14. Greenfield BH, Donatelli R, Wooden MJ, Wilkins J: Isokinetic evaluation of the shoulder rotational strength between plane of scapula and functional plane. *Am J Sports Med* 18:124–127, 1990.
15. Hellwig EV, Perrin DH: A comparison of two positions for assessing shoulder rotator peak torque: The traditional frontal plane versus the plane of scapula. *Isokinetic Exerc Sci* 1(4):202–206, 1991.
16. Inman VT, Saunders JR, Abbott JC: Observations of the function of the shoulder joint. *J Bone Joint Surg* 26:1–30, 1944.
17. Jobe FW, Tibone JE, Perry J, et al: An EMG analysis of the shoulder in throwing and pitching. A preliminary report. *Am J Sports Med* 11:3–5, 1983.
18. Jobe FW, Moynes DR, Tibone JE: An EMG analysis of the shoulder in pitching. A second report. *Am J Sports Med* 12:218–220, 1984.
19. Jobe FW, Moynes DR: Delineation of diagnosis criteria and a rehabilitation program for rotator cuff injuries. *Am J Sports Med* 10:336–339, 1982.
20. Johnston TB: Movements of the shoulder joint: Plea for use of "plane of the scapula" as plane of reference for movements occurring at the humeroscapula joint. *Br J Surg* 25:252–260, 1937.
21. Knott M, Voss D: *Proprioceptive Neuromuscular Facilitation.* New York, Harper & Row, 1968, pp 84–85.
22. Light LE, Nuziks, Personins W, Barstrom A: Low load prolonged stretch vs high load brief stretch in treating knee contractures. *Phys Ther* 64:330, 1984.
23. Moseley JB, Jobe FW, Pink M, et al: EMG analysis of the scapular muscles during a shoulder rehabilitation program. *Am J Sports Med* 20:128–134, 1992.
24. Rhu KN, McCormick J, Jobe FW, et al: An electromyographic analysis of shoulder function in tennis players. *Am J Sports Med* 16:481, 1988.
24a. Rockwood CA, Young DC: Disorders of the acromioclavicular joint. In Rockwood CA, Matsen FA (eds): *The Shoulder.* Philadelphia, W. B. Saunders, 1990, pp 413–424.
25. Saha AK: Mechanism of shoulder movements and a plea for the recognition of "zero position" of the glenohumeral joint. *Clin Orthop* 173:3–10, 1983.
26. Shapiro R, Stine RL: *Shoulder Rotation Velocities.* Technical report submitted to the Lexington, KY, Lexington Clinic, 1992.
27. Soderberg GJ, Blaschek MJ: Shoulder internal and external rotation peak torque production through a velocity spectrum in differing positions. *J Orthop Sports Phys Ther* 8:518–524, 1987.
28. VanGheluwe B, Hebbelinck M: Muscle actions and ground reaction forces in tennis. *Int J Sport Biomech* 2:88, 1986.
29. Warren CG, Lehman JF, Koblanski NJ: Elongation of rat tail tendon effects of load and temperature. *Arch Phys Med Rehabil* 52:465, 1971.
30. Wilk KE, Arrigo CA, Andrews JR: Rehabilitation of the throwers' elbow. *J Orthop Sports Phys Ther* 17(6):305, 1993.
31. Wilk KE, Arrigo CA: Current concepts in the rehabilitation of the athletic shoulder. *J Orthop Sports Phys Ther* 18(1):365, 1993.
32. Wilk KE, Arrigo CA: An integrated approach to upper extremity exercises. *Orthop Phys Ther Clin North Am* 1:337, 1992.
33. Wilk KE, Voight ML, Keirns MA, et al: Stretch- shortening exercises for the upper extremity. *J Orthop Sports Phys Ther* 17(5):225, 1993.
34. Wilk KE, Andrews JR, Keirns MA, et al: The strength characteristics of internal and external rotator muscles in professional baseball pitchers. *Am J Sports Med* 21:61, 1993.

Chapter 5

SWIMMING INJURIES:
Diagnosis, Treatment, and Rehabilitation

Frank Y. Wei, MD

Renewed interest in health and fitness has resulted in increased participation in recreational and competitive sports. It has been estimated that 120 million individuals participate in recreational swimming annually.[36] Early participation and continuation into adult life through such groups as United States Masters Swimming (USMS) have contributed to the growing popularity of organized swimming. By 1989 there were approximately 28,600 athletes registered with USMS. It is the national governing body for swimmers, age 19 years or over, who participate in noncollegiate organized competition.[66]

The benefits of swimming have long been recognized. In addition to its aerobic benefits, it has gained popularity as a mode of cross-training. Swimming is one of the few aerobic sports that emphasizes upper body conditioning and also improves flexibility. Because gravity is eliminated, there is less potential for injury to lower extremity joints, muscles, and tendons. Hydrotherapy has long been used for exercise by individuals with rheumatologic, neuromuscular, and skeletal disorders.

Growing enthusiasm has led to new records in competitive swimming. The sport has developed a science of its own: new technologies, training regimens, equipment, and adaptations in stroke mechanics have allowed swimmers to move through the water faster and more efficiently. It is not unusual for an elite competitor to swim up to 20,000 yards a day, 5 to 6 days/week.[47] Estimates of the number of arm strokes range between 1.2 million[47] to 2 million/year.[14] This translates into a metabolic equivalent of 30 to 45 miles of

running per day.[36] This training intensity, however, takes its toll. Approximately 50% of participants in organized swimming experience shoulder pain. The knee and lower leg are the next two most frequently cited areas of musculoskeletal injuries. Swimmers may also experience elbow and back complaints.[23]

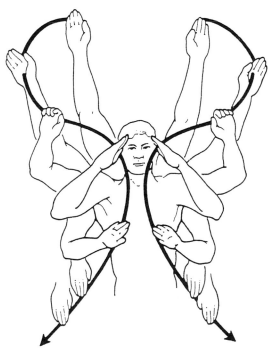

FIGURE 1. Basic arm movement of swimming during the pull-through phase. (From Pink M, et al: The normal shoulder during freestyle swimming. *Am J Sports Med* 19(6):569–576, 1991; with permission).

Swimming is a sport that requires power through a wide range of joint motion, especially in the shoulders. Travelling through a medium with much greater resistance than air places continuous stress on the joint as it moves through its arc. Technique is extremely important, because streamlining improves speed and efficiency. A balance has to be struck between maximal forward thrust and minimal drag.

Because of the highly repetitive demands of swimming, maintenance of good technique is vital to injury prevention. A knowledgeable coach and athletic trainer can prevent and reduce the incidence of chronic problems. Good communication with the physician allows the most expedient treatment with minimal interruption of the swimmer's training regimen. For a review of the roles of physician, coach, and athletic trainer, see Donnelly,[20] Counsilman,[17] and Becker.[2]

Frequency and type of injury correlate with intensity of training and type of stroke. Richardson et al.[65] looked at 137 high-level participants at the U.S. Olympic training camp and the International Amateur Swimmers World Championships in 1978. Forty-two percent of the swimmers had shoulder problems. A direct relationship was seen between the caliber of the swimmer and the incidence of shoulder injuries. Freestyle and butterfly swimmers had the highest incidence of shoulder pain, followed by backstrokers and then breaststrokers. Ciullo and Guise[12] noted that 80% of swimmers with shoulder pain swam the freestyle. Kennedy et al.[39] found the incidence of foot and calf problems to be equally divided across the four competitive strokes. Knee complaints, however, were isolated to breaststrokers.

SHOULDER

With the exception of the breaststroke, the shoulders provide the primary source of forward propulsion. The arms can contribute up to 90% of the work performed.[36] To appreciate the mechanism of injury, the basics of stroke mechanics must be understood. All four swimming strokes (breast, butterfly, freestyle, and backstroke) use the same basic arm movement (Fig. 1). The differences lie in the position of the swimmer (prone or supine), the length of pull through the water, whether the arms exit the water, and whether the arms alternate or move in unison (Fig. 2).

The arm stroke is easily divided into a pull-through or propulsive phase and a recovery phase.[19] The purpose of the recovery phase is to reposition the arm in preparation for the arc of movement in which the body is pushed forward as the hand moves backward or caudally against the water. Anterior shoulder pain occurs most frequently at the mid pull-through phase; the arm is near 90° of abduction and passes from an externally into an internally rotated position (Fig. 3).

Shoulder adduction and internal rotation are the major movements from which propulsion is derived. For this reason, the "high-elbow" position is coached[18] (Fig. 4). As the arm is drawn down from an overhead position, the proximal arm is adducted in a plane nearly parallel to an imaginary line connecting both shoulders; this allows generation of maximal force with internal rotation (Fig. 5). Unfortunately, this arc of motion can lead to degenerative changes if good technique, appropriate flexibility, or strength is lacking.

Anatomy

The shoulder is best appreciated as a complex of multiple joints, muscles, and ligaments (Fig. 6). The humeral head sits in the shallow glenoid fossa, which is made slightly deeper by the glenoid labrum. The glenoid concavity covers only a quarter of the surface of the articulating humeral head.[69] Overlying the humerus is the coracoacromial arch, which consists of the acromion, the coracoacromial ligament, and the coracoid process. Full abduction and flexion of the arm to 180° are allowed by pivoting of the scapula on the thoracic wall. Rotation and protraction of the scapula are guided by the acromioclavicular and sternoclavicular joints.

Passive glenohumeral stability is provided by numerous structures in addition to the glenoid labrum. The coracohumeral ligament, the superior portion of the anterior capsule, and the tendon of the long head of the biceps also suspend the humeral head within the joint. Because the shoulder joint is an encapsulated structure, negative intraarticular pressure has been found to provide a stabilizing force to inferior translation.[8] Anterior stability is provided by the middle and inferior glenohumeral ligaments, the long biceps tendon, and the subscapularis muscle. The capsule, the inferior glenohumeral ligament, and the tendons of the infraspinatus and teres minor provide posterior support. Selective cutting studies of the inferior

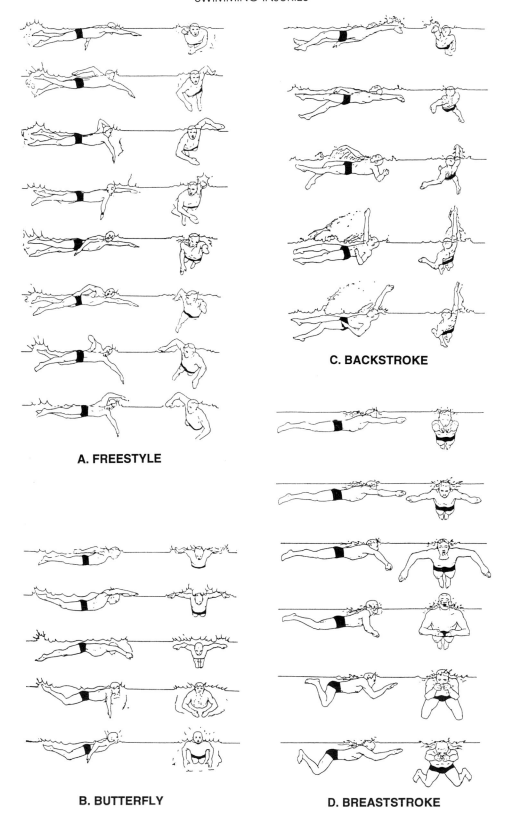

FIGURE 2. The four competitive strokes: **A.** freestyle; **B.** butterfly; **C.** backstroke; **D.** breaststroke. (Modified and reprinted from Counsilman JE: *The Science of Swimming.* Englewood Cliffs, NJ, Prentice-Hall, 1968, with permission.)

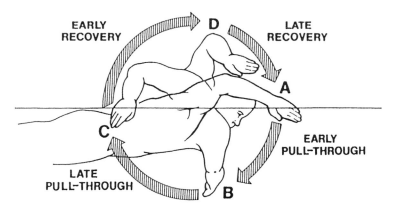

FIGURE 3. Phases of arm movement during the freestyle stroke. (From Pink M, et al: The normal shoulder during freestyle swimming. *Am J Sports Med* 19(6): 569– 576, 1991; with permission.)

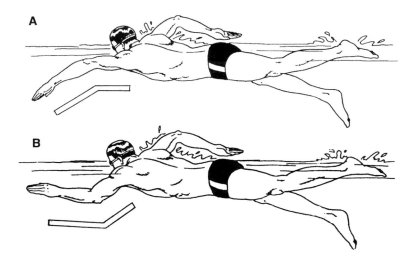

FIGURE 4. *A,* "High-elbow" position during the freestyle pull-through phase. *B,* "Dropped elbow" pull, a serious defect.

glenohumeral ligament have revealed importance to stability greater than initially realized.

The anatomy of this ligament is best described as a thickened anterior and posterior band separated by an axillary pouch. It assists in providing inferior stability to the joint; the anterior and posterior edges provide significant resistance to anterior-posterior translation, depending on the degree of abduction and internal and external rotation.[8] Most importantly, however, studies of the shoulder illustrate the complexity of its stability: depending on position, different static stabilizers may have variable responsibility in controlling the joint.

Shoulder Mechanics

Shoulder movements revolve around four separate sites of articulation, the gle-nohumeral, scapulothoracic, acromioclavicu-lan, and sternoclavicular joints. Motions are controlled by 19 primary muscles of the shoulder girdle and arm (Table 1). Movements about the glenohumeral joint include abduction, adduction, flexion, extension, and internal and external rotation. Scapular motion includes elevation, depression, rotation, protraction, and retraction. Further specifics of these movements and muscles involved are detailed by Hollinshead and Jenkins.[30] Swimming strokes require all of these motions. Thus, the muscles must provide not only power for propulsion but also stability to the shoulder complex.

The importance of proper coordination of movement within the shoulder complex cannot be overemphasized. The concept of scapulohumeral rhythm was originally described by Codman[15] and advanced by Inman et al.[31]

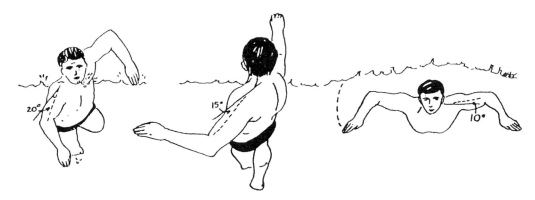

FIGURE 5. Position of the arm during the freestyle, backstroke, and butterfly. The humerus is nearly parallel with the shoulders at mid pull-through. (From Richardson AR: The biomechanics of swimming: the shoulder and knee. *Clin Sports Med* 5(1):103–114, 1986; with permission.)

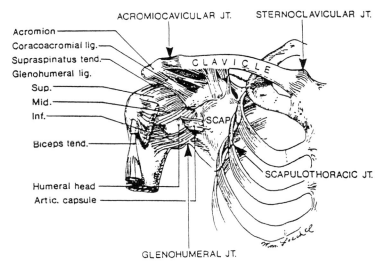

FIGURE 6. Anatomy of the shoulder. (From Ciullo JV, Stevens GG: The prevention and treatment of injuries to the shoulder in swimming. *Sports Med* 7:182–204, 1989; with permission.)

TABLE 1. Muscles of the Shoulder Girdle

Levator scapula	Biceps
Trapezius—upper	Triceps
Rhomboid minor	Teres minor
Rhomboid major	Teres major
Latissimus dorsi	Subscapularis
Pectoralis minor	Supraspinatus
Pectoralis major	Infraspinatus
Deltoid—anterior	Serratus anterior
middle	Coracobrachialis
posterior	

During the first 30° of abduction, motion occurs primarily at the glenohumeral joint, whereas the scapulothoracic joint may or may not move as it finds a position of stabilization (called the "setting phase"). During further abduction the glenohumeral joint accounts for two-thirds of abduction and the scapulothoracic joint for one-third. The remaining 150° of abduction is accounted for by 100° of humeral abduction and 50° of scapular rotation.

The deltoid is the primary mover of the humerus in abduction. Below 90°, however, it requires the assistance of the supraspinatus and the other rotator cuff muscles to depress the humeral head and to maintain good glenohumeral contact. Otherwise, humeral impingement upon the undersurface of the coracoacromial arch would occur; the axis of rotation would then be at the point of contact. Maximal shear and compressive forces occur at the glenohumeral joint at 90° of abduction, making it the most vulnerable to instability at this angle.[14]

The concept that certain groups of muscles, such as the deltoid and rotator cuff, always work together in a standard uniform pattern has not held true. Electromyography combined with high-speed cinematography has allowed more specific and detailed analysis of the forces and mechanics involved in shoulder movements. Bradley and Tibone[9] reviewed several studies involving swimmers, golfers, and pitchers. Each of these sports had a different firing pattern, as might be expected.

Swimming Technique

Nuber et al.[54] looked at muscles of the shoulder during performance of three strokes: the freestyle, butterfly, and breaststroke. The muscles primarily involved in propulsion are the pectoralis major and latissimus dorsi. The pectoralis major is activated at early pull-through; the latissimus has peak activity at approximately 90° of humeral abduction, which is the beginning of late pull-through. Only in the breaststroke is the pectoralis active in recovery. The arms are brought together in the midline and flexed forward during this phase. The primary recovery muscles are the middle deltoid, supraspinatus, and infraspinatus. The arm is abducted and externally rotated as it is drawn out of the water. The serratus anterior, which is responsible for scapular rotation, is very active during recovery. Full scapular rotation and protraction are necessary to obtain full abduction as the hand reenters the water.

Pink et al.[61] studied the freestyle stroke in more detail. At hand entry, the upper trapezius, rhomboids, supraspinatus, and anterior deltoid are active to achieve maximal scapular rotation, protraction, and glenohumeral abduction. The initial pull is by the pectoralis major, with the teres minor providing a balancing, antagonistic, externally rotating force. As the humerus becomes more extended and internally rotated, the latissimus dorsi becomes the major propulsive muscle. During the pull-through phase, the serratus anterior assists in pulling the body over the outstretched arm by scapular retraction and rotation. Pulling stops when the hand reaches the thigh.

During early recovery, the shoulder is lifted and abducted out of the water by the middle deltoid and supraspinatus. This movement is assisted through scapular retraction by the rhomboids. As the arm is brought forward, the humerus is internally rotated, primarily by the subscapularis. The infraspinatus is then activated as the arm is flexed more forward to rotate the humerus externally, depress its head, and stabilize the glenohumeral joint.

During the freestyle stroke, Pink et al.[61] found the subscapularis and serratus anterior to be active throughout all phases of pull-through and recovery. The infraspinatus has a function separate from the teres minor. The infraspinatus assists during recovery with humeral depression and external rotation. The teres minor is primarily active at pull-through (during activation of the pectoralis major) to prevent excessive internal rotation.

Pathology

There are multiple potential causes of shoulder pain in a swimmer (Table 2). The

TABLE 2.   Potential Causes of Shoulder Pain in the Swimmer

Neck
Congenital anomalies
Thoracic outlet syndrome
Disc disease
Facet arthropathy
Pulmonary tumor
Nerve entrapment
Skeletal tumors
Spinal cord pathology
Clavicle
Acromioclavicular arthritis
Acromioclavicular meniscal injury
Sternoclavicular arthritis
Shoulder
Inflammatory
Bursitis
Tendonitis
Synovitis
Mechanical
Subluxation
Dislocation
Muscle imbalances (instability)
Impingement
Capsular adhesions
Structural
Rotator cuff tear
Loose body
Labral damage
Osteochondrosis
Skeletal tumor

Adapted from McMaster WC: Painful shoulder in swimmers: A diagnostic challenge. *Phys SportsMed* 14(12):108–22, 1986.

three major mechanisms of pain are impingement, instability, and acromioclavicular arthritis.

Impingement

The term *swimmer's shoulder* is most commonly applied to pain in the anterior shoulder associated with impingement. This often involves the development of inflammation within the local tissues—the subacromial bursa, the tendons of the rotator cuff, and the long head of the biceps. The mechanism of injury, however, is debated.

Rathbun and Macnab[62] performed injection studies on the microvasculature of the rotator cuff and biceps. The supraspinatus exhibited an area of hypovascularity within its tendon between the site of insertion on the greater tuberosity and 1 cm proximally. This finding was consistent in all cadavers studied, even those younger than age 20 years. Unlike "round" tendons, which are supplied by vasculature within the paratendon that perforates the substance of the tendon at intervals, "flat" tendons, such as those of the rotator cuff, contain their primary vasculature within the tendon itself. The blood vessels run the length of the structure.[62] Compression of these vessels by the humeral head occurs when the arm is adducted (Fig. 7).

A similar phenomenon is found in the infraspinatus and in the intracapsular portion of the long biceps tendon. This area of diminished blood flow is therefore predisposed to degenerative changes. Breakdown occurs first within the center of the tendon.[43] Cell death causes an inflammatory reaction that leads to an initial response of neovascularization, actually increasing blood flow. As degeneration progresses, however, attenuation and hypovascularity ensue. Swiontkowski et al.[73] have confirmed this vascular blush phenomenon by examining arterial flow intraoperatively on patients with known impingement and tears of the rotator cuff. Increased intraarticular pressure has been found in cadavers as well as in volunteers when the arm is placed in forward flexion, as reported recently in pressure catheter work by Sigholm et al.[71] and Regan and Richards.[63] Several possible mechanisms predispose this portion of the tendon to injury and impaired healing: microvascular anatomy, susceptibility to increased external capillary pressure, and limited volume below the coracoacromial arch.

The overriding coracoacromial arch can pinch the soft-tissue structures between it and the underlying humerus, mainly at the greater tuberosity, the site of attachment of the rotator cuff. Maximal impingement occurs at 90° of abduction.[39] Neer[49] explained that most functional movements occur in the forward flexed position (Fig. 8). Therefore, it is the anterior inferior third, not the lateral aspect of the acromion, that contacts the underlying structures most frequently and causes impingement. Repetitive impingement leads to bony spurring and eburnation on the underside of the anterior third of the acromion, thus accelerating the degenerative changes in the tendons (Fig. 9). Bigliani and associates[5] correlated acromial shape to rotator cuff pathology. Three basic shapes were identified: flat, curved, and hooked. The greatest incidence of rotator cuff tears was associated with a hooked acromion; the least with a flat architecture.

Neer and Welsh[50] categorized trauma from impingement into three stages. **Stage I,** the development of edema and hemorrhage within the rotator cuff, is reversible and is typically seen in young athletes, primarily be-

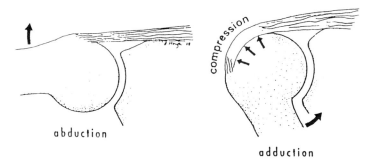

FIGURE 7. Compression of the intratendinous vessels with shoulder adduction. (From Rathbun JB, Macnab I: The microvascular pattern of the rotator cuff. *J Bone Joint Surg* 52B(3):540–553, 1970; with permission.)

low 25 years of age. **Stage II,** which results from continued irritation that leads to fibrosis and thickening of the subacromial bursa, usually occurs between the ages of 25 and 40 years. **Stage III,** which presents with tears of the rotator cuff secondary to osteophytosis and tendon attenuation, is seen most commonly in persons over 40 years of age. At each stage, the functional space between the coracoacromial arch becomes smaller due to the edema or overgrowth of the involved structures. Hawkins and Kennedy[28] believe that two processes result in swimmer's shoulder: repetitive extension and adduction at the end of the pull-through phase, and the abduction, flexion, and internal rotation during recovery and pull-through phases.

Risk Factors. Richardson et al.[65] looked at risk factors for shoulder problems in elite swimmers. The average age of prevalence was 18 years. Most had been swimming competitively since the age of 8 years. Freestyle and butterfly were the two strokes most commonly associated with shoulder pain; 81% of swimmers with bilateral pain listed butterfly as their best or second-best stroke. Of those with shoulder symptoms, 60% had pain on the side on which they breathed. Middle distance or sprint athletes had increased incidence of complaints compared with distance swimmers. Shoulders were most problematic in early and middle season. Hand paddles, which increase resistance of pull, have been associated with worsening of symptoms.[26] Weight training has not been found to significantly affect the occurrence of shoulder pain.[26,65]

History. A good history is essential in making the correct diagnosis and instituting appropriate therapy. In typical swimmer's shoulder, pain is worst during combined forward flexion and internal rotation. This motion,

ARC OF ELEVATION

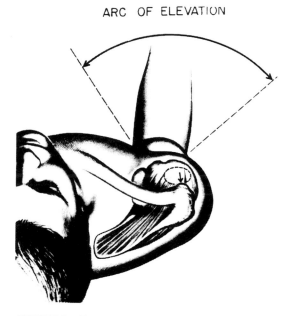

FIGURE 8. Functional arc of motion of the shoulder predisposing impingement to occur at the anterior inferior third of the acromion. (From Neer CS II: Anterior acromioplasty for the chronic impingement syndrome in the shoulder. *J Bone Joint Surg* 54A(1):41–50; 1972; with permission.)

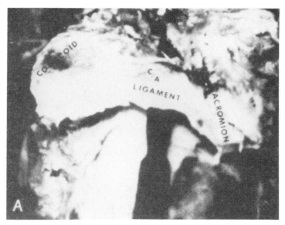
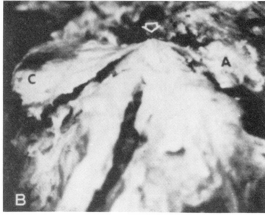

FIGURE 9. **A,** With the arm adducted, there is a small amount of clearance between the rotator cuff and the coracoacromial arch. **B,** With abduction such as at hand entry during the freestyle, the supraspinatus tents the coracoacromial arch *(arrow)*. A = acromion, C = coracoid. (From Ciullo JV: Swimmer's shoulder. *Am J Sports Med* 5(1):115–138, 1986; with permission.)

which drives the greater tuberosity beneath the acromion, occurs in the pull- through phase, most frequently after hand entry.[21,64] The pain typically occurs along the coracoacromial ligament or at the acromion. Pain in the back, especially the periscapular area and trapezius, is more likely to be related to fatigue.[21]

The history should include whether prior episodes of shoulder pain have occurred during other sports or activities. It is important to learn the current yardage, which strokes aggravate the discomfort, whether hand paddles are used, and during which part of the swim season the pain occurs. Changes in swimming technique, increase in distance, or early season practice can provoke bouts of shoulder pain. Recent recovery from febrile illnesses, such as the flu or other viral illnesses, often results in periscapular pain that may take 3 to 6 weeks to resolve.[21]

Clinical Signs. Several clinical signs indicate involvement of the supraspinatus tendon and/or rotator cuff:[13,28,33,38,39,50]

1. Well-localized tenderness over the greater tuberosity and occasionally over the anterior acromion;
2. Pain with abduction between 60° and 120° that is usually the worst at 90°;
3. A positive impingement sign: pain with maximal forward flexion and internal rotation (Fig. 10A) and relief of pain with the injection of 10 mL of 1% lidocaine into the subacromial bursa;
4. Pain with forced internal rotation when the arm is forward flexed to 90° (Fig. 10B);
5. A positive supraspinatus test: pain and/or weakness when the arms are abducted 90°, 30° anterior to the coronal plane, with maximal internal rotation (Fig. 10C).

Acute involvement of the bursa can be demonstrated by pushing the humeral head superiorly into the coracoacromial arch while palpating the bursa. Tenderness is the expected positive sign[13] (Fig. 11). When the bursa becomes fibrotic secondary to chronic irritation, crepitation is often felt. This can be demonstrated by internal and external rotation while the arm is abducted 90°.

Bicipital tendinitis may occur in the swimmer either alone or in conjunction with rotator cuff tendinitis. This may be due either to repeated extension of the humerus which causes a "wringing out" of the tendon over

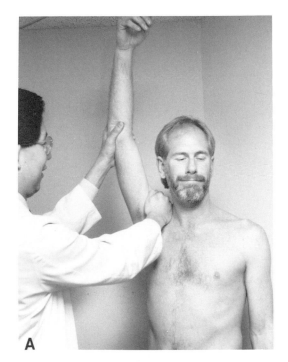

A

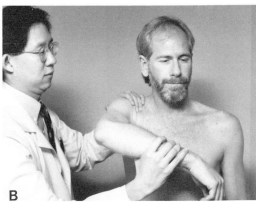

B

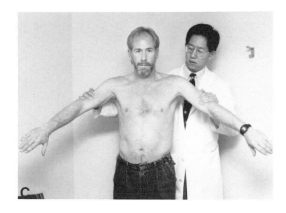

C

FIGURE 10. Tests of the supraspinatus tendon and/or rotator cuff. **A,** Impingement sign popularized by Neer.[49] **B,** A second impingement sign from Hawkins and Kennedy.[28] **C,** Supraspinatus test.

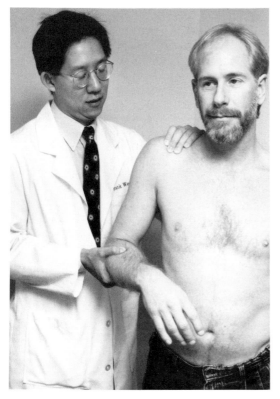

FIGURE 11. Bursal sign.

the humeral head or to impingement of the rotator cuff. Involvement is indicated by

1. Tenderness is the bicipital groove.
2. Pain in area of the tendon or bicipital groove with forced forward flexion of the humerus while the forearm is supinated and the elbow extended (Fig. 12A);
3. Pain with forced forearm supination with the elbow flexed at 90° (Yergason's test) (Fig. 12B).[14,28,39]

Symptoms of impingement have been correlated with the physiologic stages of impingement[14,28] defined by Neer and Welsh.[50] In stage I, the pain is a dull ache initially present after activity. This may progress to pain with activity, possibly affecting performance. In stage II, the pain may be present all the time and may be worse at night. The shoulder often becomes stiff, with tenderness of the acromioclavicular joint. A painful catching sensation, due to scar formation, may occur as the arm is brought down from an abducted position. By stage III, there may or may not be associated weakness; the pain continues to be everpresent and may awaken the individual at night, radiating down the lateral arm to the elbow.[14]

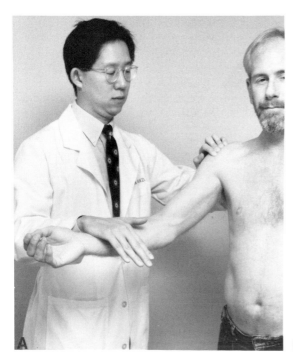
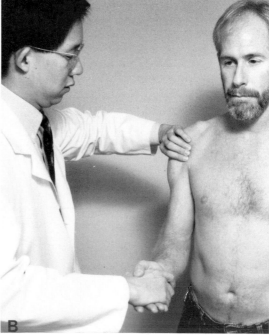

FIGURE 12. Biciptal tendinitis tests. **A,** Demonstrates tenderness over the tendon, especially when it is "rolled" under the examiner's fingers. The patient flexes the humerus while the arm is supinated and the elbow extended. **B,** Yergason's test for bicipital tendinitis. The examiner resists the patient's supination and flexion.

Instability

Inferior and multidirectional instability have been found to cause problems in swimmers.[51] Poor shoulder control can cause overtaxing of the rotator cuff, which may lead to tendinitis or result in impingement at the coracoacromial arch. It should be stressed that laxity does not imply instability. Anterior translation may be up to 25% of the glenoid surface in normal persons; posterior and inferior translation may be up to 50%.[1] Matsen et al.[44] compared normal volunteers with patients who had clinically unstable shoulders and who were about to undergo surgical stabilization. Up to 2 cm of translation occurred in both groups, with no significant difference between the two. The importance of an accurate history, assessment of laxity, and demonstration of discomfort during simulation of shoulder movement cannot be overemphasized in determining whether instability is present.

Anterior glenohumeral instability ("apprehension shoulder") is most commonly seen in the backstroker. The arm is fully abducted and externally rotated above the head as the outstretched arm contacts the wall to help with deceleration and turning (Fig. 13). Because the subscapularis is no longer in an anterior position to assist in preventing anterior subluxation, the anterior capsule and inferior glenohumeral ligament provide the stabilizing force.

In examining for clinical instability, it is important to obtain information about any previous shoulder injuries. Clinical evidence of hyperlaxity in other joints often accompanies multidirectional instability.

Several clinical maneuvers are used to assess shoulder laxity. To detect the "apprehension sign," the patient's shoulder is abducted to 90° and external rotation is applied to the humerus. Anxiety in the patient or resistance to the maneuver is suggestive of anterior instability (Fig. 14A). A positive Fowler's sign, a reduction in pain or apprehension when the humeral head is directed posteriorly in conjunction with the above maneuver, is more sensitive for subtle instability.[48] A "sulcus sign" is present when distraction is applied to adducted arm. Formed by the humeral head being pulled from the acromion, the sulcus, or step-off, is indicative of inferior laxity and is often seen in multidirectional instability (Fig. 14B).

Anterior-posterior translation can be tested by the "load and shift" test.[4] With the patient supine or sitting, the humeral head is grasped with one hand while the other hand stabilizes the scapula. A mild compressive load is applied through the glenohumeral joint as the humeral head is pushed in all three directions (Fig. 14C). Comparison with the opposite arm is made.

Gerber and Ganz[24] describe an anterior and posterior drawer sign, which is much akin to the drawer test of the knee, to evaluate laxity of the shoulder. The patient is examined while supine (Fig. 15). They found the anterior drawer sign to be more helpful when the shoulder was painful and felt that it provided evidence of subluxation even when the apprehension test was negative. The posterior drawer sign was believed to be reliable for posterial subluxation as well (Fig. 16). Norwood and Terry[54] described a different tech-

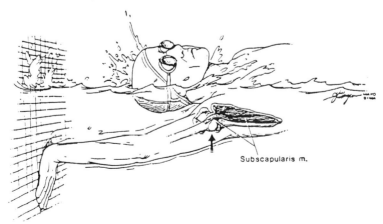

Subscapularis m.

FIGURE 13.   Position of the shoulder during the backstroke when the hand contacts the wall. The subscapularis is no longer in a position to prevent anterior translation of the humeral head. (From Johnson JE, et al: Musculoskeletal injuries in competitive swimmers. *Mayo Clin Proc* 62:289–304, 1987; with permission.)

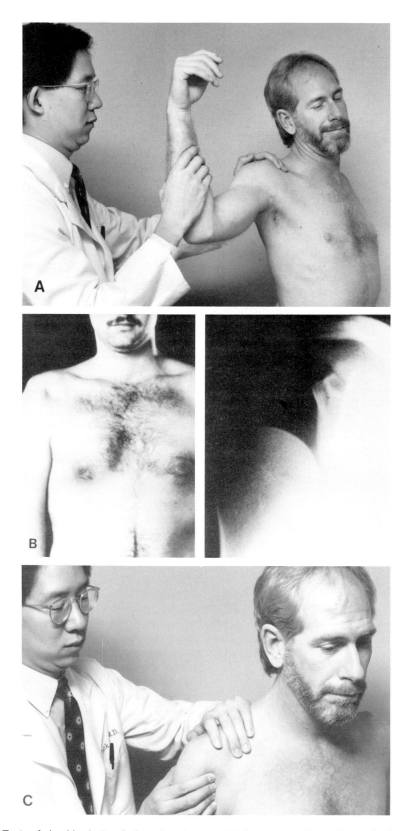

FIGURE 14. Tests of shoulder laxity. **A,** Apprehension sign. **B,** Sulcus sign. (From Gerber C, Ganz R: Clinical assessment of instability of the shoulder. *J Bone Joint Surg* 66B(4):551–556, 1984; with permission.) **C,** Load and shift test.

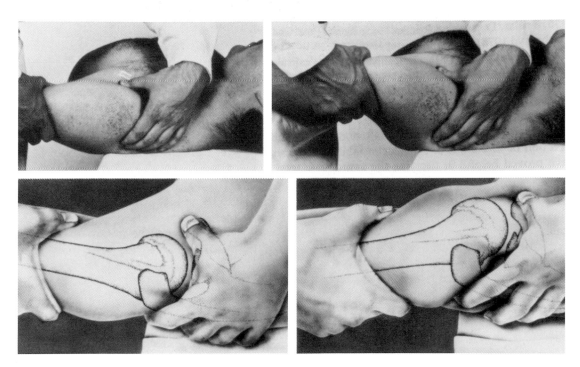

FIGURE 15. Anterior drawer test. The scapula is fixed while the humerus is drawn forward. The bottom panels show a schematic depiction of the test. (From Gerber C, Ganz R: Clinical assessment of instability of the shoulder. *J Bone Joint Surg* 66B(4):551–556, 1984; with permission.)

nique for assessing posterior subluxation. The patient is supine and the arm is abducted to 90° with the humerus in neutral. The arm is then brought to a forward-flexed position. A positive test is a palpable posterior displacement of the humeral head as the arm is put through this arc of motion (Fig. 17).

McMaster[46] described another possible etiology of shoulder pain in the swimmer— anterior labral tears. Swimmers with anterior labral tears often feel the shoulder lock or catch, with a sensation of being unable to control the arm. Pain is most prominent immediately after hand entry. A click when the arm is adducted and internally rotated indicates that anterior labral damage has occurred and that the torn fragment is interposed between the articulating surfaces of the glenohumeral joint. This locking phenomenon has been defined as functional instability by Pappas.[59] Interposition of hypertrophic flaps, bucket-handle tears, or free fragments may result. This phenomenon is different from anatomic instability in which labral defects or capsular laxity allows subluxation or dislocation to occur. A positive apprehension test and anterior instability may be present with this entity.

Acromioclavicular Arthritis

Although uncommon in the young athlete, pain may originate in the acromioclavicular joint. Angulation at the acromioclavicular joint occurs in the first 30° of abduction and between 135° and 180°. In addition, clavicular rotation of up to 50° occurs at this joint.[42] Examination of the acromioclavicular joint should be included in the evaluation of the shoulder. Swelling and point tenderness may be present over the joint. Compression of the joint may elicit pain, as with horizontal adduction: the arm is brought across the chest from a 90° abducted position (Fig. 18). Crepitation over the joint or pain with full flexion can also be useful indicators of acromioclavicular pathology.

Imaging

In the competitive swimmer who is less than 25 years of age and otherwise healthy, plain radiographs are of little value in assessing shoulder pain.[21] They may be useful, however, if osseous pathology is suspected or if

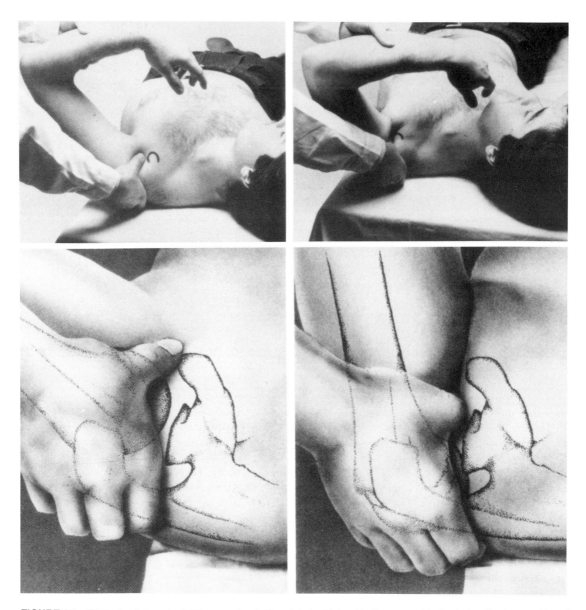

FIGURE 16. Posterior drawer test. The examiner's thumb is just lateral to the coracoid, displacing the humeral head posteriorly. The bottom panels show a schematic depiction of the test. (From Gerber C, Ganz R: clinical assessment of instability of the shoulder. *J Bone Joint Surg* 66B(4):551–556, 1984; with permission.)

there is a history of an antecedent acute trauma. Standard views include anteroposterior projections with internal and external rotation and an axillary view. Variations have been developed to allow better visualization of specific structures: the Grashey view,[14] the West Point view,[67] the Ciullo axillary view,[11] and the Stryker notch view.[53]

Fluoroscopic evaluation with or without anesthesia is helpful in documenting instability.[58] Shoulder arthrotomography and computed tomographic (CT) arthrograms assess labral pathology and define the bony relationships of the glenohumeral joint. Arthrograms have long been used to assess rotator cuff pathology; they are limited, however, in detecting partial thickness tears. Ciullo and Stevens[14] found that arthrograms have a false negative rate of 20% compared with arthroscopy. Magnetic resonance imaging (MRI) has been extremely helpful because of its ever-improving resolution and ability to format images in various planes. It also provides information on the osseous and capsular

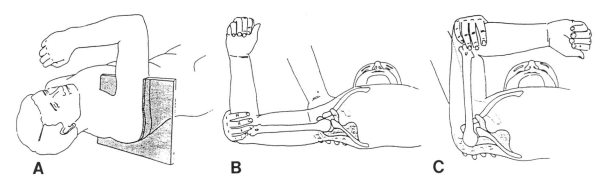

FIGURE 17. **A,** Plane of section through the shoulder joint demonstrating the anatomy depicted in B and C. **B,** The examiner stabilizes the scapula by resting his hand between the scapula and the examination table, allowing detection of scapular thoracic motion. Placing his hand posterior to the scapula, the examiner palpates the scapular neck and humeral head, and controls the patient's upper extremity with his opposite hand. For patient comfort, balance, and control, the examiner controls the arm at the olecranon and proximal forearm. The examiner moves the extremity to 90° of abduction and external rotation. The patient's arm rests in the neutral position between flexion and extension. The examination begins with the humeral head resting in the normal position in the glenoid. The examiner then brings the arm into forward flexion. **C,** If posterior subluxation is present, the examiner can feel the humeral head slip posteriorly to the glenoid. The patient verifies the familiar sensation and associated discomfort experienced during athletics. The arm is then returned to the neutral position in 90° of abduction. Both the patient and the examiner feel the humeral head relocate to the reduced position. Some patients are more uncomfortable when the humeral head leaves the glenoid; others are more symptomatic when the humeral head relocates. If the initial examination does not indicate subluxation, then the humeral rotation and degree of abduction are changed, and the examination is repeated. (From Norwood LA, Terry GC: Shoulder posterior subluxation. *Am J Sports Med* 12(1):25–30, 1984; with permission.)

structures. Nelson et al.[52] compared MRI, CT arthrography, and ultrasound with intraoperative shoulder pathology. MRI was found to be the most accurate in regard to partial thickness rotator cuff tears and was as accurate as CT arthrograms in evaluating the glenoid labrum. The authors acknowledged that MRI accuracy was technique- and operator-dependent. Poor positioning of the patient, obesity, and previous shoulder surgery resulted in less than optimal studies. Ultrasonography has been found to be useful in evaluating the soft tissues of the shoulder, including the rotator cuff, biceps tendon, and even the coracoacromial arch. Its utility, however is limited in assessment of the glenoid labrum, subacromial space, glenohumeral ligaments, joint capsule, and bone.[75] This method of evaluation is also heavily operator-dependent.

Initial radiologic evaluation in an otherwise healthy swimmer with shoulder pain should be a rare occurrence. A good clinical history and examination should be the mainstays of diagnosis and subsequent treatment. Refractoriness to a rehabilitation program and ascending age may be indications for earlier use of imaging studies.

Other Diagnostic Aids

Selective injections with anesthetic, such as into the acromioclavicular joint, may help to define more precisely the etiology of a swimmer's complaint. Isokinetic testing can quantify areas of weakness and pain during range-of-motion testing, particularly in strong individuals. Electromyography and nerve conduction studies assist in evaluating protential nerve injury. Circulatory causes of shoulder pain may require arteriography.

Rehabilitation

Shoulder injuries in the swimmer usually result from repetitive cumulative trauma. Management in the acute period is therefore important in preventing chronic injury. Grading of clinical severity helps to direct treatment. Blazina et al.'s[7] scale of jumper's knee can be conveniently applied to swimmer's shoulder. Stage 1 pain occurs only after swimming; stage 2, pain during and after workouts of a nondisabling nature; and stage 3, disabling pain during and after workouts. A fourth category proposed by Johnson et al.[36] is pain sufficiently severe to interfere with competitive swimming. Fowler[22] defines a fourth category as pain that occurs with daily activities. The mainstay of treatment for stages 1 and 2 consists of rest, change in training regimen, technique adjustments, nonsteroidal antiinflammatory agents, modalities, and conditioning. Complete rest of the shoulder

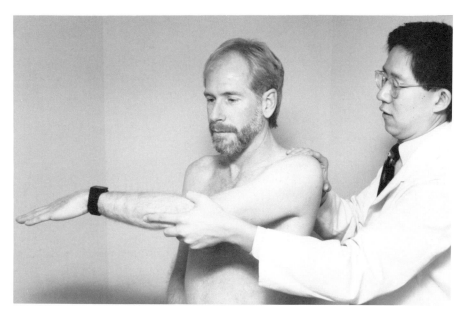

FIGURE 18. Horizontal adduction test for acromiclavicular (AC) joint pathology.

should occur if the swimmer's symptoms are stage 3 or 4.

Rest

In the young swimmer who is less than 12 years old, Dominguez[21] recommends that the patient should abstain from swimming until the symptoms resolve. However, as the competitive swimmer gets older, this becomes more difficult to do. State and national level swimmers need to train 9 to 10 months of the year to remain in top form. The high demands of the sport, especially in the shoulder girdle, result in rapid deconditioning when training is halted.[16]

Training Regimen

The training regimen can often be varied to accommodate the injured shoulder. Cooperation with the coach and athletic trainer is invaluable in this aspect of treatment. Total yardage can be decreased. Avoidance of the pain-eliciting stroke or limiting the yardage with that stroke often allows recovery without jeopardizing the swimmer's conditioning. Yardage should be limited to pain-free distances. Changing the event of a competitive swimmer may also help to reduce shoulder symptoms.

If the individual is unable to swim comfort-

ably because of shoulder pain, rest is appropriate but should not imply time out of the water. A kickboard with or without fins can be used to maintain endurance and conditioning during rehabilitative efforts. To avoid a position of impingement, the board should be held not at arm's length but with the elbows bent. Swimming fins may also be advantageous in providing greater propulsive force, decreasing the effort needed by the arms to maintain the same speed.[36]

An adequate time period for preswim stretching should be enforced. Avoidance of partner stretch activities is recommended.[17,47] Improper technique as well as overstretching to the point of pain can aggravate symptoms, particularly if instability is present. A warm-up swim of 20 to 30 minutes with several different strokes is suggested prior to hard training.[28,39] Hand paddles should be avoided during the early rehabilitative period.[36,47] Weight training should be assessed to ensure proper technique and avoidance of exercises that induce pain.[47] Greipp[25] felt that weight training itself could lead to shoulder pain by causing tendon hypertrophy of the rotator cuff and the bicipital tendon, thereby increasing the potential for impingement.

Stroke Technique

Close examination of stroke technique is crucial. A "high elbow" during recovery can help to prevent impingement by limiting excessive abduction at the shoulder.[47] Fowler[22] noted that swimmers with higher-arm recoveries had fewer shoulder problems (Fig. 19). Greipp[25] linked anterior shoulder tightness to the incidence of shoulder pain. The greater the flexibility, the less the body roll in such strokes as the freestyle or backstroke. The normal amount of side-to-side roll is between 70° and 100°.[19] Roll allows for easier recovery of the arm as it is drawn out of the water and better mechanical advantage to the opposing arm as it is pulled through the water. With less body roll, greater abduction occurs at the shoulder, possibly increasing impingement.[66] This agrees with the observation of Greipp,[25] who found the highest incidence of shoulder pain in butterfliers. There is no body roll involved in this stroke.

Temporary stroke modifications may be necessary to reduce shoulder pain if impingement or supraspinatus tendinitis is present. In addition to increased body roll, earlier arm recovery and less internal rotation of the arm at hand entry will result in less time in adduction and reduce the likelihood of impingement.[60] Swimmers tend to make these changes in their stroke pattern naturally. Scovazzo et al.[70] correlated electromyographic and cinematographic data on freestylers with shoulder pain. The serratus anterior, which normally assists in bringing the body over the arm at pull-through, was not as active in the injured swimmer. This allows the scapula to maintain a protracted and upwardly rotated orientation that translates into greater humeral clearance beneath the coracoacromial arch. Abnormally increased activity in the supraspinatus, near the end of pull-through limits internal rotation and causes an earlier recovery phase. Decreased subscapularis activity, seen during recovery, minimized the

position of impingement. In anterior shoulder instability aggravated by the backstroke, modification of the turning technique may be tried. Depending on the extent of the modifications, the swimmer may risk disqualification in a competitive meet.[38]

Medical and Therapeutic Modalities

Temporary reduction in activity, a short course of a nonsteroidal antiinflammatory agents, and judicious use of ice often allows the symptomatic swimmer to return to full training in a short period of time. If ice massage is performed, application should be limited to 10 minutes over the painful area. Otherwise ice packs may be used for 20 minutes. Application is recommended after practice and several times per day.[21] Full shoulder range of motion should be practiced immediately after icing.[39]

Ultrasound may be helpful for tendinitis. Treatment to the biceps tendon is 0.8 to 1.2 W/cm² for 10 minutes daily for 10 days. The dosage for the supraspinatus is 1.2 to 1.5 W/cm².[38] Treatment may be repeated at 3- to 6-month intervals.[39]

An upper arm strap, akin to the strap used for tennis elbow, has been found to be helpful in impingement.[6] Placed at the level of the deltoid insertion, it exerts a tenodesis effect on the biceps muscle, making it a more effective humeral head depressor when the arm is elevated above shoulder level.

Transcutaneous electric nerve stimulation (TENS) can be useful for pain management in refractory cases. Application is for 30 minutes prior to workouts.[39] TENS has been found to be particularly beneficial in swimmers under the age of 20 with acromioclavicular joint symptoms.[14] It is perhaps most appro-

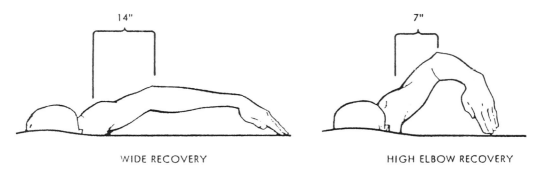

FIGURE 19. Elbow position during the recovery phase of the freestyle. (From Counsilman JE: *The Science of Swimming.* Englewood Cliffs, NJ, Prentice-Hall, Inc. 1968, with permission.)

priately used near the end of the season as finals approach and rest from competition is expected shortly.

Indications for corticosteroid use are controversial. Their antiinflammatory properties decrease the pain and edema of injured tissues, but the unwanted side effect of weakening tissue has made many practitioners cautious. Kennedy and Willis[40] found that direct injection of steroid into a normal rabbit tendon resulted in collagen necrosis and weakening. Restoration of tensile strength did not occur until 14 days after injection as amorphous material was deposited. Return to normal arrangement and appearance of collagen fibrils, however, did not occur until 6 weeks after injection. Glucocorticoids have also been found to reduce synthesis of protein, collagen, and proteoglycan in articular cartilage.[3] Kennedy and Hawkins[38] and Penny and Smith[60] limit injections to elite swimmers who have not responded to conservative measures and who are approaching a vital meet. Ciullo[14] opposes steroid injections into the acromioclavicular joint if osteolysis of the distal clavicle is present because they can retard healing.

Therapeutic Exercise

Restriction of arm motion should be closely watched by the coach and athletic trainer. Ciullo and Guise[12] found that 80% of adolescent swimmers in the Detroit area who swam over 12,000 yards daily exhibited symptoms of impingement. After a simple stretching program (Fig. 20), the overall incidence dropped to 14.6% in 3 years. Unfortunately, this program has been found to be less successful in Masters swimmers (55%), probably because of more advanced degenerative changes.[13] The goal of stretching is to obtain balanced flexibility of the shoulder muscles, thus increasing the functional room within the subacromial space.

Shoulder extension and internal rotation provide propulsive force. As a result, the internal rotators and extensors (the pectoralis major, latissimus dorsi and, to a lesser extent, the subscapularis) become relatively stronger and are more prone to tightening than the flexors and external rotators. A program of stretching of the internal rotators is important, particularly in individuals with impingement symptoms (Fig. 21).

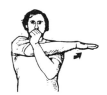

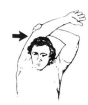

STRETCHING
to stretch supraspinatus ligament, fibrotic muscle and shoulder capsule.

FORCED HORIZONTAL FLEXION:
sustained stretch for 20 seconds; 4 reps.

FORCED HYPERABDUCTION:
sustained stretch for 20 seconds; 4 reps.

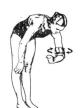

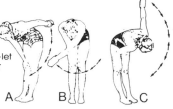

WEIGHTED FLEXIBILITY
to increase clearance under C/A arch—let gravity assist in swinging motion rather than actively using muscles.

A   B   C

WEIGHTED CODMAN:
2½-5# ankle weight on elbow; 20 rotations clockwise, 20 counter-clockwise.

WEIGHTED PENDULUM:
2½-5# ankle weight around wrist. (A) front-to-back; (B) side-to-side; (C) up over shoulder from opposite knee. 20 each.

FIGURE 20. Stretching routine to reduce the risk of impingement. (From Ciullo JV: Swimmer's shoulder. *Clin Sports Med* 5(1):115–138, 1986; with permission.)

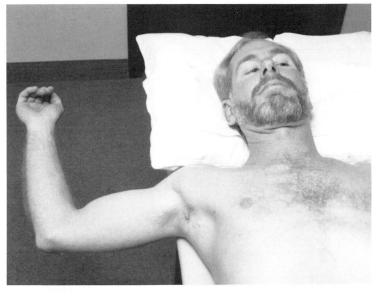

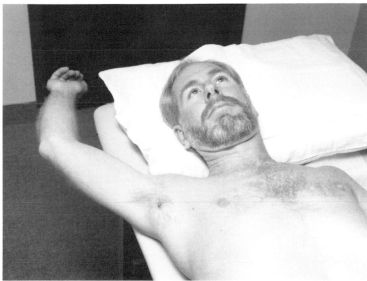

FIGURE 21. Internal rotator (*top*) and adductor (*bottom*) stretching exercises. The degree of abduction of the humerus should be varied to emphasize different muscles and portions of a given muscle.

Strengthening of the external rotators and humeral head depressors is also important and should be undertaken when the specific arc of motion is pain-free. Internal and external rotation can be performed with the aid of rubber tubing, Theraband, or free weights (Fig. 22). Bradley and Tibone[9] performed electromyographic (EMG) analysis on exercises used by professional baseball teams for shoulder rehabilitation. "Scaption"—i.e., abduction of the arm in the plane of the scapula (30° anterior to coronal) with internal rota-

tion—was found to be the most effective exercise in strengthening the subscapularis and supraspinatus (Fig. 23A). Horizontal abduction with external rotation was the best exercise for conditioning both the infraspinatus and teres minor (Fig. 23B).

The importance of the scapular stabilizers and rotators in shoulder movements and prevention of injury has recently been emphasized. Appropriate strength and flexibility in the levator scapulae, trapezius, rhomboids, pectoralis minor, and serratus anterior help

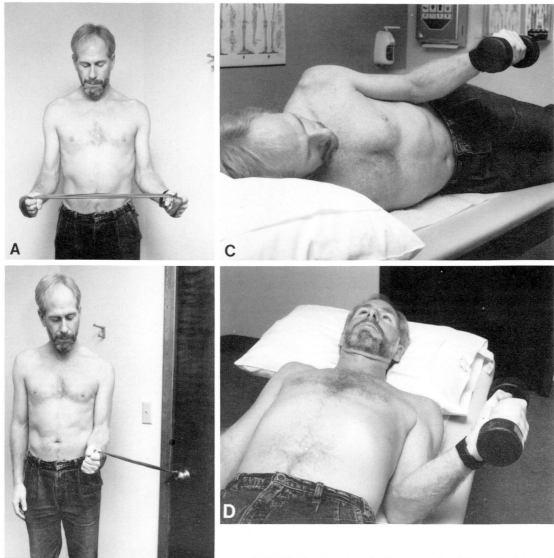

FIGURE 22. Exercises for the external and internal rotators of the shoulder with Theraband (A and B) and with free weights (C and D).

to minimize instability and impingement and to maintain a normal scapulohumeral rhythm. Electromyographic studies in swimmers show that the serratus anterior is particularly susceptible to fatigue, because it is involved in both the recovery and pull-through phases of the stroke.[55,61,70] Weakness in this muscle prevents full protraction and rotation of the scapula as the arm is abducted and flexed; thus the risk of impingement is increased. EMG analysis has revealed that the most effective exercises to strengthen the

scapular stabilizers include scaption with thumbs up, horizontal rowing, push-up with a plus (scapular protraction), and press-ups[9] (Fig. 24). Closed-grip bench press and vertical rowing have also been found to be helpful in strengthening the serratus and rhomboids while minimizing impingement positions and stress on the anterior capsular structures.[1]

When instability is the etiology of shoulder complaints, stretching should not be overlooked. Laxity in one direction may be fos-

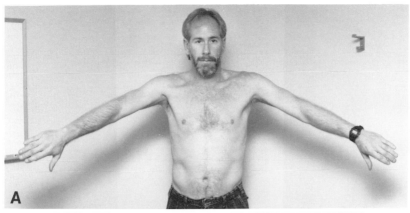

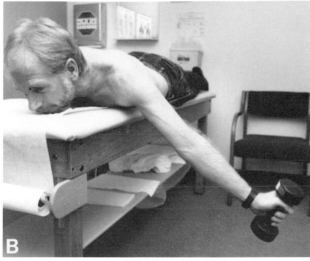

FIGURE 23. *A,* "Scaption" to strengthen the supraspinatus and subscapularis. *B,* Horizontal abduction to strengthen the infraspinatus and teres minor.

tered by tight or shortened structures on the side opposite to the increased translation.[51] Muscular stabilization primarily occurs by strengthening the internal and external rotators. Because functional activities require strength with minimal bulk, high repetition with low resistance is preferable; a goal of 20 to 30 repetitions per exercise is appropriate.[45]

Advancement to isokinetic exercises, if the equipment is available, can be very helpful in strengthening an athlete with sport-simulating movements (Fig. 25). These techniques allow the synchronous development of power and coordination.

Swimming involves a balance of flexibility, strength, and technique. When any one of these three components is impaired, the individual is prone to injury. Proprioceptive neuromuscular facilitation, as developed by Kabat, may be useful to the injured swimmer.

Janda and Loubert[32] describe the application of this technique to throwing athletes. Applied resistance through diagonal and spiral motions of the arm develop strength, endurance, and the proprioceptive skill necessary to perform the throwing motion. Isometric and isotonic maneuvers—with maximal resistance to develop function-specific strength and control—are currently used as a preventive measure by Janda and Loubert. Application to the swimmer with shoulder pain may be promising whether for correcting improper technique or for reconditioning.

In the older or posttraumatic swimmer with acromioclavicular joint arthritis, activity above the shoulder level should be limited. Strengthening the deltoid and rotator cuff may help to stabilize the joint, and a stretching program may help to improve motion and to deter further degenerative changes.[14]

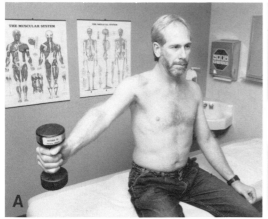

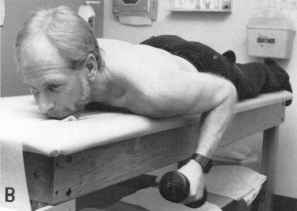

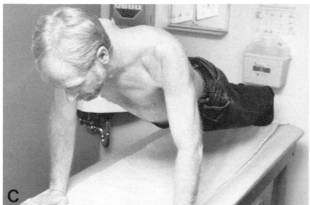

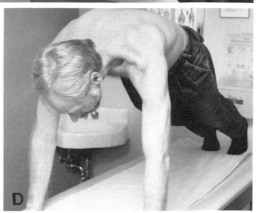

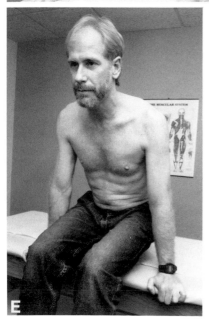

FIGURE 24. Exercises for the scapular stabilizers: **A,** scaption with external rotation; **B,** horizontal rowing; **C and D,** push-up with a plus (scapular protraction); **E,** press-up.

Surgery

As a rule, surgery should be considered only after a year of conservative therapy has been tried.[21,28,39] Ciullo and Stevens[14] feel that in the instance of anterior instability, surgery may be indicated after 3 months of aggressive therapy. However, they note that if the surgery occurs at the peak of a swimmer's career, a return to previous levels of perfor-

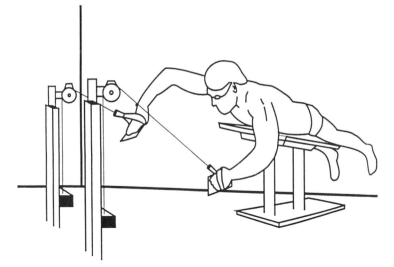

FIGURE 25. Diagrammatic representation of the freestyle stroke on an isokinetic swim bench. (Artist: Kevin Gormley)

mance is unlikely. Anterior reconstruction can lead to limitation of external rotation and the development of impingement.[27] Depending on the procedure performed, the pathologic defect may not be corrected, and normal anatomy and movement is disturbed.[76] Capsular shift procedures for multidirectional instability have allowed swimmers to return to competition, but attainment of previous performance levels is uncertain.[36] Coracoacromial ligament splitting and acromioplasty for impingement have not been successful in allowing elite swimmers to return to prior levels of competition.[36] The Mumford procedure—surgical resection of the distal clavicle—may be indicated in the Masters-level swimmer with severe arthritis in the acromioclavicular joint.[14] Prior to consideration of surgery, temporary or permanent discontinuation of swimming should be discussed.

KNEE

Kicking Technique

The kicking action of the legs serves as a secondary propulsive force in the backstroke, freestyle, and butterfly. It provides a balancing force to the arm movements, making forward progression in the water smoother and straighter. During kicking, knee flexion can be as great as 90°.[64]

The whip kick of the breaststroke is unique in that it provides much more forward force than the flutter kick or the dolphin kick of the butterfly. An externally rotating force is ap-

plied through the knee and foot. The knee also flexes more, up to 130°.[64]

In the whip kick the legs are initially fully extended and together with the feet plantar-flexed (Fig. 26). Recovery begins when the knees are dropped toward the bottom of the pool as the heels are brought toward the buttocks. Just prior to the initiation of the push phase, the feet are everted and dorsiflexed. The knees lie within the distance separating the ankles. As the legs are thrust caudally, water is pushed backward by the medial aspect and sole of the foot as well as the medial leg. The legs are extended and adducted synchronously. At the finish the hips and knees are fully extended, and the feet return to their original plantar-flexed position.

Mechanism of Pathology

There are several potential causes of knee pain in the swimmer (Table 3). Older swimmers may experience patellofemoral problems. Because of the significant amount of knee flexion in the flutter, dolphin, and whip kicks, further irritation to this joint may ensue. Tenderness along the patellar facets or respective intercondylar surfaces can be found on examination. Patellofemoral compression reproduces the symptoms, and crepitus may be present.

Most knee pain in swimmers occurs medially. Kennedy et al.[39] found knee pain to be limited to breaststrokers in their cross-Canada survey of 2,496 swimmers. They attribute medial knee pain to pathology of the tibial collateral ligament, as does Counsilman.[19] This ligament passes from the adductor tubercle of

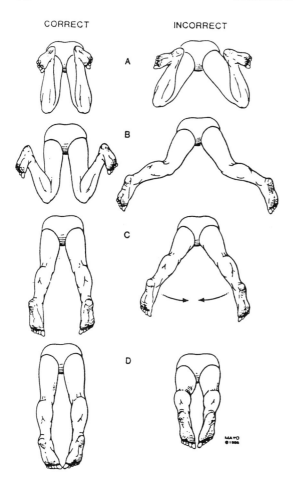

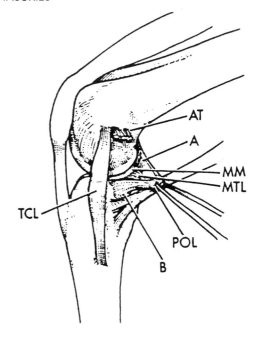

FIGURE 27. Anatomy of the medial knee. TCL=tibial collateral ligament, AT=adductor tubercle, A=posterior capsule, MM=medial meniscus, POL=posterior oblique ligament. (From Sisk TD: In Crenshaw AH (ed): *Campbell's Operative Orthopaedics*, 8th ed. St. Louis, Mosby, 1992, pp 1494; with permission.)

FIGURE 26. Correct and incorrect whip kick. (From Johnson J, et al: Musculoskeletal injuries in competitive swimmers. *Mayo Clin Proc* 62:289–304, 1987; with permission.)

TABLE 3.   Potential Causes of Medial Knee Pain in the Swimmer

Patellofemoral syndrome
Tibial collateral ligament strain
Medial synovial plica syndrome
Medial meniscal tear
Osteochondritis dessicans

the femur to the anteromedial tibia 4–5 cm distal to the joint line (Fig. 27). Examination often reveals tenderness at the adductor tubercle or along the course of the ligament, particularly as it crosses the tibial margin. Pain with a valgus and externally rotating force at the knee while in 20° to 30° of flexion is suggestive of the disorder.

Application of strain gauges to the tibial collateral ligaments of cadavers by Kennedy et al.[39] demonstrated the tension generated by the movements of the knee during the whip kick. Tibial collateral tension increased when the knee was extended, when a valgus moment was applied across the knee, and when an externally rotating force occurred during terminal extension. The knee passes through each of these movements during the performance of the whip kick. The externally rotating force was found to generate the most tension on the ligament.

Stulberg et al.[72] described the faulty mechanics of an improperly performed whip kick that led to the development of tibial collateral pain. In these swimmers the thighs are abducted widely during recovery, and the legs are then extended with the knees apart. At the end of the propulsive phase the legs are forcibly adducted (Fig. 26).

A second etiology for medial knee pain was also explored by Stulberg et al.[72] They found that a medial patellofemoral syndrome could cause such pain. Analysis of symptomatic breaststrokers revealed wide abduction of the knees during the recovery phase. However, on extension of the legs they maintained the everted and externally rotated position of the feet. At full extension they allowed the legs to

drift together. No derotation of the legs occurred with knee extension. Swimmers found
to have both patellofemoral pain and tibial
collateral pain had a combination of both
technical flaws. These findings were in swimmers who exhibited a hybrid kick, which is a
combination of the scissors kick of the side-
stroke and the classic whip kick.[37] This may
explain the occurrence of patellofemoral
pain.

Medial synovitis has also been described as
a potential cause of "breaststroker's knee."
Keskinen et al.[41] arthroscopically examined
breaststrokers with medial knee complaints.
The only abnormality noted was medial synovitis. No ligamentous or patellofemoral pathology was seen. Rovere and Nichols[68] suggest that breaststrokers experience medial
synovial plica syndrome. As the knee is extended, the plica snaps over the medial femoral condyle, resulting in inflammation, thickening, and eventual fibrosis (Fig. 28).

Risk Factors

In all instances, medial knee pain occurs
during knee extension in the propulsive
phase. Ligamentous laxity has not been associated with this disorder.[41,68,72] Stulberg et
al.[72] examined 23 symptomatic breaststrokers.
The onset of knee pain was usually within 3
years after beginning the whip kick. No consistent relationship was found between the
incidence of medial knee pain and patella
alta, patellar hypermobility, knee hyperextension, increased genu valgus or varus, internal
femoral torsion, external or internal tibial torsion, or an increased Q angle. Relative muscle
weakness also showed no correlation with medial knee complaints.

Rovere and Nichols[68] evaluated 36 competitive breaststrokers to correlate range of motion
with medial knee pain. The only significant
finding was diminished hip internal rotation in
symptomatic swimmers. This lack of internal
rotation makes proper technique—knees adducted with the ankles more laterally flexed—
difficult and encourages poor form (Fig. 26).
Onset of knee pain most commonly resulted
from increased yardage. Breaststrokers who
were older, swam more years competitively, and
trained more yards with the whip kick were
more likely to have knee pain. The repetitive
nature, along with the high torque generated
across the knee, makes breaststroker's knee an
injury of overuse.

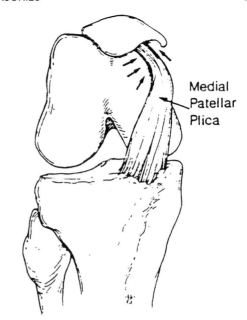

FIGURE 28. Medial patellar plica can cause a synovitis
due to friction against the medial femoral condyle. (From
Rockwood CA Jr., Green DP, Bucholz RW (eds): *Rockwood and Green's Fractures in Adults,* 3rd ed. Philadelphia, J.B. Lippincott, 1991; with permission.)

Rehabilitation

As with the shoulder, treatment involves
analysis and correction of technique, training
modifications, nonsteroidal antiinflammatory
agents, and therapeutic modalities. Less external tibial rotation may benefit the swimmer.[39] Reduction of breaststroke yardage and
increased variety of strokes is recommended.
As preventive measures, a minimum of 1,000
to 1,500 yards of warm-up should be completed prior to hard breaststroke training.[68] A
minimum of 2 months of rest each year is
recommended by Kennedy and associates[39]
for competitive breaststrokers. Attention to
improving hip internal rotation is also important.[68]

A short course of a nonsteroidal antiinflammatory agent, along with icing, can be very
beneficial. Application of ice for 10 minutes
after exercise is recommended.[39] Treatment
with courses of ultrasound may be performed
every 1 to 2 months. Dosage should be 0.2 to
0.5 W/cm^2 for 5 minutes daily for 10 days.[39]
Injection therapy with corticosteroids has
been advocated only in the presence of the
medial plica syndrome. Injection should occur only into the irritated plica and not in-
traarticularly.[68] For refractory cases, partial

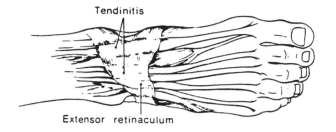

Tendinitis

Extensor retinaculum

FIGURE 29. The repetitive nature of the kick can cause tendinitis beneath the extensor retinaculum in the swimmer. (From Kennedy JC, et al: Orthopaedic manifestations of swimming. *Am J Sports Med* 6(6):309–322; 1978; with permission.)

synovectomy or arthroscopic resection of the plica may be indicated.[68]

CALF AND FOOT

Calf and foot problems are the third major area of swimming injuries. They most commonly involve the extensor tendons of the foot. The repetitive nature of the flutter and dolphin kick makes these structures prone to irritation beneath the extensor retinaculum (Fig. 29). This malady occurs less frequently in breaststrokers, for whom ankle dorsiflexion is encouraged. Butterfliers, freestylers, and backstrokers actively try to improve plantar flexibility to add power to their kick. Competitive swimmers frequently attain 90° of plantar flexion.

Pain over the extensor surface of the ankle and foot, along with crepitus at the ankle, is diagnostic of extensor tendon pathology. Temporary reduction in the intensity of the kick and avoidance of swim fins may help to alleviate the symptoms and allow healing to occur. In the case of the freestyle, switching from a 6-beat kick (3 kicks/arm stroke) to a 2-beat kick can also reduce the irritation to the involved tendons.[39] Ice, ultrasound, and a nonsteroidal agent for symptomatic management are again useful. Wrapping the ankle in neutral position at night may allow more rapid healing.[39] Injection of corticosteroid beneath the retinaculum and around the tendon sheaths is much more of an accepted practice than in the shoulder or knee. Kennedy et al.[39] consider an injection if significant crepitus is present or if a major swim meet is pending.

CONCLUSIONS

Swimming enjoys increasing popularity as a recreational and competitive sport. For the youngster or the older individual it has several benefits and advantages over other athletic activities. To become competitive, however, requires long hours and many yards of training in the water. Practice schedules frequently run 10 months out of the year. As a result, most swimming injuries are overuse disorders secondary to chronic repetitive trauma.

Prevention and early detection of injuries are the mainstays of treatment. The goal is to prevent the development of a chronic problem. Gradual increase in training intensity, maintenance of proper flexibility and strength, and attention to proper technique are instrumental in avoiding injury. Addressing symptoms early and minimizing their effect on training reduces the chance of recurrence. A knowledgeable coach and athletic trainer are the first line of defense against injury.

Once a swimmer presents to a physician with a problem, it is important that the practitioner have a fundamental understanding of stroke mechanics and training demands. Good communication with the coach, trainer, and/or parent can often aid in rapid diagnosis and treatment.

REFERENCES

1. Abrams JS: Special shoulder problems in the throwing athlete: Pathology, diagnosis and non-operative care. *Clin Sports Med* 10:839–862, 1991.
2. Becker TJ: The athletic trainer in swimming. *Clin Sports Med* 5(1):9–24, 1986.
3. Behren F, Shepard N, Mitchell N: Alterations of rabbit cartilage by intraarticular injections of glucocorticosteroids. *J Bone Joint Surg* 57A(1):70–76, 1975.
4. Bell RH, Noble JS: An appreciation of posterior instability of the shoulder. *Clin Sports Med* 10:887–900, 1991.
5. Bigliani LU, Ticker JB, Flatlow EL, et al: The relationship of acromial architecture to rotator cuff disease. *Clin Sports Med* 10:823–838, 1991.
6. Blatz D: Upper arm strap. *Swimming World* 27:43–44, 1985.
7. Blazina ME, Kerlan RK, Jobe FW, et al: Jumper's knee. *Orthop Clin North Am* 4:665–678, 1973.
8. Bowen MK, Warren RF: Ligamentous control of

shoulder stability based on selective cutting and static translation experiments. *Clin Sports Med* 10:757–782, 1991.

9. Bradley JP, Tibone JE: Electromyographic analysis of muscle action about the shoulder. *Clin Sports Med* 10:789–806, 1991.

10. Chansky HA, Iannotti JP: The vascularity of the rotator cuff. *Clin Sports Med* 10:807–822, 1991.

11. Ciullo JV, Koniuch MP, Tietge RA: Axillary shoulder roentgenography in clinical orthopaedic practice. *Orthop Trans* 6:451–452, 1982.

12. Ciullo JV, Guise ER: Adolescent Swimmer's Shoulder. *Orthop Trans* 7:171, 1983.

13. Ciullo JV: Swimmer's shoulder. *Clin Sports Med* 5:115–138, 1986.

14. Ciullo JV, Stevens GG: The prevention and treatment of injuries to the shoulder in swimming. *Sports Med* 7:182–204, 1989.

15. Codman EA: *The Shoulder: Rupture of the Supraspinatus Tendon and Other Lesions in or about the Subacromal Bursa.* Boston, Thomas Todd, 1934.

16. Costill DL, Fink WJ, Hargreaves M, et al: *Med Sci Sports Exerc* 17:339–343, 1985.

17. Counsilman JE: The role of the coach in training for swimming. *Clin Sports Med* 5:3–8, 1986.

18. Counsilman JE: *The Complete Book of Swimming.* New York, Athenium/Macmillan, 1977.

19. Counsilman JE: *The Science of Swimming.* Englewood Cliffs, NJ, Prentice-Hall, 1968.

20. Donnelly WH, Indelicato PA: The physician to a swimming team. *Clin Sports Med* 5:25–32, 1986.

21. Dominguez RH: Shoulder pain in swimmers. *Phys Sports Med* 8(7):37–42, 1980.

22. Fowler P: Swimmer problems. *Am J Sports Med* 7(2):141–142, 1979.

23. Fowler PJ, Regan WD: Simming injuries of the knee, foot and ankle, elbow, and back. *Clin Sports Med* 5(1):139–148, 1986.

24. Gerber C, Ganz R: Clinical assessment of instability of the shoulder. *J Bone Joint Surg* 66B:551–556, 1984.

25. Greipp JF: Swimmer's shoulder: The influence of flexibility and weight training. *Physician Sportmed* 13(8):92–105, 1985.

26. Hall G: Hand paddles may cause shoulder pain. *Swimming World* 21(10):9–11, 1980.

27. Hawkins RH, Hawkins KJ: Failed anterior reconstruction for shoulder instability. *J Bone Joint Surg* 67B:709–714, 1985.

28. Hawkins RJ, Kennedy JC: Impingement syndrome in athletes. *Am J Sports Med* 8(3):151–158, 1980.

29. Hay JG: *The Biomechanics of Sports Techniques.* Englewood Cliffs, NJ, Prentice-Hall, 1985, pp 343–394.

30. Hollinshead WH, Jenkins DB: *Functional Anatomy of the Limbs and Back.* Philadelphia, W.B. Saunders, 1981.

31. Inman VT, Saunders M, Abbott LC: Observations on the function of the shoulder joint. *J Bone Joint Surg* 26:1–30, 1944.

32. Janda DH, Loubert P: A preventative program focusing on the glenohumeral joint. *Clin Sports Med* 10:955–972, 1991.

33. Jobe FW, Jobe CM: Painful athletic injuries of the shoulder. *Clin Orthop Rel Res* 173:117–124, 1983.

34. Jobe FW, Moynes D: Delineation of diagnostic criteria and a rehabilitation program for rotator cuff injuries. *Am J Sports Med* 10(6):336–339, 1982.

35. Jobe FW, Pink M: Shoulder injuries in the athlete: The instability continuum and treatment. *J Hand Ther* 4:69–73, 1991.

36. Johnson JE, Sim FH, Scott SG: Musculoskeletal injuries in competitive swimmers. *Mayo Clin Proc* 62:289–304, 1987.

37. Kennedy JC: Commentary. *Am J Sports Med* 8(3):170, 1980.

38. Kennedy JC, Hawkins RJ: Swimmer's shoulder. *Phys Sports Med* 2(4):35–38, 1974.

39. Kennedy JC, Hawkins R, Krissoff B: Orthopaedic manifestatiions of swimming. *Am J Sports Med* 6(6):309–322, 1978.

40. Kennedy JC, Willis RB: The effects of local steroid injections on tendons. A biomechanical and microscopic correlative study. *Am J Sports Med* 4:11–21, 1976.

41. Keskinen K, Eriksson E, Komi P: breaststroke swimmer's knee. *Am J Sports Med* 8(4):228–231, 1980.

42. Lucas DB: Biomechanics of the shoulder joint. *Arch Surg* 107:425–432, 1973.

43. Macnab I: The painful shoulder due to rotator cuff tendinitis. *Rhode Island Med J* 54(7):367–374, 388, 1971.

44. Matsen FA III, Harryman DT II, Sidles JA: Mechanics of glenohumeral instability. *Clin Sports Med* 10:783–788, 1991.

45. Matsen FA III, Kirby RM: Office evaluation and management of shoulder pain. *Orthop Clin North Am* 13:453–475, 1982.

46. McMaster WC: Anterior glenoid labrum damage: A painful lesion in swimmers. *Am J Sports Med* 14(5):383–387, 1986.

47. McMaster WC: Painful Shoulder in Swimmers: A diagnostic challenge. *Phys Sports Med* 14(12):108–122, 1986.

48. Mohtadi NGH: Advances in the understanding of anterior instability of the shoulder. *Clin Sports Med* 10:863–870, 1991.

49. Neer CS II: Anterior acromioplasty for the chronic impingement syndrome in the shoulder. *J Bone Joint Surg* 54A:41–50, 1972.

50. Neer CS II, Welsh RP: The shoulder in sports. *Orthop Clin North Am* 8:583–591, 1977.

51. Neer CS II, Foster CR: Inferior capsular shift for involuntary inferior and multidirectional instability of the shoulder. *J Bone Joint Surg* 62A:897–908, 1980.

52. Nelson MC, Leather GP, Nirschl RP, et al.: Evaluation of the painful shoulder: A prospective comparison of magnetic resonance imaging, computerized tomographic arthrography, ultrasonography and operative findings. *J Bone Joint Surg* 73A:707–716, 1991.

53. Norris TR: *Diagnostic Techniques for Shoulder Instability: Vol 34. AAOS Instructional course lecture.* St. Louis, Mosby, 1985, pp 239–257.

54. Norwood LA, Terry GC: Shoulder posterior subluxation. *Am J Sports Med* 12:25–30, 1984.

55. Nuber GW, et al: Fine wire electromyography analysis of muscles of the shoulder during swimming. *Am J Sports Med* 14(1):7–11, 1986.

56. O'Brien SJ, Warren RF: Anterior shoulder instability. *Orthop Clin North Am* 18:395–408, 1987.

57. Pande P, Hawkins R, Peat M: Electromyography in voluntary posterior instability of the shoulder. *Am J Sports Med* 17:644–648, 1989.

58. Papilion JA, Shall LM: Fluoroscopic evaluation for subtle shoulder instability. *Am J Sports Med* 20:548–552, 1992.

59. Pappas AM, Goss TP, Kleinman PK: Symptomatic shoulder instability due to lesions of the glenoid labrum. *Am J Sports Med* 11(5):279–288, 1983.
60. Penny JN, Smith C: The prevention and treatment of swimmer's shoulder. *Can J Appl Sports Sci* 5:195–202, 1980.
61. Pink M, Perry J, Browne A, et al: The normal shoulder during freestyle swimming. *Am J Sports Med* 19:569–576, 1991.
62. Rathbun JB, Macnab I: The microvascular pattern of the rotator cuff. *J Bone Joint Surg* 52B:540–553, 1970.
63. Regan W, Richards R: Subacromial pressure measurement: A pilot study in a cadaveric model. In Post M, Morrey BF, Hawkins RJ (eds): *Surgery of the Shoulder.* St. Louis, Mosby-Year Book, 1990, pp 181–185.
64. Richardson AR: The biomechanics of swimming: The shoulder and knee. *Clin Sports Med* 5(1):103–114, 1986.
65. Richardson AR, Jobe FW, Collins HR: The shoulder in competitive swimming. *Am J Sports Med* 8(3):159–163, 1980.
66. Richardson AR, Miller JW: Swimming and the older athlete. *Clin Sports Med* 10:301–316, 1991.
67. Rokous JR, Feagin JA, Abbott HG: Modified axillary roentgenogram. *Clin Orthop* 82:84–86, 1972.
68. Rovere GD, Nichols AW: Frequency, associated factors, and treatment of breaststrokers's knee in competitive swimmers. *Am J Sports Med* 13(2):99–104, 1985.
69. Saha AK: Mechanisms of shoulder movements and a plea for the recognition of zero position of the glenohumeral joint. *Clin Orthop* 173:3–10, 1983.
70. Scovazzo ML, Browne A, Pink M, et al: The painful shoulder during freestyle swimming. *Am J Sports Med* 19:577–582, 1991.
71. Sigholm G, Styf J, Korner S, et al: Pressure recording in the subacromial bursa. *J Orthop Res* 6:123–128, 1988.
72. Stulberg SD, Shulman K, Stuart S, Culp P: breaststroker's knee: Pathology, etiology and treatment. *Am J Sports Med* 8:164–171, 1980.
73. Swiontkowski MF, Iannotti JP, Boulas HJ, et al: Intraoperative assessment of rotator cuff vascularity using laser doppler flowmetry. In Post M, Morrey BF, Hawkins RJ (eds): *Surgery of the Shoulder.* St. Louis, Mosby-Year Book, 1990, pp 208–212.
74. Uhthoff Hk, Sarkar K: Classification and definition of tendinopathies. *Clin Sports Med* 10:707–720, 1991.
75. Vellet AD, Munk PL, Marks P: Imaging techniques of the shoulder: Present perspectives. *Clin Sports Med* 10:721–756, 1991.
76. Zarins B, Rowe CR: Current concepts in the diagnosis and treatment of shoulder instability in athletes. *Med Sci Sports Exerc* 16(5):444–448, 1984.

Chapter 6

BASKETBALL INJURIES AND REHABILITATION

Sanford S. Kunkel, M.D.

HISTORY OF THE GAME

In 1891, at a YMCA in Springfield, Massachusetts, James Naismith used a large round ball and a peach basket to invent a game that is now the great sport of basketball. Nearly 100 years later, basketball is played by nearly 42 million people in the United States. Naismith's concept of elevating the goals was to promote fitness and agility over the brute strength associated with football. Over the next 100 years, arguably some of the greatest athletes in the world have embraced the game of basketball for recreation or profession.

The game of basketball as we know it today requires nearly an equal amount of upper-extremity and lower-extremity coordination. This fact alone sets it apart from many other highly skilled games. Over the past 10 years, the professional game of basketball has been represented by athletes with incredible quickness and stamina and superb overall conditioning. The physique of a professional basketball player is no longer long and lanky, but rather resembles that of a well-developed body builder who can leap 10–11 feet into the air.

Unfortunately, as size, speed, and strength have increased, the injuries that athletes sustain, particularly contact injuries, have become more severe. And although none of us has watched the game for entire last 100 years, intuition tells me that it has become more physical as well.

As the interest in basketball increases, so does the opportunity for the young basketball player to become a multi-millionaire in the National Basketball Association (NBA). With potential professional careers at stake, the importance of diagnosing and properly treating basketball injuries also has increased. This chapter focuses on the most common injuries and their treatment and rehabilitation.

EPIDEMIOLOGY OF INJURIES

Over the past 19 years, the National Basketball Trainers Association has employed an injury surveillance system.[1] Although the reported injuries apply to professional basketball, they are similar in all age groups and at all levels of competition.

The lower extremity is the most common injury site, followed by the upper extremity and torso (Fig. 1). The most common injury is an ankle sprain, followed by patellar tendinitis and lumbar spine strain (Fig. 2). Injuries that result in the most time lost from play are knee injuries, followed by wrist, hand, and ankle injuries (Table 1). The most common fractures involve the hand or wrist, followed by the foot and toes (Fig. 3).

Approximately one-fourth of the reportable problems seen by medical staff are due to nonathletic-related conditions, 72% of which involve the respiratory system. In contrast, only 3% are orthopedic.

INJURIES BY ANATOMIC SITE

Ankle (Sprains)

Ankle sprains (see also chapter on ankle sprains and bracing) are the most frequent

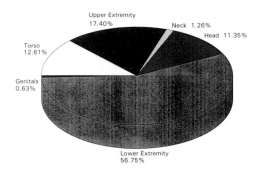

FIGURE 1.   Percentage of injuries by body area.

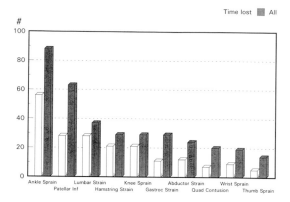

FIGURE 2.   The top ten most commonly occurring injuries are presented. Overall frequency is compared with the frequency of time-lost occurrences. The injuries presented in this figure represent 43% of all athletic-related injuries reported for the season.

acute musculoskeletal injury in basketball at all levels of play. The most common mechanism of injury is an inversion sprain which results when one player lands on the dorsum of another player's foot. The injury can involve the anterior talofibular ligament, the calcaneofibular ligament, and the posterior talofibular ligament in a sequential injury. Sprains of the deltoid ligament, which are much less common but significantly more debilitating, occur from forceful eversion of the ankle. Injuries to the tibiofibular syndesmosis and interosseous membrane occur with extreme dorsiflexion or inversion and also are particularly debilitating.[2] The mechanism of injury is extremely helpful in diagnosing the specific structures involved.

Medial and lateral ankle sprains can be diagnosed by palpation and stress testing. A positive anterior drawer test indicates injury to the anterior talofibular ligament; laxity to inversion indicates injury to the calcaneofibular ligament and the anterior talofibular ligament. The uninjured ankle should always be

evaluated for comparison. Radiographs should include anteroposterior, lateral, and mortise views to rule out fracture or ligamentous avulsion injuries.

Early treatment involves **R**est, **I**ce, **C**ompression, and **E**levation (RICE). If the injury is minor (grade I or II), elastic or tape wrap can be used, followed by nonsteroidal anti-inflammatories and a period of rest. When a player has active peroneal and ankle muscle function, full weight-bearing and muscle-strengthening can begin, followed by proprioceptive exercises and stretching. Often athletes can return to play after several days with the use of an ankle brace or taping to prevent excessive inversion.

If the sprain is diagnosed as major (grade III), a walking cast molded in dorsiflexion can be used for approximately 3 weeks. Smith[3]

TABLE 1.   Frequency of Time-Lost Injuries by Major Body Areas*

Body Area	Number	Days Missed	Frequency Rank	Time-Lost Rank
Ankle	72	732	1	3
Elbow	4	36	15	15
Femur	50	333	5	7
Foot and toes	41	558	6	6
General medical	60	203	2	9
Head (eyes, ears, etc.)	24	102	10	13
Hip	12	108	13	12
Knee	51	1406	4	1
Lower leg	35	584	8	5
Lumbosacral	54	588	3	4
Neck	7	170	14	11
Patellofemoral	34	319	9	8
Shoulder	17	75	11	14
Thorax	16	178	12	10
Wrist and hand	39	814	7	2

*1992–1993 league results.

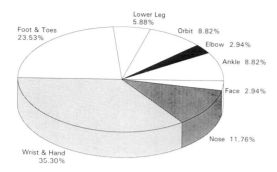

Foot & Toes 23.53%
Lower Leg 5.88%
Orbit 8.82%
Elbow 2.94%
Ankle 8.82%
Face 2.94%
Nose 11.76%
Wrist & Hand 35.30%

FIGURE 3. Proportion of fractures occurring by structure.

demonstrated that the use of cast immobilization with the ankle in dorsiflexion approximates the edges of the disrupted talofibular ligament and reduces anterior subluxation in the ankle region. Cast removal is followed by muscle-strengthening and proprioceptive training. A tilt board or biomechanical ankle platform system (BAPS) is helpful for proprioception, strengthening, and confidence.

Preventive measures include routine taping for practice and games or use of commercial ankle braces.

If chronic ankle instability is diagnosed and has not responded to taping and bracing, stress radiographs can help to determine the extent of instability. Lateral ligament reconstruction should be undertaken if the instability interferes with the player's ability to perform despite nonoperative measures. Special care should be taken to differentiate ankle instability from subtalar instability. This distinction is made with radiographic evaluation under anesthesia.

Knee

Injuries to the knee are second in occurrence to ankle injuries, but are the number-one reason for missed practices and games. The most common knee condition is patellofemoral pain, followed by ligament sprain and meniscal tear.[1]

Patellofemoral Pain

Patellofemoral pain is usually caused by two main conditions: patellofemoral malalignment, which may be subtle or gross, and tendinitis. The malalignment can be attributed to the biomechanics of the lower extremity. Athletes with excessive femoral anteversion, valgus knees, and pronating feet (miserable malalignment syndrome) are more susceptible to patellofemoral problems and instability. Treatment should be based on correcting the biomechanics, starting with orthotics to correct pronation and heel valgus. Femoral anteversion and genu valgum are difficult to correct, and if the instability is gross, surgical intervention for realignment of the extensor mechanism is considered (Fig. 4).

Patellar Tendinitis

Patellar tendinitis is usually chronic and related to the age of the athlete, the amount of playing time, and the number of games played.[4] Patellar tendinitis can be caused or exacerbated by abnormal biomechanics. Athletes should be examined for hamstring tightness, Achilles tightness, and overall lower-extremity flexibility. Treatment first should address flexibility deficits of the lower extremity, followed by local measures, including ultrasound and phonophoresis of the involved area, and patellar bracing. On rare occasions, the problem is surgically addressed. In chronic refractory patellar tendinitis, the athlete is found to have a build-up of fibrous tissue at the inferior pole of the patella.[5] This

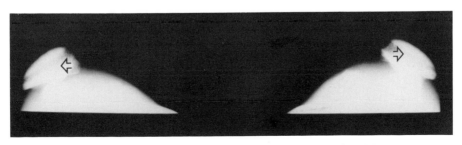

FIGURE 4. Radiograph demonstrates bilateral patellar instability.

tissue may be excised and the patellar tendon reattached to a healthy bed of bleeding bone at the inferior pole of the patella. Rehabilitation and recovery time after reconstruction of the patellar tendon for a high-level athlete is 6–12 months.

Sprains

Sprains are the second most common knee injury. The medial collateral ligament (MCL) is the most commonly affected, followed by the anterior cruciate ligament (ACL). MCL injury usually results from a valgus injury to the knee, which may or may not be due to contact. Athletes complain of pain near the medial joint line, often with a minor effusion and pain on valgus stressing of the knee. Injuries should be graded I–III, depending on the integrity of the ligament. If a complete rupture of the MCL is detected, the knee should be evaluated specifically for an ACL tear. First- and second-degree tears can be treated with weight-bearing as tolerated and are mobilized as quickly as pain allows. The athlete should be braced to avoid valgus injury to the knee. Third-degree MCL tears are braced at 20–30° of flexion for approximately 2 weeks until the ligament begins to heal and early stability is regained. Most third-degree tears are due to a disruption either at the femoral or tibial insertion of the ligament. The disruption can be detected on physical examination. Once early stability has been restored with good end-point-to-valgus stress, full weight-bearing and range-of-motion exercises with resistance may begin. A prophylactic knee brace to prevent valgus injury, either single or double upright, may be advisable in the first several months of return to play. Recent studies indicate that MCL tears rarely, if ever, need to be addressed surgically.[6,7] If the integrity of the ACL is in doubt, magnetic resonance imaging can be helpful to assess its status. If the MRI is inconclusive, arthroscopy of the knee should be used for diagnostic and prognostic purposes.

Injuries to the ACL deserve special consideration because of their debilitating nature. The mechanism is often noncontact, with a decelerating valgus and external rotation injury to the lower extremity.[8] The athlete often recalls a popping sensation or audible pop, followed by swelling in the next 1–2 hours. Immediately after the injury, athletes may attempt to resume playing, which often results in a second episode of instability. Early physi-

cal examination reveals minimal swelling or point tenderness. A positive Lachman examination (Fig. 5) is the most sensitive indicator of ACL rupture.[9,10] Anterior drawer and pivot shift tests are also useful in diagnosis.[11] Once a hemarthrosis has developed, muscle guarding may preclude reliable evaluation.

If an ACL tear is suspected, the athlete should be withheld from play until further evaluation is undertaken. Initial treatment should include ice, compression, evaluation, and partial weight-bearing. Once the diagnosis of an ACL tear is made, the status of the menisci must be determined. Approximately 50% of ACL tears are accompanied by meniscal tear at the initial injury. There is some controversy as to whether an athlete should be returned to play after an ACL tear. When a concurrent meniscal tear has been diagnosed, further injury to the knee may extend the damage and perhaps make a reparable tear irreparable. The greatest concern about returning an athlete to play with an ACL-deficient knee is the occurrence of a second giving-way episode, which can lead to significant injury to the articular cartilage and menisci. Recent MRI studies suggest an 80% incidence of occult fractures after ACL ruptures.[13] Athletes may be at the greatest risk of

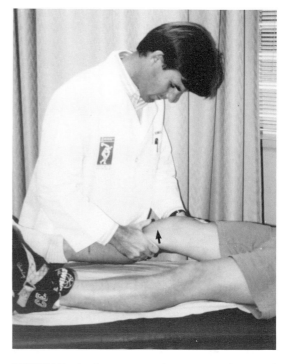

FIGURE 5. Lachman exam demonstrates increased tibial translation with ACL rupture.

developing future degenerative changes if they are allowed to return to full weight-bearing and sports activities without a period of protection.

Many athletes have been able to return to their sport after an ACL tear without suffering further giving-way episodes. Unfortunately, those who sustain a second (or more) giving-way episode have been known to suffer significant secondary injuries to the knee.[14-18] Our approach to the ACL-deficient athlete is individual evaluation of both player and sport for potential for reinjury. Many factors go into this decision, including the player's eligibility and time of the season. Players with an ACL-deficient knee can learn to compete in a brace but rarely at their preinjury level. If the injury involves a meniscal tear or combined damage (ACL and MCL or ACL and lateral side disruption), surgical reconstruction is the treatment of choice.

Surgical reconstruction of the ACL uses the central one-third of the patellar tendon with a bone-tendon-bone construct.[19] The ligament is actually reconstructed and not repaired (Fig. 6). Alternative sources for ligament graft may be considered if the athlete's anatomy precludes autologous patellar tendon tissue. The reconstruction is carried out arthroscopically, using 1 and at times 2 incisions to secure the graft. Secure graft fixation and isometric placement of the graft allow an early and aggressive rehabilitation program (Fig. 7).

Our current rehabilitation protocol begins with early partial weight-bearing and an emphasis on full extension and hyperextension. Quadriceps function and control are stressed, and flexion is gradually regained over the first

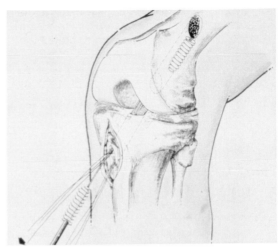

FIGURE 7. Isometric placement of ACL graft with screw fixation at femoral and tibial ends.

1–2 weeks. When swelling and pain permit, closed-chain kinetics are started, including the use of a stair stepper, leg press, step-ups, and partial squats (Fig. 8). Henning[20] has shown that functional rehabilitative (closed-chain kinetics) exercises put significantly less stress on the ACL graft than open-chain kinetic exercises. Sport-specific exercises are

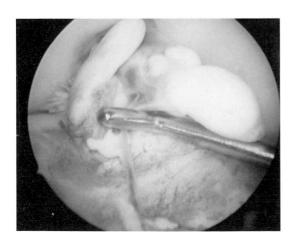

FIGURE 6.   Arthroscopic view of ACL rupture.

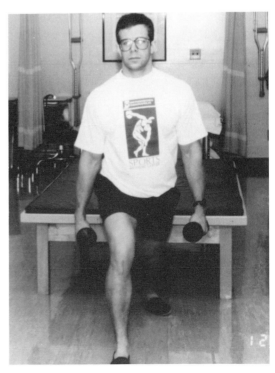

FIGURE 8.   One-legged squat with dumbbells for early closed-chain ACL rehabilitation.

started at 6–12 weeks postoperatively, when the patient has demonstrated good control of the extremity with little pain and swelling. We use a prophylactic knee brace after ACL reconstruction for the first postoperative year. Although no good scientific studies demonstrate the efficacy of brace use in preventing ACL tears or reinjury, many patients have a greater sense of security with a brace.[21,22] Often patients choose to wear a neoprene knee sleeve, which provides good proprioception, instead of a bulky-hinged knee brace. Complete rehabilitation after ACL surgery often requires 1–2 years before the athlete has complete confidence and function in the leg.[24] Although athletes may be allowed to return to play as early as 3 months after reconstruction, they are advised that rehabilitation is not complete and that they need to adhere to a maintenance program indefinitely.

Injury to the posterior cruciate ligament (PCL) is uncommon in athletes and very rare in basketball.[25–27] The PCL is the largest ligament of the knee and the primary stabilizer in posterior translation of the tibia.[28,29] The mechanism of injury to the PCL is usually a fall on the anterior aspect of the proximal tibia with the foot in a plantarflexed position.[30] The force is then translated through the proximal tibia to the PCL. If the foot is in dorsiflexion, the force is transmitted to the patella rather than the PCL. Despite the size and importance of the PCL, athletes have little functional problems after a PCL injury.[31–34] Clancy et al.,[30] however, showed significant disability after PCL injuries, with degenerative changes in the patellofemoral and medial knee joint compartments.

The diagnosis of a PCL tear is best made by evaluating the posterior drawer test and the passive posterior sag (Fig. 9) sign. Surgery is rarely indicated for an isolated injury. Rehabilitation should emphasize quadriceps strengthening to prevent excessive posterior translation of the tibia. Athletes are usually unable to return to play for 3–6 months after injury. Return to play is often accompanied by pain and swelling. A PCL brace may be used, but its value is questionable. Athletes should be evaluated closely for injuries to the posterolateral capsule of the knee.

Meniscal Tears

Meniscal tears represent a fairly common injury in the basketball player. The injury is

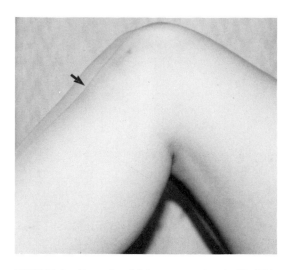

FIGURE 9. Posterior tibial sag associated with PCL injury.

often a noncontact, twisting injury. The player may recall a popping or tearing sensation and often is initially able to resume playing. An effusion develops over the ensuing 24–48 hours. If the tear is small, it may be asymptomatic for a prolonged period of time. If the tear is large and unstable, jointline pain and repeated effusions develop. Initial treatment is with ice, elevation, and anti-inflammatories. Physical examination usually reveals an effusion and jointline pain over the torn meniscus. We have found that Steinmann's test[35] (forceful rotation of the tibia with the knee flexed 90°) is highly reliable in detecting meniscal tears. In the older athlete the meniscal tear may be accompanied by articular cartilage injury to the femoral condyle, which may present with crepitus in the involved compartment. MRI examination may be useful in detecting small tears or a tear that is minimally symptomatic.

As with tears of the ACL, the decision to allow an athlete to return to play with a meniscal tear should be individualized. Because certain meniscal tears can be repaired, we are more reluctant to allow athletes to return to play for fear of making a reparable tear irreparable.[36] In a review of 105 patients with a minimal 2-year follow-up, we had a retear rate of less than 5%.[37] Meniscal tears that are in the peripheral third, greater than 1.5 cm in length, and unstable are considered for repair. Recent studies show that healing may be enhanced with the insertion of a fibrin clot into the tear at the time of repair.[38] Numerous studies demonstrate the debilitating long-term effects of meniscectomy.[39–42] We believe that the inconvenience and lost time from a meniscal repair are greatly outweighed by the potential degenerative problems in the knee that accompany a meniscectomy.

Rehabilitation after a meniscal repair is individualized, depending on the tear itself. Weight-bearing is limited in the first 2 weeks, after which full weight-bearing is allowed. Closed-chain rehabilitation[43] is begun in the first week, with avoidance of pivoting, twisting, and turning. Patients should avoid full squatting for the first 12 weeks postoperatively. When they demonstrate full range of motion with no effusion and 80% normal strength, return to play is allowed. If the return is accompanied by mechanical symptoms or recurrent effusions, the athlete is removed from play. Bronstein et al.[44] demonstrated that meniscal tears heal with fibrous scar tissue rather than replication of meniscal tissue. Meniscal repair may take many years to heal completely. Many meniscal tears may be clinically silent, but second-look arthroscopy may demonstrate incomplete healing.

Rehabilitation after partial meniscectomy for tears that are not reparable progresses on the basis of the athlete's pain and function. Weight-bearing and closed-chain kinetic exercises may begin the first postoperative day. Water running and resistance exercises can be used in the first postoperative week with water-occlusive bandages. Return to sport-specific activities can begin as early as 1 week postoperatively. Full play can be resumed when the player has a full painless range of motion of the joint and good functional control. Nonsteroidal anti-inflammatories are helpful in the early postoperative period to treat swelling and inflammation.

Thigh

Contusions

The most common injury to the thigh is a quadriceps contusion. Because of variations in height, players are particularly susceptible to thigh contusion from another player's knee. Physical examination reveals point tenderness at the area of contact, and spasm may be present. Swelling is due to hemorrhage and edema in the muscle. Pain is elicited with passive stretching and contraction of the muscle. Early treatment consists of ice for 20-

minute intervals and compression with an elastic wrap. Deep massage should be avoided acutely, and local steroid injections should be avoided to prevent development of infections in the posttramatic hematoma. The athletes can return to play when they have a relatively full and painless range of motion. Studies show that the time to recovery is directly proportional to the initial range of motion after injury.[45]

Strains

Hamstring injuries are usually a noncontact injury due to violent contraction of the muscle. The muscle is usually injured during eccentric contraction. The athlete experiences sudden severe pain or a popping sensation. Physical examination shows a local tenderness in the hamstring area, usually at the proximal musculotendinous junction. Massive tears may involve a palpable gap. Initial treatment is the RICE regimen. Prevention includes a good warm-up period and stretching.

Lumbar Spine

Injuries to the lumbar spine rank third in frequency behind ankle and knee injuries. They usually consist of sprains, strains, contusions, and disc herniations. The mechanism of injury usually involves a mechanical predisposition. The athlete may present with a leg-length discrepancy that leads to mechanical low back problems or with a genetic predisposition. Such conditions include spondylolysis, spondylolisthesis, stenosis, and scoliosis.

Strains

The majority of injuries are due to muscle strain. Muscle strain and rupture usually result from excessive stress or torque on the lumbar spine. Minor ruptures of the fasiculi in the erector spinae occur. Physical examination shows point tenderness in the lumbar spine. There are no radicular symptoms or signs, and the neurovascular examination is normal. The erector spinae is often in spasm, and back range of motion is limited. Chronic sprains often result from excessive tension on the lumbar spine due to inadequate rehabilitation from injury. Treatment involves reduction of inflammation by physical therapy modalities, including phonophoresis and ultrasound, and nonsteroidal anti-inflammatories. Gradual muscle strengthening and conditioning is essential to prevent further injury.

Disc Herniation

Disc herniation is secondary to excessive pressure in the disc, often due to heavy lifting or a fall. The athlete presents with radicular pain below the knee with or without low back pain.[46] Neurologic examination may reveal positive straight leg-raising and motor and sensory changes. Initial treatment involves rest from pain-producing activities, but avoidance of total bed rest. Gentle range-of-motion exercises, stretching, ultrasound, and phonophoresis are helpful in the first several weeks. Routine radiographs should be taken to rule out spondylolysis and spondylolisthesis. If radicular signs persist, computed tomographic (CT) scan or MRI is indicated to evaluate further the extent of disc herniation. Electromyography may help in diagnosing the radiculopathy as well. Epidural steroids may be indicated for radicular symptoms not responsive to conservative treatment. If radicular symptoms persist beyond 4–6 weeks, surgical intervention for excision of herniated or protruded disc fragments may be indicated. Studies indicate that most patients report similar pain relief and function 1 year after injury, regardless of operative versus nonoperative treatment. Operative treatment is therefore indicated for patients with intolerable pain or failure to improve with time.

Spondylolysis and Spondylolisthesis

Spondylolysis is a defect in the pars interarticularis that is thought to be due to stress fracture.[47] Physical examination reveals unilateral pain in the lumbar spine as well as pain with hyperextension and twisting. Neurologic examination is normal. Plain radiographs reveal a defect in the pars interarticularis on oblique views. Bone scan can be helpful in diagnosing acute versus chronic pars defect. Brace treatment is indicated in the presence of a positive bone scan, which suggests an acute defect with greater healing potential. The brace should be used for up to 3 months to assure healing.

Spondylolisthesis may be due to spondylolysis or degenerative changes in the lumbar spine.[48] Treatment of spondylolysis or low-grade spondylolisthesis with less than 50% slippage is usually restriction from activity until the athlete is asymptomatic. Rehabilitation then should address strength deficits, and an exercise program emphasizing flexibility should be instituted. Athletes presenting with persistent low back pain and a spondylolisthesis of greater than 50% that is not responsive to conservative treatment may be candidates for spinal fusion.[48]

Foot and Toe Injuries

Injuries to the foot and toes accounted for approximately 9% of total practices and games missed in the NBA in the 1992–1993 season. The most common condition was foot sprain, followed by inflammatory conditions and fractures. Sprains to the metatarsophalangeal joint and midfoot are common and often result from landing on another player's foot or a dorsflexion injury.

Plantar Fasciitis

Plantar fasciitis is usually a chronic condition due to a biomechanical imbalance in the heel and midfoot.[49] In the cavus foot, the windlass mechanism of the plantar fascia may cause a repetitive stretching at its attachment to the calcaneal tuberosity. With dorsiflexion of the metatarsophalangeal joints, the height of the longitudinal arches is increased and causes a subsequent shortening of the plantar fascia at the calcaneal turberosity or just distal to the insertion.

Conversely, excessive heel valgus and pronation also may put increased stress on the plantar fascia because of instability of the longitudinal arch. Most often plantar fasciitis responds to nonoperative measures such as a heel cup or heel pad, nonsteroidal anti-inflammatories, or corticosteroid injection at the insertion of the plantar fascia into the calcaneal tuberosity. Night splints also are an effective treatment for patients who experience severe pain and stiffness on arising in the morning. A night splint positions the foot and ankle at 90° or more of dorsiflexion to prevent shortening of the plantar fascia during sleeping hours. Prevention includes stretching of the plantar fascia and heel cord on a routine basis.

Tendinitis

The most common inflammatory condition of the foot in the basketball player involves Achilles tendinitis, which can be divided into insertional and noninsertional types.[49] Noninsertional Achilles tendinitis may be classified as (1) pure peritendinitis, (2) peritendinitis and tendinosis, and (3) tendinosis. The condition of tendinosis may lead to later rupture. Rupture usually occurs in a segment of tendon between 2 and 6 cm above its insertion on the calcaneus.[50] Tendinosis is characterized by tenderness and thickening of the tendon. The thickening represents areas of mucoid degeneration or fibrosis.

Peritendinitis involves only the tendon sheath and is not associated with tendon enlargement. Initial treatment should involve heel wedges to decrease the strain on the Achilles tendon, nonsteroidal anti-inflammatories, ice massage, and orthotic devices. The player may need to be removed from basketball for several seeks if pain persists. Clancy[51] suggested that surgical intervention should be considered if pain persists 6–8 weeks after athletic activities have been stopped. In chronic cases, surgical excision of the diseased tissue can be augmented with the flexor hallucis longus to gain additional strength.

Insertional Achilles tendinitis may be due to local pressure from shoe wear. Athletes with a large bony prominence at the posterior superior aspect of the calcaneus may be more prone to this condition. Early treatment may involve use of a heel lift with stretching exercises and the use of a "donut" to relieve local pressure on the bony prominence. Evaluation of different basketball shoe styles may be helpful. Surgical management of insertional Achilles tendinitis includes extensive debridement of the bony prominence at the posterior superior calcaneus and removal of intratendinous calcification and fibrosis.

Fractures

Fractures of the foot and toes may be acute or chronic. Calcaneal beak fractures are acute injuries that may occur among basketball players. Fracture of the beak of the os calcis occurs when the foot is inverted and plantarflexed, as in landing on another player's foot. The patient complains of pain and has local point tenderness in the area of the sinus tarsi. The fracture may be missed on routine radiographs and should be suspected in injuries in which pain persists for several weeks (Fig. 10). Treatment is with a short-leg, non–weight-bearing cast for 4 weeks, followed by a walking cast for 4 weeks. Chronic pain may require surgical removal of the fragment.

Avulsion fractures at the base of the fifth metatarsal are often due to an inversion injury. Often a player lands on another player's foot, causing inversion injury. The mechanism involves a violent contraction of the peroneus brevis and subsequent bony avulsion at its insertion on the fifth metatarsal. The injury can be treated initially with a walking cast or short leg brace for a period of 4–6 weeks. Radiographic healing may take 2–3 months, but players can be allowed to return to play when they are able to bear full weight without pain and have good peroneal strength and function.

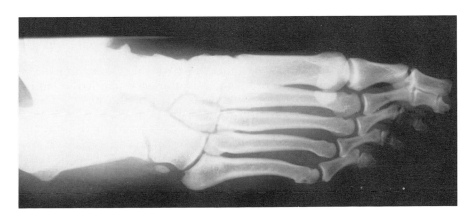

FIGURE 10.   Oblique radiograph demonstrates fracture of the anterior process of the calcaneus.

Two common stress fractures in basketball players are the Jones fracture and fracture of the tarsonavicular. The Jones fracture involves the proximal metaphyseal-diaphyseal junction of the fifth metatarsal (Fig. 11).[52,53] This fracture has a high rate of nonunion and a high incidence of refracture after nonoperative treatment.[52,54,55] The mechanism of injury involves abnormal loading of the lateral part of the foot where the heel is elevated and the metatarsophalangeal joints are hyperextended. Initial radiographs may be negative, but physical examination demonstrates point tenderness over the proximal metatarsal shaft–metaphyseal junction. Early bone scanning may demonstrate a stress fracture even after negative plain radiographs.

Treatment of acute Jones fractures is controversial.[52,54,55] Torg recommends nonoperative treatment with a non–weight-bearing, short leg cast for an average of 7 weeks.[55] In the highly competitive or professional athlete, many authors recommend early operative treatment, including intramedullary screw fixation.[53,54] In a study by DeLee et al.,[53] 10 athletes treated with screw fixation healed at a mean of 7.5 weeks. Once healing has occurred and the athlete has returned to play, the screw should be left in place to prevent late fracture after removal.

Stress fractures of the tarsonavicular are uncommon but can be significantly debilitating. This fracture is most often found in basketball players. Torg[56] found a mean interval of 7.2 months from onset to diagnosis. The patient may complain of a vague pain over the dorsum or medial aspect of the foot. Pain is usually worse with activity and relieved with rest. The fracture may be difficult to detect on plain radiograph. If a fracture is suspected, a bone scan should be helpful. If the bone scan is normal, CT may be helpful. The fracture is usually in the sagittal plane through the middle third of the navicular. Treatment usually involves initial non–weight-bearing immobilization for 6–8 weeks. Fractures that appear to be nonunions should be treated with curettage and bone grafting and internal fixation. Surgical treatment is followed by non–weight-bearing immobilization for 6–8 weeks.

Wrist and Hand

The sport of basketball requires players to perform both fine and gross motor movements with their hands. Hand injuries are common in basketball at all levels of play. Players can injure their hand in several different ways, including contact with another player, the ball, or the rim of the basket. Hand injuries can be trivial or serious with long-lasting consequences.

Thumb Injuries

The thumb is a frequent site of injury in the hand because of its unprotected position. The most common soft-tissue injury is rupture of the ulnar collateral ligament of the thumb (gamekeeper's thumb).[57,58] Injury may occur from a fall on an outstretched hand or from an aberrant pass that catches the thumb metacarpal and forces it into hyperabduction and hyperextension. The ligament may be par-

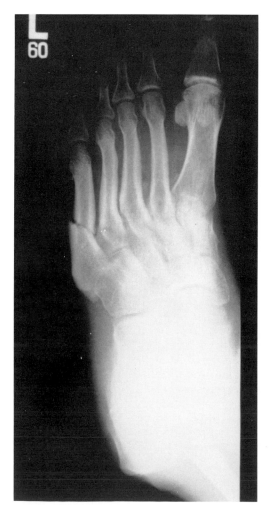

FIGURE 11. Radiograph demonstrates Jones fracture of the proximal fifth metatarsal.

tially or completely ruptured and should be evaluated with a stress examination and stress radiographs. Failure to diagnose this injury my lead to chronic instability and degenerative arthritis of the joint. First- and second-degree tears can be treated with anti-inflammatories, ice. and a protective brace or cast.

Complete ruptures are detectable on examination and stress radiographs. The metacarpophalangeal (MP) joint is at least 35° more unstable to radial stress in comparison with the contralateral MP joint.[59,60] This stress test should be performed in full extension and in 30° of flexion. Stress radiographs support the instability detected on examination. The radiographs are also helpful in detecting a small fragment of bone that may be avulsed with the ligament from the articular surface of the thumb metacarpal. If the bony fragment is greater than 10–15% of the articular surface and displacement is ≥2 mm or rotated, operative repair should be considered. Nondisplaced fragments may be treated with a cast for 4–6 weeks. Treatment of a complete rupture without a bony fracture is controversial.[61] Some authors advise immobilization in a well-molded thumb spica cast. Most, however, believe that nonoperative treatment is unpredictable and that surgical repair of the ligament results in a more predictable outcome. In the professional athlete, a complete rupture may be treated with taping or a brace under extenuating circumstances. The athlete is advised that the longer the tear is left untreated, the less likely a repair can be accomplished. Chronic injuries may be treated with ligament reconstruction, but results are less predictable. Little can be done to prevent rupture of the ulnar collateral ligament (UCL). With sports such as downhill skiing, in which the incidence of UCL injuries is high, protective splints can be used. Protective splints are obviously quite cumbersome for the basketball player, but protective taping is a possibility.

Metacarpophalangeal Injuries

Injuries to the MP joints are also common in basketball players. Injuries to collateral ligaments are frequent, particularly in the little and index fingers because of their exposed positions. Diagnosis is made by demonstrating tenderness over the ligament itself. With a complete rupture, instability is present with stress testing when the joint is held in full flexion. Radiographs may demonstrate a small bony avulsion.

Acute injuries should be treated with immobilization at 45° of MP flexion for 3 weeks, followed by "buddy taping" for the next 3 weeks or, most often, the rest of the season. Open repair should be performed when an intraarticular fracture involves 10% or more of the articular surface and is displaced 3 mm or more.[62]

A chronic MP ligament injury can be treated with taping and corticosteroid injections. If pain persists, surgical reconstruction of the ligament should be considered.

Finger Injuries

Injuries of the proximal interphalangeal (PIP) joint are also quite common in basketball. Injuries may include dislocation, tendon ruptures, or capsuloligamentous injury. Evaluation focuses on history of the mechanism of injury and initial deformity. Physical examination should evaluate the point of maximal tenderness, and radiographs should be obtained. Once the injured structure has been identified, the degree of instability is determined. Instability is divided into 3 grades, depending on range of motion and deformity within that range of motion. Grade 1 injuries are stable, with full range of motion, and do not angulate more than 20° compared with the opposite side on stress testing; they are treated with a splint for comfort.

Grade 2 injuries do not deform with active range of motion, but stress testing reveals greater than 20° angulation compared with the opposite hand. Treatment involves a splint for protection for 2–4 weeks and then buddy taping for 6–8 weeks.

Grade 3 injuries demonstrate deformity with active range of motion, which is limited to less than 75% of the opposite hand when evaluated under anesthetic block. This finding is consistent with compete disruption of greater than 50% of the entire capsule, and surgical repair is considered.

Isolated collateral ligament injuries are due to a pure angulatory stress. Grade 1 and 2 injuries are treated with immobilization in 15–20° of flexion for 2–3 weeks, followed by buddy taping. Most grade 3 injuries are treated with open ligamentous repair.

Dislocations may be treated with a extension block at 20° of flexion. Radiographs are obtained to assure congruent reduction of the joint.

Boutonniere deformity results from rupture of the insertion of the central extensor tendon slip into the base of the middle phalanx. The mechanism of injury is a sudden, forceful flexion of the extended PIP joint.[58,63] Physical examination reveals tenderness dorsally over the joint. The athlete experiences dorsal pain and weakness on resisted extension. Treatment involves splinting the PIP joint in full extension while leaving the distal joint free for active flexion. The splint is maintained for 6 weeks continuously and during play for an additional 4 weeks. Untreated injuries may lead to chronic boutonniere deformity, which involves a stiff PIP joint and degenerative arthritis. Treatment is aimed at early diagnosis and treatment with splinting of the PIP joint.

The most common injury to the distal interphalangeal joint is a mallet finger.[63,64] The injury involves a rupture of the extensor tendon insertion into the base of the distal phalanx. The mechanism of injury involves a sudden flexion force on an extended distal interphalangeal (DIP) joint, which often occurs in basketball when a player is hit on the tip of the finger.

Treatment involves splinting the distal joint in full extension for 6 weeks while leaving the PIP joint free. The athlete is then weaned from the brace over the following 2–4 weeks. If at any point during the weaning process the distal joint droops, the splint is then reapplied for 3 more weeks.

Wrist Injuries

Wrist injuries are less common than finger injuries in the basketball player, but they may be serious. The most common serious wrist injury involves a fracture of the scaphoid,[58,65] which is often due to a fall on an outstretched hand. The player presents with radial-sided wrist pain in the anatomic snuff box. This injury is complicated by the fact that fractures are not always diagnosed initially; in addition the rate of nonunion is high. Almost all scaphoid fracture are treated initially with cast immobilization; the length of time varies, depending on the location of injury. Occasionally displaced fractures are treated with open reduction and internal fixation. The use of a playing cast may not provide sufficient immo-

bilization, and the rate of nonunion may be unacceptably high.[66,67]

The most common wrist ligament injury is a scapholunate dissocation, which usually involves a fall on an outstretched hand. Diagnosis may be difficult because of relatively minor changes on static radiographics. If a scapholunate dissociation is suspected, a posteroanterior view of the wrist should be evaluated. Clinched-fist radiographs may also demonstrate an increase in the scapholunate interval. Lateral radiographs may demonstrate rotation of the lunate in association with dorsal intercalary segmental instability (DISI).

Treatment of acute scapholunate dissociation involves closed reduction and pinning or open reduction with ligamentous repair. Partial ligament injuries may be treated in a thumb spica cast for 6 weeks. Chronic or unrecognized injuries may lead to a pattern of instability characteristic of scapholunate advanced collapse (SLAC) and arthritis in the wrist.

Prevention of late complications involves thorough evaluation and diagnosis of fractures and instability patterns as well as appropriate initial treatment.

Shoulder Injuries

Rotator Cuff Injuries

Shoulder injuries in basketball players are relatively rare. The most common shoulder condition that requires treatment is rotator cuff tendinitis.[68] This condition is often due to an off-season weight-training program; it is unlikely to result from basketball play. Tendinitis often responds to a period of rest, nonsteroidal anti-inflammatories, and ultrasound. As the pain and inflammation subside, emphasis should be placed on rotator-cuff strengthening and flexibility. Prevention should include the avoidance of repetitive overhead lifting and resistance exercises in pure abduction.

Instability

Occasionally basketball players present with shoulder instability. If the instability is due to a basketball injury, it commonly results from an abduction/external rotation injury or from attempting to block another player's shot. The instability may present as a subluxation or dislocation. Physical examination reveals apprehension in abduction and external rotation, and the athlete often reports that the instability occurs in this position. Multidirectional or posterior instability of the shoulder in a basketball player is rare in our experience.[69]

Treatment of anterior instability begins with a muscle-strengthening program, including the rotator cuff, subscapularis, and anterior deltoid muscles (Fig. 12). Avoidance of abduction and external rotation should be considered, but often it is not feasible in a competitive basketball player. For chronic, recurrent instability of the shoulder, anterior reconstruction should be considered. As with any overhead athlete, surgical reconstruction must involve a retensioning of the anterior capsule, with or without repair of a Bankart lesion, while leaving the subscapularis tendon undisturbed, if possible. Even a minor degree of loss of external rotation affects performance. Postoperative rehabilitation should emphasize full range of motion in the first 6 weeks, followed by a vigorous strengthening program, particularly of the rotator cuff, deltoid, and scapular stabilizers.

CONCLUSION

Evaluation and treatment of the basketball player are a privilege and a challenge. The basketball player represents one of the most skilled and talented athletes. Although many minor injuries may be treated with little concern or skillful neglect, all injuries need to be completely evaluated and a course of treatment instituted. Nothing is more disheartening than to see the career of a talented athlete shortened because of a preventable injury or a treatable condition.

REFERENCES

1. *Injury Surveillance System.* NBTA 1992–1993 Season Summary.
2. Hopkinson WJ, St. Pierre P, Ryan JB, et al: Syndesmosis sprains of the ankle. *Foot Ankle* 10:325–330, 1990.
3. Smith RW, Reischl S: The influence of dorsiflexion in

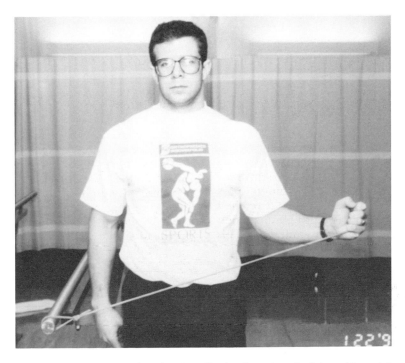

FIGURE 12.   Resistance exercises for strengthening the external rotators of the rotator cuff.

the treatment of severe ankle sprains: An anatomical study. *Foot Ankle* 9:28–33, 1988.

4. Herring SA, Nilson KL: Introduction to overuse injuries. *Clin Sports Med* 6:225, 1987.

5. Bodne D, Quinn SF, Murray WT, et al: Magnetic resonance images of chornic patellar tendinitis. *Skelet Radiol* 17:24, 1988.

6. Kannus P: Long-term results of conservatively treated medial collateral ligament injuries of the knee joint. *Clin. Orthop.* 226:103, 1988.

7. Indelicato PA: Nonoperative management of complete tears of the medial collateral ligament. *Orthop Rev* 18:947–952, 1989.

8. Feagin JA, Lambert KL: Mechanism of injury and pathology of anterior cruciate ligament injuries. *Orthop Clin North Am* 16:41, 1985.

9. Torg JS: Who is John Lachman? *Contemp Orthop* 20:139, 1990.

10. Gurtler RA: Lachman test revisited. *Contemp. Orthop* 20:145, 1990.

11. Galway HR, MacIntosh DL: The lateral pivot shift: A symptom and sign of anterior cruciate ligament insufficiency. *Clin Orthop* 147:45, 1980.

12. Lynch MA, Henning CE, Glick KR: Knee joint surface changes. Long-term follow-up meniscus tear treatment in stable anterior cruciate ligament reconstructions. *Clin Orthop* 172:148–153, 1983.

13. Anterior cruciate ligament and posterior cruciate ligament injuries of the knee. American Association of Orthopedic Surgeons Meeting, San Francisco, 1992.

14. Jackson RW: The torn ACL: Natural history of untreated lesions and rationale for selective treatment. *In* Feagin JA Jr (ed): *The Crucial Ligaments.* New York, Churchill Livingstone, 1988, pp 341–348.

15. Arnold JA, Coker TP, Heaton LM, et al: Natural history of anterior cruciate tears. *Am J Sports Med* 7:305–313, 1979.

16. Feagin JA Jr, Curl WW: Isolated tear of the anterior cruciate ligament: 5-year follow-up study. *Am J Sports Med* 4:95–100, 1976.

17. Fetto JD, Marshall JL: The natural history and diagnosis of anterior cruciate ligament insufficiency. *Clin Orthrop* 147:29–38, 1980.

18. McDaniel WJ, Dameron TB: Untreated ruptures of the anterior cruciate ligament: A follow-up study. *J Bone Joint Surg* 62A:687–695, 1980.

19. Beck CL, Paulos LE, Rosenberg TD: Anterior cruciate ligament reconstruction with the endoscopic technique. *Orthop* 2:86–98, 1992.

20. Henning CE, Lynch MA, Glick KR: An in vivo strain gauge study of elongation of the anterior cruciate ligament injury. *Am J Sports Med* 13:22–26, 1985.

21. Grace TG, Skipper BJ, Newberrry JC, et al: Prophylactic knee braces and injury to the lower extremity. *J Bone Joint Surg* 70A:422–427, 1988.

22. Teitz CC, Hermanson BK, Kronmal RA, Diehr PH: Evaluation of the use of braces to prevent injury to the knee in collegiate football players. *J Bone Joint Surg* 69A:2–9, 1987.

23. Reference deleted.

24. Steadman JR, Forster RS, Silferskiold JP: Rehabilitation of the knee. *Clin Sports Med* 8:605–627, 1989.

25. DeHaven KE: Diagnosis of acute knee with hemarthrosis. *Am J Sports Med* 8:9–14, 1980.

26. Loos WC, Fog JM, Dlazinga ME, et al: Acute posterior cruciate ligament injuries. *Am J Sports Med* 9:86–91, 1981.

27. Torg JS, Barton TM, Pavlov H, et al: Natural history of the posterior cruciate ligament deficient knee. *Clin Orthop* 246:208–215, 1989.

28. Gollehon DL, Torzilli PA, Warren RF: The role of the posterolateral and cruciate ligaments in the stability of the human knee. *J Bone Joint Surg* 69A:233–242, 1987.

29. Butler DL, Noyes FR, Grood ES: Ligamentous restraints to anterior-posterior drawer in the human knee. *J Bone Joint Surg* 62A:259–269, 1980.

30. Clancy WG, Shelbourne KP, Zoellner GB, et al: Treatment of knee joint instability secondary to rupture of the posterior cruciate ligament. *J Bone Joint Surg* 65A:310–322, 1983.

31. Cross MJ, Powell JF: Long-term follow-up of posterior cruciate ligament rupture—A study of 116 cases. *Am J Sports Med* 12:292–297, 1984.

32. Fowler PJ, Messich SS: Isolated posterior cruciate ligament injuries in athletes. *Am J Sports Med* 9:107–113, 1981.

33. Parolie JM, Bergfeld JA: Long-term results of nonspecific treatment of isolated posterior cruciate ligament injuries in the athlete. *Am J Sports Med* 14:35–38, 1986.

34. Torg JS, Barton TM, Pavlov H, et al: Natural history of the posterior cruciate ligament deficient knee. *Clin Orthop* 246:208–215, 1989.

35. Ricklin P, Ruttiman A, del Buono MS: *Meniscal Lesions. Practical Problems of Clinical Diagnosis, Arthroscopy, and Therapy.* New York, Grune & Stratton, 1971.

36. Jackson RW, Kunkel SS: Arthroscopic meniscal repair. In Bentley G, Greer RB III (eds): *Orthopaedics.* Oxford, Butterworth Heinemann, 1991, pp 1056–1061.

37. Kunkel SS: Presented at Garceau-Wray Lectures, 1991.

38. Arnoczky SP, Warren RF, Spivak JM: Meniscal repair using an exogenous fibrin clot. An experimental study in dogs. *J Bone Joint Surg* 70A:1209–1217, 1988.

39. Fairbank TJ: Knee joint changes after meniscectomy. *J Bone Joint Surg* 30B:664–670, 1948.

40. Johnson RJ, Kettlekamp DB, Clark W, Leaverton P: Factors affecting late results after meniscectomy. *J Bone Joint Surg* 56A:719–729, 1974.

41. Jackson JP: Degenerative changes in the knee after meniscectomy. *BMJ* 2:525–527, 1968.

42. Dandy DJ, Jackson RW: The diagnosis of problems after meniscectomy. *J Bone Joint Surg* 57B:349–352, 1975.

43. Gray GW: *Chain Reaction.* Wynn Marketing, 1990, p 16.

44. Bronstein R, Kirk P, Hurley J: The usefulness of MRI in evaluating menisci after meniscus repair. *Orthop Sports Med* 15:149–152, 1992.

45. Jackson DW, Feagin JA: Quadriceps contusion in young athletes: Relation of severity of injury to treatment and prognosis. *J Bone Joint Surg* 55A:95–101, 1973.

46. Jackson DW, Wiltse L: Low back pain in athletes. *Physician Sports Med* 2:53, 1974.

47. Hensinger R: Spondylolysis and spondylolisthesis. In Evarts CM (ed); *AAOS Instructional Course Lectures,* vol 32. St. Louis, C.V. Mosby, 1983, pp 132–151.

48. Brown Mark, Lockwood John: Spondylolysis and spondylolisthesis. In Evarts CM (ed); *AAOS Instructional Course Lectures,* vol 32. St. Louis, C.V. Mosby, 1983, pp 162–169.

49. McDermott E: Basketball injuries of the foot and ankle. *Clini Sports Med* 12:373,1993.

50. Hansen S: Trauma to the heel cord. *In* Jahss MH (ed): *Disorders of the Foot and Ankle.* Philadelphia, W. B. Saunders, 1991, pp 23–55.

51. Clancy WG, Neilhard D, Brand RL: Achilles tendinitis in running: A report of five cases. *Am J Sports Med* 4:41, 1976.

52. Dameron TB: Fracture and anatomical variations of the proximal portion of the fifth metatarsal. *J Bone Joint Surg* 57A:788–1975.

53. DeLee JC, Evans JP, Julian J: Stress fractures of the fifth metatarsal. *Am J Sports Med* 11:349, 1983.

54. Kavanaugh JH, Brower TD, Mann RV: The Jones fracture revisited. *J Bone Joint Surg* 60A:776, 1979.

55. Torg JS, Baulduini FC, Zelko RR, et al: Fracture of the base of the fifth metatarsal distal to the tuberosity: Classification and guidelines for non-surgical and surgical management. *J Bone Joint Surg* 66A:209, 1984.

56. Torg JS, Pavlov H, Cooley LH, et al: Stress fractures of the tarsal navicular: A retrospective review of twenty-one cases. *J Bone Joint Surg* 64A:700, 1982.

57. Campbell CS: Gamekeeper's thumb. *J Bone Joint Surg* 37B:148, 1955.

58. Culver JE, Anderson TE: Fractures of the hand and wrist in the athlete. *Clin Sports Med* 11:101, 1992.

59. Bowers WH, Hurst LC: Gamekeeper's thumb evaluation by arthrography. *J Bone Joint Surg* 59A:519, 1977.

60. Lamb DW, Angarita G: Ulnar instability of the metacarpophalangeal joint of the thumb. *J Hand Surg* 10B:113, 1985.

61. Arnold DM, Cooney WP, Wood MB: Surgical management of chronic ulnar collateral ligament insufficiency of the thumb metacarpophalangeal joint. *Orthop Rev* 21:583, 1992.

62. Barton NJ (ed): *Fractures of the Hand and Wrist.* New York, Churchill Livingstone, 1988.

63. Doyle JR: Extensor tendons: Acute injuries. In Green DP (ed): *Operative Hand Surgery* vol 3, 2nd ed. New York, Churchill Livingstone, 1988, p 777.

64. Bowers WH (ed): *The Interphalangeal Joints.* New York, Churchill Livingstone, 1987.

65. Burton RI, Eaton RG: Common hand injuries in the athlete. *Orthop Clin North Am* 4:809, 1973.

66. Bergfeld JT, Werker GG, Andrish JT: Soft playing splint for protection of significant hand and wrist injuries in sports. *Am J Sports Med* 10:293, 1982.

67. Riester J, Baker B, Mosher J, et al: A review of scaphoid fracture healing in competitive athletes. *Am J Sports Med* 13:159, 1985.

68. Hawkins RJ, Kunkel SS: Rotator cuff tears. In *Current Therapy in Sports Medicine,* 2nd ed. Toronto, B. C. Decker, 1990, pp 395–399.

69. Hawkins RJ, Kunkel SS: Multidirectional instability of the shoulder; the technique of inferior shift. Chicago, American Association of Orthopedic Surgeons, 1990, [videotape].

Chapter 7

EVALUATION AND TREATMENT OF INJURIES IN COMPETITIVE DIVERS

Steven J. Anderson, MD, and Benjamin D. Rubin, MD

With few exceptions,[2,12,18] the sport of competitive diving has received relatively little attention in the medical literature. Many of the reviews occur as subheadings under more general discussions of aquatic sports.[8,15] The unique medical aspects of competitive diving are more difficult to appreciate when the sport is lumped together with skin diving, scuba diving, or swimming. Similarly, the assumption that diving is simply an aquatic version of gymnastics or dance can be misleading.

Much of the medical attention focused on diving has dealt with the recreational version of the sport. An unacceptably high number of serious head and neck injuries has plagued recreational diving.[10,19] Despite the absence of similar injury patterns in organized diving, the safety issues of competitive and recreational diving are often inadvertently linked. As a result, the medical literature on diving may be arguably unfocused or inappropriately focused on an activity considered distinct from competitive diving.

This chapter provides a clearer medical perspective on the sport of competitive diving. Background information on the sport of springboard and platform diving is provided as well as a review of the physical demands of training and competition. In the discussion of common injuries, emphasis is placed on how the pathomechanics of injury serves as the basis for the diagnosis, treatment, and ultimate prevention of diving-related injuries.

BACKGROUND

The evolution of diving can be traced to the 17th century when gymnasts in Germany and Sweden were first observed to perform acrobatics over water in what was known as "fancy diving." Springboard diving became an Olympic sport at the 1904 games in St. Louis. Platform diving became an Olympic event at the 1908 games in London. The United States has long been a dominant force in diving, but increasingly competitive programs from China and the former Soviet Union testify to the international growth and development of the sport.

The standard format for diving competitions involves a 1-m springboard, 3-m springboard, and 10-m platform event for both men and women.[24] Olympic competition involves 3- and 10-m events only. A diver must perform from 8 to 11 dives, depending on the event. A dive must be selected from six types of dives (Fig. 1): forward, backward, reverse, inward, twisting, and handstand (for platform only). The dives are performed in a straight, pike, or tuck position (Fig. 2). Each dive is assigned a degree of difficulty that ranges from 1.2 to 3.5.

Approximately half the dives are voluntary and half are optional. The voluntary dives (formerly called "required" or "compulsory") are chosen from a representative sample of the six different types of dives. The total degree of difficulty of the voluntary dives must not exceed a predetermined maximal number. The optional dives have no limit on

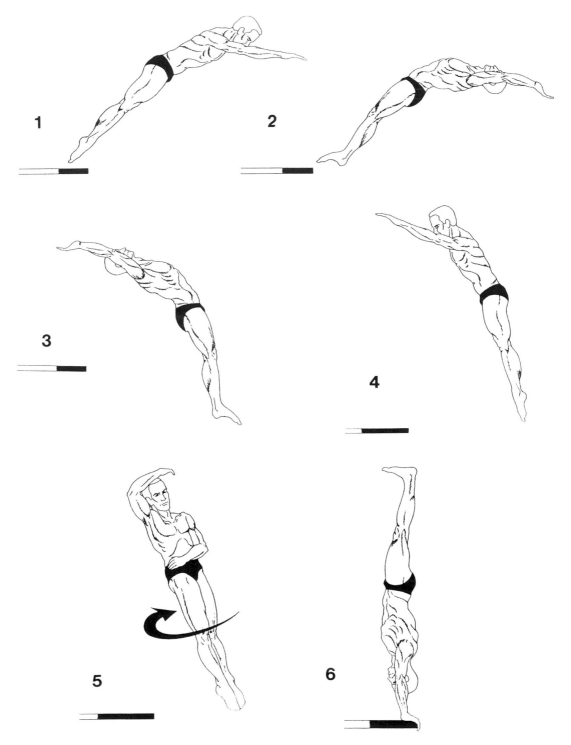

FIGURE 1. Basic diving positions: (1) **Forward group:** The diver faces the front of the board and rotates toward the water. Dives in this group vary from the simple front dive to the difficult forward 3½ somersault. (2) **Backward group:** Dives begin with the diver on the end of the board with back to the water. The direction of rotation is from the board. (3) **Reverse group:** Formerly called "gainers," these dives begin with the diver facing the front of the board (using a forward approach) and rotating toward the board. (4) **Inward group:** The diver stands on the end of the board with back to the water and rotates toward the board or opposite the backward group's movement. The earlier term for these dives was "cutaways." (5) **Twisting group:** Any dive with a twist is included in this group. There are four types: forward, backward, reverse and inward. Because of the many possible combinations, this group includes the most dives. (6) **Armstand group:** The diver assumes a handstand position on the edge of the platform before diving. (Adapted from Shatkowski D (ed): *1992 US Diving Media Guide Record Book.* Indianapolis, US Diving, 1992.)

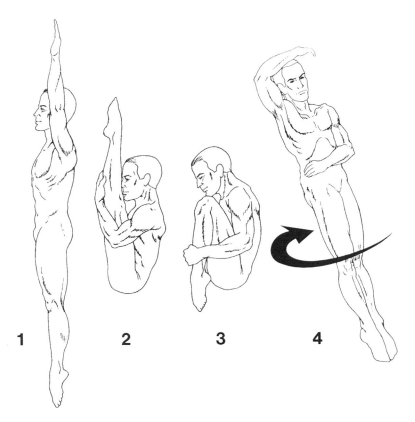

FIGURE 2.   Body positions. (1) **Straight:** This position requires no bend at the waist or knees. Arm placement is the diver's choice or is defined by the dive performed. (2) **Pike:** The legs are straight with the body bent at the waist. Like the straight position, arm placement is dictated by the particular dive or by the choice of the diver. (3) **Tuck:** The body is bent at the waist and knees, with thighs drawn to the chest and heels kept close to the buttocks. (4) **Twisting:** The diver initiates a twisting motion by throwing one arm down and across the body and one arm up and away from the body. Rotation occurs around the long axis of the body. (Adapted from Shatkowski D (ed): *1992 US Diving Media Guide Record Book*. Indianapolis, US Diving, 1992.)

cumulative degree of difficulty. The list of voluntary and optional dives must be declared prior to competition. The divers structure their lists to feature individual strengths as well as to demonstrate proficiency in all types of dives.

The dives are scored by a panel of judges who analyze the approach, take-off, elevation, execution, and entry. Scores range from 0 to 10, with 10 the best possible score. The high and low scores are eliminated, and the total award is calculated by using the degree of difficulty as a multiplier.

Participant Profile

The exact number of participants in competitive diving is unknown, although approximately 10,000 athletes (5,500 women, 4,500 men) are registered with U.S. Diving, and many more are nonregistered participants in YMCA, club, and high-school programs. The typical age of a diver of world-championship caliber varies from 12 years to the late 20s. The average age for the US national diving team is 23.5 years for women and 25 years for men.[21] Divers at the national team level have competed for an average of 11 years for women and 13 years for men. National team divers train an average of 4.5 hrs/day, 6 days/ wk. Most national team members began diving between age 11 and 12 years. Many have prior competitive experience as gymnasts.

Epidemiology of Injuries

Given the extraordinary training demands for serious divers, it is no surprise that injuries occur. Detailed epidemiologic studies of diving injuries are not available. Many of the reports on diving safety have centered on catastrophic injuries to the cervical spine.[10] Despite the fact that such injuries have occurred exclusively in the recreational setting,[3] competitive diving has been the unfortunate victim of guilt by association.

In an effort to determine the problems most relevant to the competitive diver, a survey was distributed to a limited number of elite divers in 1980.[17] Of the 37 divers (16 men, 21 women) who responded, 34 (92%) reported an injury that interrupted training for at least 1 week. In this group, 61% reported back injuries, 61% reported upper-extremity injuries, and 40% reported neck problems. The respondents ranged in age from 11 to 26 years with a trend toward a higher injury rate with increasing years in competition.

In 1991 a medical and injury history was distributed to all divers participating in a National Junior Olympics competition.[25] The survey was administered as part of a talent identification battery that minimized any response bias based on injury status. For the most part, the divers were able to consult their parents regarding details of their health history. Medical personnel were available to clarify terminology and to answer medical questions. A total of 172 divers (78 boys, 94 girls) responded; 90% of the respondents were 18 years of age or younger. The subject profile and most common injuries are listed in Table 1. Fractures (48%), back pain (47%), and muscle strains (42%) were the most frequently mentioned problems. Shin splints, ligament sprains, and contusions were also common. Gender differences in the type or frequency of injury were not seen. A trend toward a higher injury rate in older, more

experienced divers was again noted. Unfortunately, precise diagnoses could not be confirmed, nor could the relation of the injury to diving be established. Nonetheless, injuries are clearly present in abundance in young divers and appear to become an increasing burden with additional years of training and competition.

INJURY PATHOMECHANICS

Rationale for a Pathomechanical Approach to Diagnosis and Treatment

Understanding the cause of a diving injury is essential for administering proper treatment, determining readiness to return to participation, and planning preventive programs. Inherent in any physical activity are forces of compression or load, tension or traction, and friction. Any of these forces applied in excess can cause injury. Rapidly applied, maximal forces can result in tissue disruption and lead to acute musculoskeletal injuries such as fractures, dislocations, sprains, and strains. Repetitive, submaximal forces can result in overuse or overload injuries such as tendinitis, periostitis, bursitis, traumatic arthritis, and stress fracture.

The likelihood of breakdown in response to maximal or submaximal forces is determined, in part, by the presence of extrinsic and intrinsic risk factors for injury[13] (Table 2). Extrinsic risk factors for diving injury may include the training regimen, coaching, facilities and/or equipment used for both wa-

TABLE 1. Injury History in Junior Olympic Divers (n = 172)*

Injury†	No. (% of total)
Broken bone/fracture	83 (48)
Back pain/injury	80 (47)
Muscle pull/strain	72 (42)
Shin splints	53 (31)
Ligament sprain	47 (27)
Deep bruise	40 (23)
Neck pain/injury	37 (22)
Painful kneecap	31 (18)

*Subjects included 78 males and 94 females: ages = ≤ 13 yrs, 30 M/32 F; 14–15 yrs, 17 M/25 F; 16–18 yrs, 23 M/27 F; senior, 8 M/10 F.

†Injury terminology is deliberately written for "lay" readership and is listed as it appeared on questionnaire.

Data from US Diving, Ad Hoc Talent Identification Committee.[25]

TABLE 2. Extrinsic and Intrinsic Risk Factors in Diving Injuries

Extrinsic Factors	Intrinsic Factors
Training	Physical characteristics
Intensity, duration, frequency	Age
quency	Maturational status
Coaching/supervision	Physical fitness
Environment	Previous injury
Facility design	Flexibility
Clearance from obstacles	Strength/power
cles	Joint motion
Water surface visibility	Joint stability
Pool depth	Malalignment
Board/platform surface	Spatial orientation, spotting ability
Equipment	ting ability
Tape, braces, splints	Skills, technique
Spotting belts	Psychosocial characteristics
Dry land training equipment	acteristics

ter and dry land training. Intrinsic risk factors for injury include individual variables such as flexibility, joint laxity, strength, alignment, and skills and technique. When a diver presents with an injury, it is helpful to identify both the pathomechanic forces involved and the extrinsic and intrinsic factors that may be contributory. This approach encourages treatment programs that address the cause as well as the symptoms of the injury.

Pathomechanics of Diving Injuries

For purposes of understanding the physical demands of executing a dive, it is useful to separate the dive into its three component parts—takeoff, flight, and entry.

The **takeoff** phase of the dive involves work on the springboard or platform. For a front dive, the takeoff includes an approach (minimum of 3 steps), a hurdle (the upward jump from one foot to the end of the board), and a press (depression of the board and upward acceleration of the body). For maximal height, divers must synchronize their descent from the hurdle with the descent of the board; this technique allows them to "ride" the board for a more efficient press. Working against the motion of the board has consequences for both performance and injury risk.

The takeoff for back or inward dives can be subdivided into the preparatory arm swing that sets the board in motion and the press. For platform dives, height is achieved by whatever spring the diver can generate from a fixed (nonflexible) surface.

The injury-producing forces during take off are related to jumping and deceleration, with the greatest physical demands and greatest injury potential placed on the extensor mechanism of the knee. The most common injuries related to this part of the dive are patellar tendinitis, quadriceps tendinitis, and patellofemoral compression syndrome. Eccentric overload to the Achilles tendon and impact to the leg from bouncing may result in injuries to these structures. Injuries to the lumbar spine may also occur during take off. If the diver is out of position while pressing the board or jumping, compensatory movements such as hyperextension of the back may lead to injury.

With handstand dives, takeoff must be initiated from a controlled, stable handstand position at the end of the platform. This position demands tremendous isometric strength and balance. The potential for injury in the handstand position stems from the use of the upper extremity for weight-bearing. The load-bearing demands on the wrist, elbow, and shoulder can be excessive—particularly when the necessary joint motion, joint stability, or muscular support is lacking.

The **flight** or **mid-air maneuver** phase of the dive begins when the diver leaves the board or platform and ends with initial water contact. During this phase, forces operate to allow the diver to spin forward, to spin backward, and/or to twist along the long axis of the body. To initiate a twisting motion, the diver throws one arm down and across the body and one arm up and away from the body[4] (Fig. 2). Irritation of the long head of the biceps tendon on the abducted and externally rotated arm has resulted from this type of movement. The potential for torsional overload to the spine also exists. Strength and control in the trunk and extremities are necessary to maintain the pike, tuck, or straight-body position required for the dive. The rapid and forced flexion of the trunk with pike dives causes increased loading of the anterior segment (vertebral body and disc) and can be a factor in injury to these structures.

Intrinsic factors such as body awareness, spatial orientation, and "spotting" ability are critical during the mid-air maneuver and, in part, determine whether or not the maneuvers results in injury. Many of the injuries that occur during flight occur as compensation for a flawed takeoff or as an attempt to save an entry. Injuries during flight may occur from striking the board. Such injuries are usually due to a mistake during takeoff on the board—not in the air.

Most diving injuries occur upon **entry** into the water. Even with a perfectly executed dive, the diver strikes the water surface with considerable impact. Additional forces occur underwater as the diver performs forceful maneuvers to facilitate a clean, splashless entry or "rip." With multiple repetitions in practice and an inevitable number of less than perfect entries, the risk for entry-related injury becomes cumulative.

The approximate velocities of entrance from various springboard and platform heights are shown in Table 3. The average force of impact for a 10-m dive varies from 20 to 24Gs (1G = 9.8 m/s^2). The challenge for the diver is to dissipate impact forces and to control deceleration in the water while still

TABLE 3.   Approximate Entrance Velocities*

Height	Springboard	Platform
1 m	8.4 m/s (18.75 mi/h)	4.4 m/s (9.82 mi/h)
3 m	10.1 m/s (22.54 mi/h)	7.7 m/s (17.19 mi/h)
10 m	—	14.0 m/s (31.25 mi/h)

*From Gabriel JL (ed): *US Diving Safety Manual.* Indianapolis, US Diving Publications, 1990, with permission.[6]

achieving a splashless entry. To dissipate impact initially and to protect the head and spine from axial loading, the diver enters with arms extended and hands in a clasped or overlapping configuration (Fig. 3). This position also serves to "punch a hole in the water" through which the body can presumably pass with minimal splash.

A proper entry requires enough strength to maintain a handstand position with the added demands created by deceleration forces on the water surface. The forces at impact initially act to cause dorsiflexion of the wrist and flexion or "buckling" of the elbow. The wrist flexors and elbow extensors must work to counteract these forces. Strains to the wrist flexors and tendinitis and/or strains to the triceps may result from overload of these supportive structures.

As impact forces are transmitted proximally, the shoulder must be prepared to absorb axial loading. Adequate scapular abduction is crucial to providing bony stability to the glenohumeral joint. Inadequate scapular abduction increases the demands on the soft-tissue structures of the shoulder to maintain support and to prevent glenohumeral instability (Fig. 4).

When a diver is short of a vertical entry at impact, he or she attempts to save the dive. The attempt involves hyperextension of the back and hyperflexion of the shoulders. This position of the shoulder markedly increases susceptibility to anterior glenohumeral subluxation. Save attempts are common in back and reverse dives—in part, because of the inherent difficulties with back-spinning dives. With back and reverse dives, the diver's vision is oriented opposite the direction of the somersault and away from the intended entry point. The diver has to initiate extension toward the water before seeing the entry point. If rotation is inadequate in a back-spinning dive, the diver has only a fraction of a second to recognize position and to make corrective maneuvers. To avoid a nonvertical entry, divers literally thrust themselves into the save position. The speed, force, and amplitude of this effort may contribute to injury. The effects of water impact on hyperflexed shoulders and hyperextended spines exceeds the already considerable impact forces associated with neutral alignment.

During the entry into the water, the diver must execute what is known as a "swim-out." As the arms and upper body enter the water, the diver forcibly pulls the arms forward or to the side in a swimming motion in an attempt to pull the hips and lower extremities into the water. The swim-out may also assist in an underwater save. The diver turns underwater in the same direction as the midair maneuver to maintain a smooth and continuous arc of motion. The timing of the underwater ma-

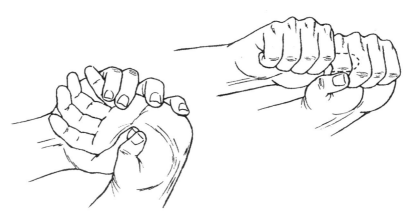

FIGURE 3.   Hand position at entry.

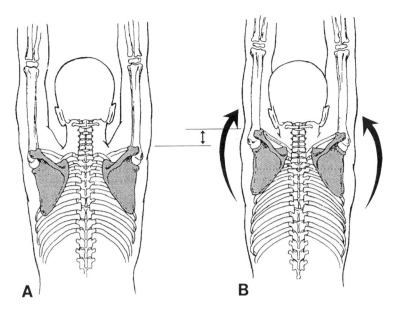

FIGURE 4.   Role of scapular abduction during entry. **A,** Shoulder girdle depression; **B,** Shoulder girdle elevation. Note comparison of shoulder girdle position with depression and elevation. Abducting the shoulder *(B)* positions the glenoid fossa behind the humeral head to better withstand axial loading at impact.

neuvers and the adequacy of strength to support sudden changes in direction and velocity are factors in production of injury and should be factors in treatment of injury.

"Dry land" training may also contribute to diving injuries. The acquisition of basic diving skills and the progression toward more complicated spinning and twisting dives may involve practice on a trampoline, a dry board with portable landing pit, or use of an overhead spotting belt. A thorough evaluation of an injured diver should include inquiries about dry land training and any risks that may result from the specific equipment and personnel involved.

COMMON DIVING INJURIES

The discussion of diving injuries is divided into those affecting the extremities and those affecting the spine. Most of the diagnoses in injured divers are also seen in nondiving settings. It is assumed that the reader has some baseline familiarity with these conditions; this discussion focuses on the aspects of diagnosis and treatment most germane to diving.

Shoulder Injuries

The most common shoulder problems affecting divers are rotator cuff impingement and glenohumeral instability. It is difficult to separate the discussion of pathogenesis of these problems because they may be interrelated.[11] The shoulder is an inherently unstable joint. This creates added demands on supportive structures (rotator cuff, glenoid labrum, capsule) when external forces are applied. Inadequacy or weakness of supportive structures may lead to subacromial impingement of the supraspinatus tendon, biceps tendon, or subacromial bursa. Failure of supportive structures can cause labral disruption as well as glenohumeral subluxation or dislocation. Increased glenohumeral laxity may, in turn, lead to further problems with impingement. Ironically, a certain amount of increased glenohumeral laxity is required for divers to perform.

Shoulder injuries appear to be related to repetitive overhead use, saving short dives, and swimming entries. Because of the continuum of shoulder problems from impingement to instability, all divers with shoulder pain should be thoroughly evaluated for problems of both stability and strength. Anterolateral shoulder pain occurring after multiple dives may be the earliest sign of injury. Recognition and treatment of pathology at this stage usually lead to an earlier and more complete recovery than if the injury is allowed to progress. Shoulder pain at rest, pain that is present with simple reaching and extension, or shoulder pain that restricts movement and function indicates a more advanced stage of disease. The presence of gross glenohumeral instability may be associated with reports of recurrent shoulder subluxations or dislocations. More subtle degrees of instability are not reliably detected by history but may be the cause of an athlete's report of popping, catching, or apprehension in positions of abduction and external rotation.

The physical examination of a diver with shoulder pain should include inspection, palpation, and assessment of range of motion, stability, and strength. The inspection should assess muscle bulk and definition, presence of scapular winging, and thoracic kyphosis. A kyphotic posture or an anteriorly tilted acromion limits forward flexion of the shoulder and results in increased risk of impingement. Systematic palpation should be carried out with particular attention to tenderness over the biceps tendon, the greater tubercle of the humerus, and the anterior glenohumeral joint line.

The assessment of shoulder range of motion can serve the dual purpose of detecting signs of impingement and signs of instability. Patients with symptomatic instability often have apprehension with passive abduction and external rotation of the humerus, whereas patients with symptomatic impingement may have pain in all directions except abduction-external rotation. Pain or restricted motion in all planes suggests a combined instability/impingement problem.

The goal of strength testing is to determine both the consequences as well as the contributing causes of injury. Isolated supraspinatus weakness usually indicates injury or disuse. Weakness of the external rotators of the humerus and the scapular stabilizers is more likely to be a risk factor for instability or impingement rather than an effect of the injury. Weakness of the deltoid, biceps, and/or triceps may indicate local injury or a referred problem from a cervical nerve root or brachial plexus injury.

The treatment for shoulder injuries should be based on specific pathomechanic changes in the injured diver. Some degree of rest is usually indicated. Relative rest may take the form of simply limiting dives from higher elevations and/or limiting back and reverse dives. With more severe symptoms, rest may require more global restrictions of activity. Inflammatory changes can be addressed with ice and nonsteroidal antiinflammatory medications. A selective strengthening regimen is essential to restore optimal strength to the downward stabilizers of the humerus and the scapular stabilizers. For patients who have impingement or instability refractory to conservative measures or evidence of significant labral pathology, surgical intervention should be considered. Arthroscopic surgery has a role in both diagnosis and treatment of chronic impingement and labral pathology. The surgical treatment of instability is more controversial. The delicate balance between having "enough" and "too much" glenohumeral laxity must be respected in surgical decision-making.

Elbow Injuries

The maximal stress on the elbow for divers occurs during water entry. Repetitive impact and hyperextension forces may be seen, particularly with platform diving. Hyperextension may result in tensile overload to the medial collateral ligament. The resultant instability may interfere with the diver's ability to maintain a handstand position on the platform and to extend and lock out the elbows during entry. Medial elbow laxity may contribute to the development of ulnar nerve irritation as well.

Triceps injuries are also seen in response to the forces at entry. Triceps strength is required to maintain full elbow extension and to resist impact forces during entry. Failure to maintain full elbow extension results in an eccentric overload to the triceps. Strains to the triceps are most commonly seen at the distal musculotendinous junction but may also occur proximally.

The assessment of an elbow problem in a diver requires an evaluation of range of motion, stability, neurologic status, and strength. Lack of full elbow extension limits the diver aesthetically and functionally. A long line is visually desirable and facilitates a cleaner entry. Inability to lock the elbow into extension markedly increases demands on the triceps to hold the entry. The lack of full elbow extension warrants a radiologic evaluation of the elbow to rule out loose bodies, bony irregularities in the olecranon fossa, and deformity of the radiocapitellar joint. Restrictions of elbow flexion or pain and weakness associated with resisted elbow extension should raise concern about a triceps injury.

Stability of the elbow should be assessed with emphasis on the medial collateral ligament. Medial instability can be checked by applying valgus stress to the elbow in a 30°-flexed position or with a stress radiograph at the same degree of flexion. Side-to-side comparison measurements should be obtained. The neurologic examination should include an assessment of irritability, instability, and/or dysfunction of the ulnar nerve. Strength testing should include not only the biceps and triceps but also the wrist flexors and extensors. Weakness or pain with resisted wrist flexion or pronation may be associated with medial elbow instability or secondary to overload of the wrist flexors from forces at entry.

The treatment of elbow injuries depends on the specific abnormalities and dysfunction present. The goals of treatment and criteria for return to activity should include restoration of full, pain-free motion, strength (especially in the triceps and wrist flexor groups), and adequate stability. Elbow taping and/or bracing may provide some protection for lax medial structures or weak dynamic stabilizers. However, taping and bracing tend to restrict motion and are generally not acceptable as a long-term solution. A simple test to determine readiness to return to full training after an elbow injury is to have the diver demonstrate the ability to maintain a handstand position.

Wrist and Thumb Injuries

Wrist injuries occur from repetitive impact and forced dorsiflexion at entry. Handstands and the act of pushing up to get from the water to the pool deck may also be contributory. Fractures may occur from the hand striking the board. Ulnar collateral ligament sprains of the thumb may occur at impact or as a result of missing a grab for the opposite hand prior to entry.

The assessment of wrist and thumb injuries in divers should include an evaluation of joint range of motion and stability. Palpation should be performed over the distal radius and ulna (including the epiphysis in skeletally immature divers), the proximal and distal carpal row, the ulnar snuff box (triangular fibrocartilage complex), the radial snuff box (scaphoid bone), and the first carpometacarpal and first metacarpophalangeal joint. Radiographs should be evaluated for evidence of fracture, stress fracture, carpal instability patterns, ulnar variance, epiphyseal widening, joint irregularity, or arthritis.[23,24]

Some of the common causes of wrist pain

that may have normal-appearing radiographs include the dorsal impaction syndrome (pain at radiocarpal joint secondary to forced wrist dorsiflexion), synovial ganglion (including occult ganglion cysts), flexor carpi ulnaris tendinitis, and milder sprains or capsulitis.

In the author's experience, volar subluxation of the lunate may underlie much of the wrist pain seen in divers. This condition can be diagnosed by careful palpation of the wrist. Volar prominence of the lunate may be seen in association with wrist pain, whereas a nonprominent or reduced lunate may correlate with decreased pain.

Selected fractures and sprains with significant instability may require casting or even surgery. The remainder of wrist or thumb conditions may be treated conservatively with rest, antiinflammatory medications, and protective taping or bracing. Many divers with injury, or even those attempting to prevent thumb and wrist injury, use a semirigid brace to provide added stability and protection against the forces of impact.

Lower-Extremity Injuries

Lower-extremity injuries in divers are less common and have fewer unique implications for diagnosis and treatment than upper-extremity injuries. Lower-extremity injuries are generally related to jumping. Like other athletes in jumping sports, divers experience patellofemoral pain. The specific diagnoses include patellofemoral compression syndrome, patellar tendinitis, and quadriceps tendinitis.

The evaluation of knee pain in a diver should include an assessment of risk factors for patellofemoral pain, including malalignment; abnormal patellar tracking; poor flexibility in the hamstrings, quadriceps, or hip flexors; and strength imbalances between the hamstrings and the quadriceps. The risk factors should serve as the basis for treatment of patellofemoral dysfunction.[11] Good eccentric quadriceps strength and adequate time for a functional training progression that includes jumping drills should precede a full return to training.[5] McConnell patellar taping may be a useful adjunct for quadriceps reeducation and to facilitate pain-free return to activity.[14]

Other jumping-related conditions include tibial periostitis (shin splints) and tendinitis in the foot and ankle, including posterior tibialis tendinitis and Achilles tendinitis. Again, assessment for malalignment, flexibility problems, and strength imbalances serves as the basis for rehabilitation.[11] Orthotics to compensate for malalignment are not a viable option for a diver during training. However, athletic taping and modification of training regimens to decrease jumping may allow an athlete to continue to train during rehabilitation.

Cervical Spine Injuries

Diving-related injuries to the cervical spine have drawn attention primarily because of the catastrophic problems seen in recreational diving.[10] Recreational divers sustaining spinal cord injuries usually have no formal training in diving and are often injured in a setting with inadequate water depth and inadequate supervision. Often they are under the influence of alcohol.[7] Fortunately, these risk factors can be and are addressed in organized diving. Catastrophic cervical spine injuries have not been reported in competitive diving or in a teaching or school environment.[3]

Although catastrophic injuries may be preventable through implementation of safety measures (*US Diving Safety Manual*[6]), the potential still exists for noncatastrophic injuries from repetitive impact-loading to the cervical spine. A frequently quoted study on the effects of recurrent spinal trauma in high diving was published by Schneider et al. in 1962.[20] Histories, neurologic examinations, and cervical roentgenograms were obtained in 6 cliff divers from Acapulco. The divers averaged over 1,000 dives/year (5,000–26,000 over career) from diving points at 100 and 135 ft above water. None of the divers had cervical abnormalities by history or neurologic examination. The radiographic changes were felt to be minor, and no diver had received prior medical treatment for the changes that appeared in the cervical spines. The greatest bony changes of the cervical spine were in divers who had longer, less heavily muscled necks *and* who struck the water with hands apart. Fewer radiographic changes were seen in divers who locked thumbs or clasped hands to break the force of the dive. Despite the small numbers in the study, the theory that a strong neck, rigid arms, and locked hands protect the spine is widely accepted and practiced today.

A review of recent medical literature has failed to reveal a pattern of specific cervical injury or degenerative process that can be attributed directly to the sport of diving.

Therefore, cervical spine problems in divers need to be considered individually with ongoing surveillance for patterns that may lead to further safety measures.

The clinical evaluation of a diver with cervical complaints should include an assessment of cervical range of motion. Pain or restriction of cervical extension should raise the possibility of a cervical facet injury or possible impingement of the interspinous ligament. Restricted cervical flexion or cervical pain associated with radicular findings should raise suspicion for a disc injury. Upper-extremity neurologic findings with a normal cervical spine examination may indicate brachial plexus injury ("stinger"). Part of the evaluation of a diver with neck pain should include radiographs to rule out instability, stenosis, and degenerative changes.

Criteria for determining a safe return to participation after cervical injury include restoration of pain-free, normal range of motion, absence of neurologic abnormalities, and restoration of normal cervical and upper extremity strength. Current investigation includes correlating cervical symptoms and physical findings with the presence of structural changes by radiographic and magnetic resonance imaging.

Lumbar Spine

The sport of diving requires both mobility and stability in the lumbar spine. When the demands for motion or stability are exceeded, injury may occur.[1]

The anterior segments (vertebral body, vertebral endplate, and intervertebral disc) are particularly vulnerable to compressive forces or increased load. Increased disc-loading would be expected at takeoff and entry and with trunk flexion during the mid-air maneuver. A flexed or rotated spine during maximal loading (at takeoff or entry) combines the forces most likely to lead to disc injury.

An anterior segment injury typically presents with low back pain that lateralizes or radiates into the buttock or hamstring area. The pain may be worsened by sitting, bending, lifting, and/or straining and relieved by standing, walking, lying prone, and/or extending the spine. Radiographic evaluation should take place to rule out compression fracture, endplate irregularities, or disc-space narrowing. A normal radiograph does not rule out a disc protrusion or a degenerative disc. Therefore, magnetic resonance imaging may be indicated for more definitive evaluation of disc pathology.[22]

Conservative treatment of an anterior segment injury includes relative rest, antiinflammatory medication, and physical therapy to restore optimal flexibility, lumbar segmental motion, trunk strength, and body mechanics. Surgery should be considered for instability, progressive bony deformity, disabling discogenic pain, or neurologic compromise. The potential for loss of lumbar motion after surgery warrants careful consideration prior to surgical intervention.

Posterior element injury (facet joints, pars interarticularis) may be a more common cause of back pain in divers. The posterior elements are subjected to overload during maximal lumbar extension or extension combined with rotation. Settings in which overload can occur include the takeoff for a back dive, an entry for a back-spinning dive when the diver is "short," or a front-spinning dive when the diver overrotates.

The diver with posterior element pain typically presents with back pain at the level of the waist that is worse with standing, walking, running, jumping, and/or lumbar extension. The pain may be relieved by sitting, forward flexion, and/or lying supine. Physical findings may include hyperlordotic posture, restricted and painful lumbar extension, tender posterior elements, and, usually, a normal neurologic examination. Radiologic evaluation is aimed primarily at ruling out spondylolysis and spondylolisthesis. Rossi[16] found that spondylolytic lesions appear with increased frequency in divers with back pain compared with symptomatic athletes in other sports (prevalence rates of 63% vs 17% respectively). Most authorities agree that diving is a sport where the rate of spondylolysis may be disproportionately high.[9,22]

The presence of a spondylolytic defect on the radiograph does not always mean that spondylolysis is the cause of back pain nor does a normal-appearing radiograph rule out a symptomatic spondylolysis. A bone scan and/or single photon emission computed tomography (SPECT) can help to reconcile differences between clinical and radiographic findings. A positive bone scan indicates that a spondylolysis is new and likely causing symptoms. A negative bone scan indicates that a spondylolytic defect on radiograph is old and suggests that other etiologies for back pain need to be pursued.

The treatment for spondylolysis requires a period of rest with restriction of lumbar extension, followed by an exercise program aimed at decreasing hyperlordosis and increasing abdominal and trunk strength and a graded return to pain-free activity. Use of a semirigid antilordotic brace (i.e., Boston brace) may be required to control extension forces and to decrease pain. Skeletally immature adolescents with spondylolysis need to be monitored during their growing years for progressive spondylolisthesis.

Lumbar facet arthropathy may also underlie a pattern of posterior element pain. The clinical findings of a facet syndrome are difficult to distinguish from spondylolysis. Accordingly, the diagnosis of a facet syndrome should not be made until spondylolysis has been ruled out.

Lumbar pain with extension may also be due to a midline disc protrusion or lateral recess stenosis. Back pain with extremes of motion in any plane may be related to segmental hypermobility. Sprains, strains, and other soft-tissue disorders may cause back pain. Such diagnoses, however, are less likely in an athlete whose symptoms have persisted for more than 2 weeks and are less valid until more specific diagnoses have been ruled out. Because treatment varies according to diagnosis, a favorable outcome depends on diagnostic precision.

SUMMARY

The preceding discussion of competitive springboard and platform diving has included a review of pertinent background information on the sport and its participants, an analysis of the pathomechanics of diving injury, and a review of the common musculoskeletal injuries. An appreciation of the physical demands of the sport is crucial to understanding the pathogenesis of injury as well as to planning treatment and prevention strategies and to determining safe return to participation after injury.

REFERENCES

1. Anderson SJ: Assessment and management of the pediatric and adolescent patient with low back pain. *Phys Med Rehabil Clin North Am* 2:157–186, 1991.
2. Carter RL: Prevention of springboard and platform diving injuries. *Clin Sports Med* 5:185–194, 1986.

3. Clement A: *Current Trends in Aquatic Litigation.* Indianapolis, IN, Council for National Cooperation in Aquatics National Conference, November 8–12, 1989.
4. Frohlich C: The physics of somersaulting and twisting. *Sci Am* (Mar):155–164, 1980.
5. Fyfe I, Stanish WD: The use of eccentric training and stretching in the treatment and prevention of tendon injuries. *Clin Sports Med* 11:601–624, 1992.
6. Gabriel JL (ed): *US Diving Safety Manual.* Indianapolis, IN, US Diving Publications, 1990.
7. Gabrielson M: Diving injuries: A critical insight and recommendations. In *Proceedings of the National Pool and Spa Safety Conference.* Co-sponsored by the US Consumer Product Safety Commission and the National Spa and Pool Institute, Arlington,VA May 1985.
8. Gater D, Rubin B: Strength and conditioning programs for sports of the Olympic Games. *NSCA J* 10:6–25, 1988.
9. Jackson DW, Wiltse LL, Dingeman RD, et al: Stress reactions involving the pars interarticularis in young athletes. *Am J Sports Med* 9:304–312, 1981.
10. Kewalramani LS, Taylor RG: Injuries to the cervical spine from diving accidents. *J Trauma* 15:130–142, 1975.
11. Kibler WB, Chandler TJ, Pace BK: Principles of rehabilitation after chronic tendon injuries. *Clin Sports Med* 11:661–671, 1992.
12. Kimball RJ, Carter RL, Schneider RC: Competitive diving injuries. In Schneider RC, Kennedy JC, Plant ML, et al (eds): *Sports Injuries: Mechanisms, Prevention, and Treatment.* Baltimore, Williams & Wilkins, 1985, pp 192–211.
13. Lysens R, Steverlynck A, van den Auweele Y, et al: The predictability of sports injuries. *Sports Med* 1:6–10, 1984.
14. McConnell J: The management of chondromalacia patellae: A long term solution. *Aust J Physiother* 32:215–223, 1986.
15. Reilly T, Miles S: Background to injuries in swimming and diving. In Reilly T (ed): *Sports Fitness and Sports Injuries.* London, Faber & Faber, 1981, pp 159–167.
16. Rossi F: Spondylolysis, spondylolisthesis and sports. *J Sports Med* 18:317–340, 1978.
17. Rubin B: Orthopedic aspects of competitive diving injuries. In Golden (ed): *Proceedings of the United States Diving Sports Sciences Seminar.* Indianapolis, IN, US Diving, 1983, pp 65–78.
18. Rubin BD: Injuries in competitive diving. *Sports Med Digest* 9:1–3, 1987.
19. Samples P: Spinal cord injuries: The high cost of careless diving. *Phys Sports Med* 17(7):143–148, 1989.
20. Schneider RC, Papo M, Alvarez CS: The effects of chronic recurrent spinal trauma in high-diving. *J Bone Joint Surg* 44A:648–656, 1962.
21. Shatkowski D (ed): *1992 US Diving Media Guide and Record Book.* Indianapolis, IN, US Diving, 1992.
22. Sward L: The thoracolumbar spine in elite athletes: Current concepts on the effects of physical training. *Sports Med* 13:357–364, 1992.
23. Weiker GC: Hand and wrist problems in the gymnast. *Clin Sports Med* 11:189–202, 1992.
24. Wood MB, Dobyns JH: Sports-related extraarticular wrist syndromes. *Clin Orthop* 202:93–102, 1986.
25. US Diving, Ad Hoc Talent Identification Committee: Anderson SJ, Gabriel J, Golden D, et al. Indianapolis, IN, US Diving, 1991.

Chapter 8

REHABILITATION OF RUNNING INJURIES

Jeffrey L. Young, MD, MA, and Joel M. Press, MD

Despite recent fitness trends that have sent people to stairclimbers, stationary ski machines, and step aerobics classes, running remains one of the most popular forms of aerobic exercise. Nearly 30 million Americans participate in running on a regular basis.[8,33] It attracts participants because it appears to require only a modest amount of skill, is frequently cited by the media as an effective method of achieving cardiovascular fitness and weight control, is relatively inexpensive, can be done alone, and in many climates may be done year round. However, errors of training, biomechanic flaws, and poor equipment selection, among other factors, can lead to musculoskeletal injury.[8,13,28,29,33,34,43,44] This chapter presents a template for evaluating and rehabilitating the injured runner and explores a few of the more common injuries associated with regular running.

EPIDEMIOLOGY

The usual definition of a running injury is a condition that makes an athlete decrease the desired mileage per week.[33] It has been estimated that from 30% to 70% of all runners will sustain an injury; numerous authors report that people running more than 30 mi/week have greater than a 50% chance of injury.[14–16,29,33,39] Other studies report no significant relationship between injury and training pace, weekly mileage, or years of running.[17,28] Much of the variability in the reported percentages of injured runners is due to methodologic inconsistencies in determining the actual population at risk for injury and variation in the length of observation periods.[15] Nevertheless, certain factors seem to be rather consistently implicated in increasing the risk of injury. These factors may be divided into two major categories: anatomic problems and errors of training.

Most authors agree that training errors account for the majority of injuries,[8,33,34,43] and one study reported that fewer than 20% of injuries were related to identified anatomic problems.[34] Common errors include changing to a harder running surface,[8] abruptly increasing mileage by more than 10% per week,[8,28,32,43] a sudden increase in running intensity,[8,33] hill running,[28] running on crowned roads, inadequate rest, and previous injury.[15]

The most common site of injury is the knee,[8,33,46] which is estimated to account for 30% to 50% of all injuries.[8,25,30,33] Typical problems include patellofemoral tracking disorders,[10,25,36] iliotibial band friction syndrome,[25,28,44] and hamstring strains.[47] The lower leg, ankle, and foot are also problematic areas. Plantar fasciitis may alter training programs severely.[20,21,28] Up to 50% of runners report having sprained an ankle at one time or another in their running career.[33] Stress fractures have been reported as the cause of up to 10% of all injuries presenting to a running clinic.[26] Achilles tendinitis is one of the most frequently identified diagnoses for which running orthotics are prescribed.[13] The hip, pelvis, and back collectively, which make up close to 20% of all injuries,[8] are frequent sites of overuse injuries as well as muscular tightness and strength imbalance.

THE ACTION OF RUNNING

Management of the injured runner requires a basic understanding of the biomechanic events that occur during running. Running is distinguished from walking by the lack of a double support phase; instead it has an airborne phase in which neither foot is in contact with the ground. Foot strike is typically made with the heel at slower speeds, but as runners increase their speed, they tend to strike with the forefoot. Sprinters virtually always exhibit a total forefoot strike pattern. Runners typically strike the ground with their feet 800 to 2000 times/mile. The ground reaction forces at the time of initial contact are usually two to four times body weight.

With a moderate running speed and initial rearfoot contact, the ankle-foot is in a supinated posture as the foot makes contact with the ground.[8,43] Supination, associated with the closed-packed position of the tarsal bones, enables the foot to be more stable and rigid at the time of heel strike. The ankle-foot rapidly assumes a pronated, or open-packed, position of the tarsal joints, which allows for shock attenuation and accommodation of irregularities in the running surface. The tibia is internally rotated upon the talus. As the runner passes through the mid-support phase and prepares to propel toward the airborne phase, the subtalar joint progresses to a supinated posture with external rotation of the tibia, thus creating a more rigid lever for propulsion. The ankle-foot remains relatively supinated through the airborne phase and forward swing of the leg and is mildly supinated when the foot is just about to strike the ground again.[8,43] Problems with the sequencing and control of ankle-foot motion can lead to foot/ankle pathology or affect any of the links in the biomechanic chain. For example, excessive pronation and midfoot collapse with sustained internal rotation of the tibia place an increased load on the medial aspect of the knee due to valgus stress.

At the level of the knee, runners typically move between 30° to 40° degrees of flexion (mid-support) to nearly full extension at toe-off.[8,43] The partially flexed knee at initial contact allows more shock absorption. The center of gravity is thus behind the knee at this point, but progressively migrates forward with eventual development of an extension moment. Rotation of the tibia at the knee is highly influenced by the amount of pronation (internal rotation of the tibia) or supination (external rotation of the tibia) at the subtalar joint. The femur rotates in the same direction as the tibia, and the femoral neck angle influences knee angle and foot position. The normally small amount of tibia varum at heel strike may be increased in runners (especially women) who cross over the midline of the body with the feet.[8,37,43] Truncal posture should be relatively erect with relaxed upper body posture, an elbow flexion angle near 100°, and loosely held hands.[8]

The amount of energy expended during running is quite variable, and the runner's natural stride length typically produces the most economical running style.[4] An increase in stride length beyond the natural limit is accompanied by an observed increase in energy expenditure for a given running speed and thus by reduced efficiency.[4]

THE RUNNER'S HISTORY

A careful history is required to identify the diagnosis and mechanism of injury.

1. **Chronology of the Injury.** How long has the runner had the pain, and when did the pain first appear? Was the onset of pain sudden or gradual? Unless a race is at stake or a major injury is involved, runners rarely show up at a physicians office when the injury or symptoms first occur. They tend to seek help when running performance and/or their training regimens are threatened.

2. **Nature of the Pain.** Is the pain constant or intermittent? What makes it more tolerable, and what exacerbates it? Is the pain associated with weight-bearing, and how soon does it appear after beginning activity? Is the pain associated with inflammation? Pain associated with superficial nerve entrapment or with compartment syndromes is often less apparent at rest and at the onset of exercise but worsens after a relatively consistent amount of activity, whereas plantar fasciitis is typically provoked with the first step of the morning. Achilles tendinitis is recognized by the runner's description of redness, swelling, and increased warmth within a painful heel cord, whereas Achilles tendinosis is described as painful but without the aforementioned cardinal signs of inflammation.[24] Exacerbation of a runner's anterior knee pain by squatting or prolonged sitting (theater sign) alerts the clinician to patellofemoral joint dysfunction.[10]

3. **Age Considerations.** The differential diagnosis of distal Achilles tendon pain in the skeletally immature runner must include calcaneal apophysitis (Sever's disease), whereas the elderly runner is much more likely to have pathology within the tendon itself.[2,3] Hip pain in the young athlete should raise suspicion of femoral stress fracture or traction apophysitis, whereas the same symptoms in the elderly runner can indicate fracture or symptomatic spinal stenosis.[2,3]

4. **Running Habits.** How long has the runner been training? How many miles per session and per week? What pace is maintained? Does the runner take days off? Has there been a sudden increase in frequency, intensity, or duration of work-outs? Does the runner routinely stretch before and/or after exercising? Which muscle groups are stretched? Does the runner train alone or with others, and who determines the running pace? Is the patient a competitive runner who regularly enters races or a recreational jogger? These questions are important in identifying potential errors of training that can cause breakdown.

5. **Equipment.** What type of shoes does the runner use? How often are new pairs purchased and old pairs discarded? Has the runner recently started wearing a new style of shoe? Does the runner wear orthotics? When were the orthotics originally constructed and for what purpose? These questions help to provide insight into potential errors of training and biomechanic imbalances. Shoes or inserts that have broken down and no longer serve their original intent are common and easily corrected problems. The reader is referred to articles by Subotnick[43] and Newell[29] for excellent reviews of evaluating the foot and the role of foot orthotics. Orthotic devices are especially useful to correct biomechanic imbalances that are not correctable by specific stretching and strengthening programs. In a survey of 347 symptomatic runners whose average training was approximately 40 miles/week, 75% reported marked improvement or resolution of symptoms with the use of the orthotic inserts.[13]

6. **Terrain.** Where does the athlete typically run? Does the runner train on a level dirt path, on a banked concrete surface, on a treadmill at a health club, or on a flat circular track? Does the runner hill train? Have any of these factors changed recently? Poor selection of running course may create imbalances at the level of the foot and ankle that are transmitted up the biomechanic chain to the more proximal structures. For example, running on a banked surface causes uphill foot pronation, which stresses the medial ankle, and creates a knee valgus force, hip abduction, and elevation of the ipsilateral hemipelvis, whereas "downhill" foot supination stresses the lateral ankle and creates a knee varus force, hip adduction, and lowering of the ipsilateral hemipelvis.[8,37]

7. **Injury Inventory.** How many other injuries have been sustained? What were the locations? Were they managed nonsurgically or surgically? These questions help to identify patterns of overtraining and provide a sense of how much the athlete is willing to endure to continue running on a regular basis.

8. **Review of Systems.** Does the runner get chest pain or palpitations during exercise? Is it harder to do the same amount of work? Has the runner started experiencing wheezing or shortness of breath during or after runs? Does the runner experience constant fatigue and difficulty in getting rid of colds or infections? Has weight loss occurred, and was it on purpose? Has a female runner stopped menstruating, and is there reason to suspect osteoporosis? What medications are being used? Are anabolic steroids being taken? Although the major focus of this chapter is musculoskeletal problems, one must not fail to identify other factors that may heavily influence the runner's overall health.

9. **Goals.** Why does the patient run? For fun and fitness or in preparation for competition? As part of a program for weight control, stress management, or health maintenance? Is the running a substitute for something that is missing in the patient's life or a reflection of a problem in the larger psychosocial context? An overweight middle-aged man who has just started running as part of a generic fitness program may be amenable to trying a new form of exercise if running causes knee pain. On the other hand, a gaunt young woman who presents with pelvic stress fractures and amenorrhea, yet whose primary concern is fear of gaining weight, raises the possibility of disordered body image and/or other emotional issues. Such issues may require the input of a psychologist or psychiatrist, so that running rehabilitation can occur.

10. **Coping Skills.** How has the loss of running affected the person's life? Can the athlete tolerate relative or complete rest? What will he or she do if running is no longer an option for an undetermined amount of time? A more holistic approach to the injured ath-

lete, with input from a sports psychologist or psychiatrist, may be essential to successful rehabilitation.

PHYSICAL EXAMINATION

Establishing a diagnosis-specific program of rehabilitation for a runner is not possible without a thorough physical examination. It is critical to adhere to the concept of the kinetic chain and to recognize that biomechanic dysfunction in one body region may cause injury at a distance. Consequently, examination of the low back, hip, knee, and ankle regions should be routine in virtually all injured runners. The basic components of a runner's physical examination are reviewed below.

Observation

The runner is evaluated at rest, while walking, and then while running. The examination at rest helps to identify such entities as limb-length discrepancy, scoliosis, excessive lordosis, pelvic asymmetry, genu varum/ valgum, tibial torsion, side-to-side differences in muscle bulk, static ankle-foot deformities, blisters and calluses, and visible evidence of inflammation. The walking examination may reveal signs of foot pronation or supination, early heel rise from a tight gastroc-soleus complex, increased knee valgus/varus, and hip abductor weakness (Trendelenburg sign). The greatest insight is achieved with direct visualization of running itself. Treadmill evaluations provide an excellent opportunity in this regard. Analysis of video recordings of the runner at varying speeds with and without shoes and with and without orthotics is recommended. This strategy enables the clinician to identify more subtle biomechanic imbalances as well as flaws in running style. Video recordings are not only a useful diagnostic aid but also a vehicle for patient education. The recording/projecting system should be capable of high resolution when played at normal, fast-forward, or slow-motion speeds.

Physical Exam Proper

At the level of the ankle and foot, the following maneuvers are considered to be the minimum: palpation of the Achilles tendon as well as the origin and insertions of the plantar fascia; ranging of the talar, subtalar, and midtarsal joints; and evaluation of laxity in the lateral and medial ligaments of the ankle. When a specific problem such as excessive pronation is identified, maneuvers such as the navicular drop test are added. If the measured vertical descent of the navicular exceeds 1.5 cm in moving from a position in which the entire foot is just touching the floor to one of full weight-bearing on the same side, pronation is believed to be excessive.[40] Goniometric measurement of the subtalar joint checks for deviation from the normal 2:1 ratio of inversion to eversion through a 45° range and, combined with evaluation of the forefoot for presence of varus/valgus, also aids in detecting areas of tightness that need stretching or regions of connective-tissue laxity in need of orthotic devices for protection, stability, and support.[29]

Assessment of range of motion in the knee is followed by evaluation of patellar position, mobility, and tracking and retropatellar pain. The Q angle (the angle formed between straight lines drawn from the anterior superior iliac spine (ASIS) to the distal femur and from the tibial tuberosity through the middle of the patella) (Fig. 1) is considered to be excessive if it measures over 20°.[7,8,22,25] The combination of hypermobility of the patella, external tibial torsion, increased Q angle, femoral neck anteversion, a broad pelvis, and pes planus with pronation defines *malalignment syndrome,* which is associated with medial knee pain.[7,17,25] Assessment of the collateral and cruciate ligaments and menisci is also routine. Ober's test (Fig. 2) is used to evaluate tightness of the tensor fascia lata. When a friction syndrome of the iliotibial band (ITB) is suspected, the ITB (Noble) compression test can be used. After positioning the knee in 90° of flexion, the examiner presses on or just proximal to the lateral epicondyle. The knee is then gradually extended. Pain occurring at about 30° (as the ITB crosses the bony prominence) is a positive finding.[31]

In cases of anterior knee pain, the examination focuses on patellar orientation (internal/ external rotation, presence of patella baja or alta, abnormal patellar tilt), defects in the medial or lateral retinacula, apprehension, increased laxity or pain with patellar mobilization, evidence of poor patellar tracking within the trochlea, retropatellar crepitus, and atrophy of the vastus medialis obliquus.

The hip and pelvic region must be evalu-

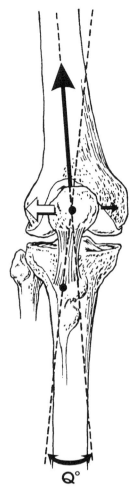

FIGURE 1. The Q-angle: The angle formed between the line of pull of the quadriceps and the center line of the patellar tendon. (From Buschbacher RM (ed): *Musculoskeletal Disorders: A Practical Guide for Diagnosis and Rehabilitation.* Stoneham, MA, Butterworth-Heinemann, 1994, with permission.)

ated for the presence of tight hip flexors, extensors, and adductors because loss of mobility in this region may be a factor in development of the runner's injury.[33,46] Stabilizing the pelvis with one hand while attempting a straight leg raise with the other gives a sense of hamstring tightness as retrotilting of the pelvis begins to occur as maximal length is approached. Having the patient bring both knees up to the chest and then trying to let one leg descend to a flat lying position on the examination table is thwarted in hip flexor tightness. (Thomas test). Tightness of the piriformis and external hip rotators can be checked with knee flexion and internal hip rotation with the patient lying prone. Placing the hip in end-range flexion plus abduction

and external rotation (FABER) (Fig. 3) stresses the hip joint itself. Gaenslen's maneuver may be used to stress the sacroiliac joint.

Certain bony prominences and landmarks should be assessed for tenderness, including the greater trochanter, posterior superior iliac spine (PSIS), anterior superior iliac spine (ASIS), and posterior inferior iliac spine (PIIS). They also need to be checked for symmetry in the evaluation of malrotation of the sacroiliac joint or pelvis. In addition, the ASIS is a fixed landmark typically used in limb-length measurement. Limb-length inequalities have been estimated to have 3 times as much an effect on the runner as on the walker.[43]

A quick but effective screen of the back incorporates all the observations from the lower body segments; again, the concept of the kinetic chain must not be overlooked. Lumbosacral spine motion is intimately related to motion at the level of the hip and pelvis. Tightness of lower-extremity muscles attaching to the pelvis can interfere with the normally smooth combination of spine flexion–pelvic rotation and spine extension–pelvic derotation (lumbopelvic rhythm), observed during trunk flexion and extension.[9] During spine flexion and extension, it is essential to identify the major motion segments—80% to 90% of the motion in the lumbosacral spine should be at L4–L5 and L5–S1.[9] Migration of the motion upward toward the thoracolumbar junction, altered tone of the paraspinal muscles, and lack of a springing sensation in the lower spine during anterior glides (placement and release of pressure along the spine while the patient is in a relaxed, prone position) suggest spinal segmental dysfunction. Weakness of abdominal muscle and thoracolumbar fascia further indicates that the spine is in need of conditioning.[38] Many individuals who appear to be otherwise highly fit from constant aerobic exercise fail to perform regular exercise that conditions the supportive musculature of the spine. In the young runner with back pain, provocative tests such as extending the spine while standing on one leg help to identify active posterior element irritation and/or symptomatic spondylolysis.

A brief neurologic exam is recommended. The elderly patient with "hip pain" may have unrecognized spinal stenosis. The young runner with a "chronic hamstring strain" may have an unrecognized S1 radiculopathy.[5] Cutaneous nerve injuries also need to be considered. Careful evaluation of a persistently

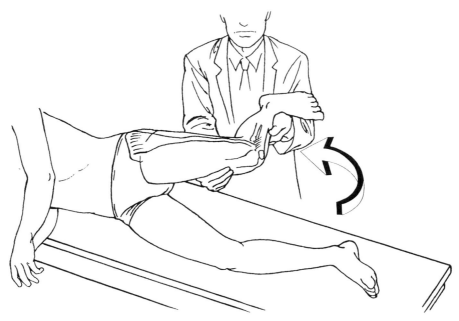

FIGURE 2. Ober's test: The leg is passively abducted and extended. Then the knee is flexed, and the examiner lets the leg drop. Failure to drop in this position is a sign of a tight tensor fascia lata. (From Buschbacher RM (ed): *Musculoskeletal Disorders: A Practical Guide for Diagnosis and Rehabilitation.* Stoneham, MA, Butterworth-Heinemann, 1994, with permission.)

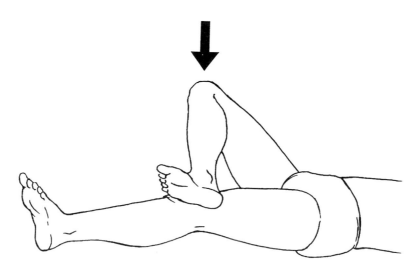

FIGURE 3. The FABER (*F*lexion, *Ab*duction, *E*xternal *R*otation) test: The leg is crossed over the opposite knee in the "figure 4" position. The examiner presses the knee towards the table. Pain in the groin or the buttock is an indication of hip or sacroiliac joint pathology respectively. (From Buschbacher RM (ed): *Musculoskeletal Disorders: A Practical Guide for Diagnosis and Rehabilitation.* Stoneham, MA, Butterworth-Heinemann, 1994, with permission.)

painful ankle with an apparently healed inversion sprain may reveal ongoing irritation of the superficial peroneal nerve. Persistent medial foreleg pain in the presence of a negative bone scan may be related to saphenous nerve irritation rather than shin splints. Finally, the running shoes should be inspected for signs of breakdown and correct fit for the runner's foot. In general, pronation is controlled better with a straight board-lasted shoe with good rearfoot control, whereas the supinator does better with a flexible and curve-lasted shoe.[8,13,43]

The initial encounter is concluded with assessment of the need for psychoemotional support. Some athletes experience considerable emotional disturbance in response to injury.[41,42] In a study using the Emotional Response to Injury Questionnaire and Profile of Mood States, elevated levels of frustration and anger were recorded early after injury. The athlete's perception of injury severity and the likelihood of recovery were direct modifiers of the response.[41,42]

REHABILITATION

Our rehabilitation scheme is based on the work of Kibler, Press, and Herring.[14,18–21,35] It requires a thorough understanding of applied anatomy and biomechanics as well as the ability to recognize the patterns of musculoskeletal adaptations and injury responses to training overload, (a substantial component of the errors of training). Description of the scheme is followed by application to a select number of common running injuries.

Step 1: Accurate Diagnosis. Inherent in this task is recognizing how muscle overload and tendon injuries may present. When the musculotendinous unit is subjected to tensile overload, damage at the cellular level impairs performance and produces symptoms of pain, dysfunction or instability.[18–20] If the extent of overload is small (microtear) and nutrition and time for healing are adequate, activity may be safely resumed. In the presence of inadequate healing or further injury (macrotear), however, subclinical adaptations such as loss of strength and flexibility, development of scar tissue, and strength imbalances develop.[18–20] This leads to further decrements in performance and biomechanic substitutions that perpetuate this "negative feedback vicious cycle" and create more overload and injury.[18–20] Muscle injury may therefore present as acute or chronic, as exacerbation of a chronic injury, or as a subclinical injury.[20] Tendon injuries present as either an inflammatory process superimposed on acute or chronic injury (tendinitis) or as a product of maladaption and intratendinous degeneration unaccompanied by mediators of inflammation (tendinosis).[19,24] In tendinitis, the immediate goal of treatment is relief of symptoms, whereas in tendinosis the immediate goal is restoration of function.[19] Identification of the components of musculotendinous injury within the vicious cycle yields an accurate diagnosis and understanding of the functional consequences that need to be addressed. The components of injury are as follows[18–21,35]:

Tissue injury complex—the area of actual tissue disruption

Clinical symptom complex—the symptoms associated with dysfunction and injury

Tissue overload complex—the tissue group subjected to tensile overload

Functional biomechanical deficit—inflexibilities and/or muscle strength imbalances that create altered mechanics

Functional adaptation complex—functional substitutions used by the athlete in an attempt to maintain performance

Step 2: Acute Management. Efforts are directed toward minimizing the effects of inflammation and controlling pain. The PRICE principle (Protection, Relative rest, Ice, Compression, and Elevation) is followed, and anti-inflammatory medications and pain-relieving modalities may be used.[14,20,35,37,47] In addition, this may be a key time to enlist the assistance of a counselor or sports psychologist to facilitate the development of coping skills and to assist with focusing on rehabilitation.

Step 3. Initial Rehabilitation. This phase continues to focus on promotion of proper healing. Restoration of motion helps to reduce the effects of immobilization; controlled tensile loading promotes ordered collagen growth and alignment. Identification of correctable biomechanic imbalances is initiated.

Step 4. Correction of Imbalances. Development of symmetric motion and strength is the goal. When the patient is pain-free and nearly full concentric strength is achieved, it is essential to initiate an eccentric strengthening program. This critical step helps to develop a musculotendinous unit that is less likely to fail in the face of future tensile stresses. Flaws in running style and training practices are identified if the patient is capable of full weight-bearing under controlled conditions. Alternative aerobic conditioning exercises are encouraged.

Step 5. Reacquisition of Endurance (return to normal function). Cross-training, aqua training, and use of stationary ski machines give way to a gradual increase in the amount of land-based activity and eventual resumption of full activity.

SPECIFIC RUNNING INJURY EVALUATION

Hamstring Strain

Strains are the most common type of hamstring injury, and the short head of the biceps femoris is the most frequent site.[37,42] Injury may occur anywhere along the course of the muscle but is more common at the proximal musculotendinous junction. Injuries are more likely to occur at higher running speeds because less time is spent in support phase. This shorter interval subjects the hamstrings to greater angular velocities and greater forces at the time of heel strike.[1] Hamstring strains are associated with inadequate flexibility, inadequate warm-up, quadriceps-hamstrings strength imbalances, previous injury, and poor muscular coordination.[1,35,37,47]

Method of presentation—acute traumatic injury[35]

Tissue injury complex—myotendinous junction disruption in the upper third of the muscle secondary to eccentric overload.

Clinical symptom complex—pain in the proximal thigh, hamstring weakness, posterior thigh ecchymosis, posterior thigh mass, difficulty sitting.

Functional biomechanical deficit—decreased knee extension, poorer hamstring to quadriceps strength ratio (normally about 0.6), increased hip flexion.[35]

Functional adaptation complex—reduced stride length

Tissue overload complex—myotendinous junction[35]

Rehabilitation

Initial treatment consists of PRICE, cane- or crutch-walking in more severe injuries, and gentle ranging of the injured leg.[35,47] Isometric strengthening is introduced when the athlete is pain-free. For full stretching of the hamstrings, the athlete must be able to maintain knee extension with the hip flexed to 90° and the ankle dorsiflexed. This is done most safely with the patient starting from a supine position. When full muscle length is achieved, alternative conditioning exercises such as bi-

cycling without toe clips (to reduce hamstring contribution to the cycling effort) may be started. Return to running is considered only with full range of motion, achievement of at least 90% of uninjured leg strength, and equalization of the quadriceps:hamstring strength ratios.[35,37,47] Full activity must not be resumed prematurely, because the risk of recurrent injury is high.

Patellofemoral Pain Syndrome

Patellofemoral pain syndrome is often cited as the most common knee problem in runners.[36] The athlete complains of pain, crepitation, and, often, swelling. Reaction forces of the patellofemoral joint are increased markedly during the single-leg support phase because the quadriceps contract vigorously while the knee is in flexion.[7,36] Previously mentioned predisposing factors include the presence of patella alta, increased Q angle, and weakness of the vastus medialis obliquus. Relative tightness of the lateral retinacula also induces a tracking problem.[7]

Method of presentation—chronic overload injury[35]

Tissue injury complex—patellar cartilage and synovium, insertion site of patellar tendon[35]

Clinical symptom complex—positive theater sign, peripatellar pain worsened with flexion, pain with descending stairs, crepitus

Functional biomechanical deficit—medial quadriceps insufficiency; inflexibility of lateral retinacula, iliotibial band, hamstrings, and gastrocnemius; abnormal patellar tracking; hamstring weakness[35]

Functional adaptation complex—flexion contracture, altered stride to avoid full loading of knee

Tissue overload complex—patellar tendon, lateral retinaculum

Rehabilitation

PRICE and antiinflammatory medications are initiated. Problems with the malalignment syndrome must be corrected. Consideration is given to fitting the runner for orthotics only if biomechanic deficits persist after achieving full flexibility of the gastroc-soleus complex, hamstrings, and iliotibial band and full strength training of the vastus medialis obliquus (VMO). Taping of the patella to simulate proper alignment, accompanied by neuromuscular reeducation of the knee musculature (McConnell technique), may also be beneficial.[27] Patellar stabilizing braces may be considered but should not be the first plan of attack. Strengthening of the VMO is facilitated via short arc (<30° flexion to full extension) quadriceps exercises.[7] Adductor squeezes, and short-arc knee extensions with closed kinetic chain also help with VMO training.

Iliotibial Band Friction Syndrome

The iliotibial band (ITB), the extension of the tensor fascia lata (TFL) down the lateral leg, inserts into Gerdy's tubercle along the lateral tibia. This syndrome is associated with painful sensation as the ITB slides back and forth over the lateral femoral condyle with knee flexion and extension.[28,31,44] Running on beveled surfaces, limb-length discrepancies, tibia vara, hyperpronation and ITB contracture are associated risk factors.[28,44]

> *Method of presentation*—exacerbation of a chronic overuse injury
> *Tissue injury complex*—ITB over the femoral condyle or at Gerdy's tubercle
> *Clinical symptom complex*—localized pain over the lateral femoral condyle, positive Ober's test and Noble compression test, worsening with running
> *Functional biomechanical deficit*—inflexible ITB
> *Functional adaptation complex*—functional pronation of the foot, external rotation at the hip, internal rotation of the leg, lateral patellar tracking[35]
> *Tissue overload complex*—varus loading on lateral knee

Rehabilitation

PRICE and antiinflammatory medications, as needed, are the initial steps, with attempts to stretch the ITB, hip flexors, and gluteus maximus. Foot pronation must be corrected, and the patient must run only on level surfaces, if at all. Swimming and stationary ski machines help to maintain fitness. Strengthening of the hip adductors, gluteus maximus, and TFL is emphasized. The adductors counter the pull of the tight ITB and the other muscles that give rise to the ITB (gluteus maximus and TFL) and must be strength-

ened to avoid overuse.[35] Symptoms may take as long as 2 to 6 months to resolve.[44] Occasionally, local injection of a combination of anesthetic agent and corticosteroid in the region of the lateral femoral condyle is helpful.[35]

Plantar Fasciitis

Plantar fasciitis consists of traction-induced microtears of the plantar fascia and associated structures at its insertion on the calcaneus.[23] Ordinarily, the fascia tightens passively with toe extension, resulting in arch elevation (windlass effect). Limited ankle dorsiflexion, a tight gastroc-soleus complex, and excessive pronation increase the chance of developing plantar fasciitis because pronation decreases the chance of achieving the rigid close-packed midtarsal joint needed to push off the ground. This subjects other support structures, such as medial portion of the plantar fascia, to greater tensile forces. Plantar fasciitis is usually seen with high or normal arches but may also be seen with flat feet. Patients present with progressively worsening pain and the "dreaded first step of the morning."

> *Method of presentation*—chronic injury
> *Clinical symptom complex*—point tenderness along the medial fascia, inability to run, painful fist step in the morning
> *Functional biomechanical deficit*—decreased plantar flexor flexibility and strength, functional pronation[21]
> *Functional adaptation complex*—forefoot running with choppy stride and attempted inversion[21,35]
> *Tissue overload complex*—eccentric overload of plantar flexor with continued running

Rehabilitation

PRICE (ice massage) and antiinflammatory medications, as needed, are the initial steps. Consideration is given to steroid injection into the calcaneal attachment.[21] Arch supports, counterforce taping, and heel pads may be helpful.[20,21,35] The critical measures are stretching of the gastroc-soleus complex, hamstrings, and plantar fascia and intrinsic strengthening of the foot, not merely support of the longitudinal arch.[21] This injury can take 3 to 4 months to resolve in chronic cases; in our experience, formulation of alternative aerobic conditioning programs (i.e., rowing, swimming, aqua running, and occasionally cycling) are well tolerated.

Achilles Tendinitis and Tendinosis

Achilles tendinitis and tendinosis are the most common injuries of the ankle-foot. Repeated episodes of microtrauma result in microtearing of the tendon in the region of least vascularity, or approximately 2 to 6 cm above the tendon insertion.[19,35] Excessive pronation, tight heel cords, and rearfoot or forefoot varus can induce this problem,[35] along with overtraining, a single excessively strenuous workout, and hill running. It is important to recognize that although the majority of patients feel that they have an acute inflammatory problem (tendinitis), in fact, they probably have a chronic problem (tendinosis), in which asymptomatic intratendinous degeneration has occurred over time.[24]

> *Method of presentation*—acute exacerbation of a chronic problem
>
> *Tissue injury complex*—myotendinous junction of the Achilles tendon
>
> *Clinical symptom complex*—pain 6 to 8 cm proximal to the insertion on the calcaneus, worsened with dorsiflexion[35]
>
> *Functional biomechanical deficit*—weak dorsiflexors, tight plantar flexors
>
> *Functional adaptation complex*—increased knee flexion and pronation
>
> *Tissue overload complex*—gastroc-soleus and Achilles tendon

Rehabilitation

PRICE and antiinflammatory medications are started immediately. The tendon is never injected. Heel lifts often provide some relief in early rehabilitation but should not be used indefinitely, because they promote shortening of the heel cord. Ultrasound may be useful in chronic cases where loosening of old, scarred connective tissue is needed and stretching is difficult.[35] Reduction in weight-bearing activity is mandatory. These patients are good candidates for aquatic-based conditioning. As pain is reduced, the patients should go through a gradual program of first concentric and ultimately eccentric strengthening of the plantar flexors. When pain continues despite all the above measures, magnetic resonance imaging of the Achilles

tendon may reveal previously unidentified partial tendon tears, musculotendinous tears, retrocalcaneal bursitis, or stress fractures.[24,35]

Stress Fractures

A stress fracture is defined as a partial or complete fracture of bone that results from the inability of the bony region to withstand a repetitively applied subthreshold and nonviolent mechanical stress.[26] Runners at risk are those who have asymmetric limb lengths, pronate excessively, or run on rigid surfaces.[11,26] The tibia is the most common site (34%), followed by the fibula (24%), metatarsals (20%), and femur (14%).[26] Pain that is relatively well localized is a major clinical feature.[26] Pain produced over the suspected fracture site with application of a vibrating tuning fork to the affected area or with percussion of the bone away from the affected site may also suggest stress fracture.[37] Because they frequently do not produce a full cortical defect, stress fractures are difficult to detect by routine radiograph early in their course.[6] Bone scans are recommended in cases of increased clinical suspicion when the plain film study is negative.[6]

> *Method of presentation*—chronic overuse injury[35]
>
> *Tissue injury complex*—local bone[35]
>
> *Clinical symptom complex*—localized pain that tends to worsen with a reproducible amount of activity and is relieved by rest[35]
>
> *Functional biomechanical deficit*—dictated by the site of fracture
>
> *Functional adaptation complex*—dictated by fracture site
>
> *Tissue overload complex*—bone

Rehabilitation

The first principle of rehabilitation is to stay below the level of activity that induces symptoms. Running on dry land is prohibited until an adequate amount of time for healing has passed—approximately 3 weeks for the fibula, 4 to 8 weeks for the tibia (although considerably longer if the tibial plateau has been affected), and months (with limited weight-bearing) for the neck of the femur.[26,35] In the past, athletes with stress fractures were primarily restricted to alternative forms of aerobic exercises, such as swimming and bicycling, which were of general conditioning value but were not particularly specific to running.

In recent years, aqua running has become available. The runner dons an inflatable vest and is placed into the deep end of the pool so that the feet are not in contact with the bottom. He or she is then tethered to a side of the pool and begins to "run." The viscosity and drag of the water provide resistance proportional to the effort, whereas the buoyancy effect maintains non–weight-bearing conditions.[45] The reader is also referred to the chapter on aqua running in this text.

The physiologic response to running in water is somewhat different from that of running on land. Because of improved venous return, an increase in central blood volume[4,45] results in an increased stroke volume and a reduced heart rate at a given level of oxygen consumption.[45] Maximal heart rate and maximal oxygen consumption values tend to be lower with aqua running, but rating of perceived exertion at a similar submaximal oxygen consumption value tends to be higher.[45] Aqua jogging can also be performed with the person touching pool bottom or on aqua treadmills in limited weight-bearing situations. This technology allows for more sport-specific rehabilitation with earlier return to preinjury form.

CONCLUSION

Running is a classic example of an activity that places constant repetitive stress on the musculoskeletal system. An understanding of training techniques, biomechanics, structures susceptible to overload injury, and factors that motivate the individual patient to run on a regular basis will lead to successful rehabilitation.

REFERENCES

1. Agre JC: Hamstring injuries: Proposed aetiological factors, prevention and treatment. *Sports Med* 2:21–33, 1985.
2. Apple DF Jr: Adolescent runners. *Clin Sports Med* 4:641–655, 1985.
3. Apple DF Jr: End stage running problems. *Clin Sports Med* 4:657–670, 1985.
4. Astrand PO, Rodahl K: *Textbook of Work Physiology*. New York, McGraw Hill, 1986.
5. Bach DK, Green DS, Jensen GM, Savinar E. A comparison of muscular tightness in runners and nonrunners and the relation of muscular tightness to low back pain in runners. *J Orthop Sports Phys Ther* 6:315–323, 1985.
6. Belkin SC: Stress fractures in athletes. *Orthop Clin North Am* 11:735–742, 1980.
7. Bourne MH, Hazel WA, Scot SG, Sim FH: Anterior knee pain. *Mayo Clin Proc* 63:482–491, 1988.
8. Brody DM: Running injuries. *Clin Symp* 39(3):2–36, 1987.
9. Cailliet R: *Low Back Pain Syndrome*. Philadelphia, F.A. Davis, 1989.
10. Cox JS: Patellofemoral problems in runners. *Clin Sports Med* 4:699–715, 1985.
11. Daffner RH: Stress fractures: Current concepts. *Skel Radiol* 2:221–229, 1978.
12. D'Ambrosia RD: Orthotic devices and running injuries. *Clin Sports Med* 4:611–618, 1985.
13. Gross ML, Dalvin LB, Evanski PM: Effectiveness of orthotic shoe inserts in the long distance runner. *Am J Sports Med* 19:409–412, 1991.
14. Herring SA, Kibler WB: Rehabilitation. In Cantu RC, Micheli LJ (eds): *ACSM's Guidelines For the Team Physician*. Philadelphia, Lea & Febiger, 1991, pp 191–195.
15. Hoeberigs JH: Factors related to the incidence of running injuries. *Sports Med* 13(6):408–422, 1992.
16. Jacobs SJ, Berson BL: Injuries to runners: A study of entrants to a 10,000 meter race. *Am J Sports Med* 14:151–155, 1986.
17. James SL, Bates BT, Osterning LR: Injuries to runners. *Am J Sports Med* 6:40–50, 1978.
18. Kibler WB: Clinical aspects of muscle injury. *Med Sci Sports Exerc* 22:450–452, 1990.
19. Kibler WB, Chandler TJ, Pace BK: Principles of rehabilitation after chronic tendon injuries. *Clin Sports Med* 11:661–671, 1992.
20. Kibler WB, Chandler TJ, Stracener ES: Musculoskeletal adaptations and injuries due to overtraining. *Exerc Sports Sci Rev* 20:99–126, 1992.
21. Kibler WB, Goldberg C, Chandler TJ: Functional biomechanical deficits in running athletes with plantar fasciitis. *Am J Sports Med* 19:66–71, 1991.
22. Kuland DN: *The Injured Athlete*, 2nd ed. Philadelphia, J.B. Lippincott, 1988.
23. Kwong PK, Kay D, Voner RT, Whitte MW: Plantar fasciitis: Mechanics and pathomechanics of treatment. *Clin Sports Med* 7:119–127, 1988.
24. Leadbetter WB: Cell-matrix response in tendon injury. *Clin Sports Med* 11:533–578, 1992.
25. Lutter LD: The knee and running. *Clin Sports Med* 4:685–698, 1985.
26. McBryde AM: Stress fractures in runners. *Clin Sports Med* 4:737–752, 1985.
27. McConnell J: The management of chondromalacia patellae: A long term solution. *Aus J Phys* 32:215–219, 1986.
28. Messier SP, Pittala KA: Etiologic factors associated with selected running injuries. *Med Sci Sports Exerc* 20:501–505, 1988.
29. Newell SG: Functional neutral orthoses and shoe modifications. *Phys Med Rehab Clin North Am* 3:193–222, 1992.
30. Newell SG, Bramwell ST: Overuse injuries to the knee in runners. *Physician Sports Med* 12:81–92, 1984.
31. Noble CA: Iliotibial band friction syndrome in runners. *Am J Sports Med* 8:232–234, 1980.

32. O'Neill DB, Micheli LJ: Overuse injuries in the young athlete. *Clin Sports Med* 7:591–610, 1988.
33. O'Toole ML: Prevention and treatment of injuries to runners. *Med Sci Sports Exerc* 24:S360–S363, 1992.
34. Paty JG Jr: Diagnosis and treatment of musculoskeletal running injuries. *Semin Arthritis Rheum* 18:48–60, 1988.
35. Press JM, Herring SA, Kibler WB: *Rehabilitation of Musculoskeletal Disorders.* United States Army (In press).
36. Putnam CA, Kozey JW: Substantive issues in running. In Vaughn CL (ed): *Biomechanics of Sport.* Boca Raton, FL, CRC Press, 1989, pp 2–33.
37. Roy S, Irvin R: *Sports Medicine.* Englewood Cliffs, NJ, Prentice-Hall, 1983.
38. Saal JA; Rehabilitation of sports-related lumbar spine injuries. *Phys Med Rehabil State Art Rev* 1:613–638, 1987.
39. Sheehan GA: An overview of overuse syndromes in distance runners. *Ann NY Acad Sci* 301:877–880, 1977.
40. Shuster R, Children's foot survey. *J Podiat Soc NY* 17:13, 1956.
41. Smith AM, Scott SG, O'Fallon WM, Young ML: Emotional responses of athletes to injury. *Mayo Clin Proc* 65:38–50, 1990.
42. Smith AM, Scott SG, Wiese DM: The psychological effects of sports injuries. *Sports Med* 9(6):352–369, 1990.
43. Subotnick SI: The biomechanics of running. *Sports Med* 2:144–153, 1985.
44. Sutker AN, Barber FA, Jackson DW, Pagliano JW: Iliotibial band syndrome in distance runners. *Sports Med* 4(7):447–451, 1985.
45. Svedenhag J, Seger J: Running on land and in water: comparative exercise physiology. *Med Sci Sports Exerc* 24:1155–1160, 1992.
46. van Mechelen W, Hlobil H, Zijlstra WP, et al: Is range of motion at the hip and ankle joint related to running injuries? *J Sports Med* 13:605–610, 1992.
47. Young JL, Laskowski ER, Rock MG: Thigh injuries in athletes. *Mayo Clin Proc* 68(11):1099–1106, 1993.

Chapter 9

PREVENTION AND TREATMENT OF BICYCLE INJURIES

Randall L. Braddom, MD

The bicycle is the most efficient means of human-powered locomotion. In underdeveloped nations, bicycling and walking remain the major forms of transportation. More people in the world ride bicycles than any other type of vehicle or animal.

In developed nations such as the United States, bicycling was one of the most popular sports until the early 1920s. With the advent of the automobile and the airplane, adults lost interest in the bicycle. Over the past few decades, bicycling has become increasingly popular once again, both for transportation and recreation. The bicycle's current resurgence of use for commuting and for general transportation is likely due to the fitness movement, the environmental movement, and recent remarkable improvements in bicycle technology.

It is estimated that there are over 85 million bicycles in the United States, and 750,000 new ones are sold each year in the state of New York alone.[11] There are 90 million to 100 million cyclists in the United States, and 20 million children ride a bicycle more than once a week.[29,34] Bicycling is more popular in Europe and Asia than in the United States. At least 82% of the population in Sweden uses bicycles, compared with 30% in the United States.[25]

Bicycling combines efficient transportation with exercise and fun, but it also can lead to many types of accidents and injuries. Trauma and overuse are the two major causes of injuries in bicyclists. The traumatic injuries can be due to falls, running into an object, or being struck by another bicycle or vehicle. Trau-

matic injuries range from minor scrapes to major trauma or even death. Overuse injuries range from minor saddle soreness to stress fractures. This chapter outlines preventive measures to reduce bicycle accidents and injuries and presents treatment alternatives for the most common bicycle-related medical problems.

SURVEY OF THE CENTRAL INDIANA BICYCLE ASSOCIATION

To gather information for this report, a survey was mailed to the first 500 members of the Central Indiana Bicycle Association (CIBA), who were listed alphabetically in the 1992 membership directory (permission granted by CIBA). The members of CIBA are on-road bicyclists; the survey was not expected to reflect the experience of off-road bicyclists. The survey consisted of 2 pages containing 21 questions. An introductory page explained the survey's purpose and provided directions. A postage-paid return envelope was included. All responses were anonymous.

Before the mailing, the survey was tested on 10 bicyclists and final revisions were made. The questions were either forced choice or open-ended. The mailing was done in late 1992, and responses were returned by 269 CIBA members. The return rate of 54% was considered excellent for a single mailing. The characteristics of the nonresponders are unknown.

Table 1 lists the ages, heights, and weights of the respondents. The broad appeal of bicy-

TABLE 1. Height, Weight and Age of the 269 Respondents of the Central Indiana Bicycle Association Survey

	Women	Men
Number	79	190
Age range (yrs)	17–63	17–76
Age mean (yrs)	40	43
Height range (in)	60–71	60–81
Height mean (in)	66	71
Weight range (lbs)	104–205	130–265
Weight mean (lbs)	138	181
Weight/height (lbs/in)	2.09	2.55

TABLE 2. Bicycling Experience in the Last 12 Months in 269 CIBA Survey Respondents

	Miles/Week	Years	Longest Ride (*mi*)
Range	10–350	1–30	5–283
Mean	87	8	76

cling is indicated by ages that ranged from 17 to 76 years. Practitioners treating bicyclists must deal with all ages, from toddlers riding passively on a bicycle to older adults in their eighth decade and beyond.

Table 2 lists the miles of cycling per week reported by CIBA members, which ranged from 10 to 350 (mean, 87). They reported serious interest in bicycling for 1 to 30 years (mean=8 years). Their longest ride in calendar year 1991 ranged from 5 to 283 miles (mean, 76 mi).

Types of Bicycles

Cyclists have never enjoyed a wider selection of types, styles, and brands of bicycles. Over the past three decades, frame materials have improved to allow lighter bikes with equal or greater frame strength. Light weight is a distinct advantage in cycling, and a relatively small increase in price greatly reduces the weight of the frame and other components. The least expensive bicycle frames are typically made of steel, whereas slightly more expensive ones are made from aluminum or an alloy of chromium and molybdenum (often called chromolly). Space-age materials such as carbon fibers and composites allow even lighter bicycles, but as yet they are too expensive for widespread use.

Bicycle gearing systems have improved dramatically in the last decade. The majority of bicycles sold currently (except racing types) have 15 to 18 speeds. Many have a very low gear ("granny gear") that permits climbing steep hills without having to stand up and pump and thus reduces stress on the knees. Modern gearing systems also have derailleurs with definite stops or clicks that allow quick shifts without the necessity of using the gear lever to search for the gear.

Racing bicycles have a light, short, stiff frame and light-weight components. Because weight is a major factor in racing success, components such as fenders, padded seats, and kickstands are not used. Thin (20–25 mm), high-pressure tires and alloy wheels are used to reduce weight and rolling resistance. Drop handlebars allow the rider to get the trunk into as much of a horizontal position as possible to lower wind resistance.

Touring bicycles (Fig. 1) are similar to racing bicycles, but have less stiff frames and a longer wheelbase to increase shock absorption. They have some loss of cornering finesse compared with a racing frame. Typical touring bike components include padded seats, kickstands, luggage racks, front and rear panniers, lights, short fenders, and water bottles. Touring bikes are designed to be comfortable on long trips and to be strong enough to carry personal gear. Tires are usually 1 to 2 inches in width.

The **mountain bike** is a relatively new type of bicycle invented for off-road use over dirt trails and other rough terrain. The main characteristic of the mountain bike is its strength, because it must withstand off-road use and intentional jumps over obstacles. It also has a relatively flattened frame designed to absorb shock. The brakes are the center-pull cantilever type that are heavier and stronger than the side-pull caliper brakes on most other types of bicycles. Mountain bikes have standard rather than dropped handlebars, and the rider sits in a relatively upright position. The tires are usually 1.5 to 2.2 in wide and have a knobby tread for off-road traction.

In the past few years a hybrid, or **city bike,** has become popular; it combines aspects of the mountain and the touring bike. Its standard handlebars allow the rider to sit fairly erect. The brakes are stronger than on a touring bike. The frame and wheels are built to withstand potholes on rough city streets, but the rolling resistance is less than for a mountain bike.

A less common type of bike is the **recumbent,** which allows the rider to sit close to the ground in a seat with a tall backrest. The bicycle is steered with levers mounted near

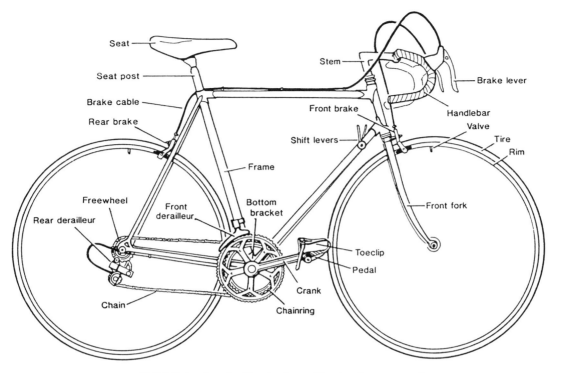

FIGURE 1. Standard touring frame bicycle with components.

the bottom of the seat. The main advantage is greater comfort for riders who have difficulty with neck pain or saddle soreness with other types of bicycles.

A common children's bicycle (especially popular with boys) is the **BMX** (Bicycle Moto Cross). This powerfully built bicycle endures acrobatic jumps and other feats that are typically seen in BMX competitions around the country.

The CIBA survey indicated that 46% of the respondents use a touring bike, 37% a racing bike, 8% a hybrid bike, 6% a mountain bike, and 3% other (Table 3). The "other" bikes were recumbents, tandems, and antique high wheelers. This list reflects the type of bicycles owned by serious on-road adult cyclists in central Indiana, which has flat terrain. Surveys in other parts of the country probably would show different statistics based on terrain and local preferences, particularly in regard to mountain bikes. Sales figures show that mountain bikes now outsell all other types. The hybrid bikes are the second most popular. The mountain and hybrid bikes now outsell other types by about a 5:1 ratio.

Bicycles for adults are usually sold now only with the "boys'" frame. The old style of "girls,'" frame (mixte frame) is inferior in most fundamental characteristics. The stan-

TABLE 3. Type of Bicycles Owned by the 269 CIBA Survey Respondents

Type of Bicycle	No.	%
Touring	130	46
Racing	105	37
Hybrid	22	8
Mountain	17	6
Other	8	3
TOTAL	282	100

dard frame is recommended for both men and women, although some manufacturers still produce a "women's" frame for the few women who prefer it. The women's frame is a relic of an age when women were socially required to wear dresses or skirts while bicycling.

BICYCLE SAFETY AND ACCIDENT PREVENTION

Statistics on Bicycle Accidents and Deaths

The statistics on cycling trauma in the United States are startling. In 1990, 580,000 bicyclists were treated in emergency rooms.[29]

Over 800 bicyclists were killed in 1989, and almost one-half were children under 14 years of age. More children are killed and injured each year on bikes than on skateboards, roller skates, big wheels, and scooters combined. Of the deaths reported in bicyclists, 400 occurred in children under the age of 14 years, and 360 were the result of motor vehicle collisions. Whereas motor vehicle collisions account for only 10% of childhood bike-related injuries, they account for 90% of bicycle-related deaths. Head injuries account for 75% of all deaths of cyclists and 70% of all hospitalizations.[29] Bicycle accidents are the leading cause of head injury in school-aged children.[37]

Bike-related deaths and injuries in children under age 14 years occur most commonly between 3 and 6 p.m. on Fridays, primarily from May to August when children are out of school. Over 50% of children's deaths are due to riding into the street from a sidewalk or driveway and colliding with a motor vehicle. It has been estimated that the total annual cost of bike-related injuries and deaths for all ages is $7.6 billion.[29]

Riders of BMX bicycles have similar accident statistics on the road,[44] but the injury rate appears to be much higher during BMX cycling competitions. A study of 976 participants in the European BMX Cycling Championship in 1989 showed that 6.3% sustained an injury. Approximately half of the injuries required medical attention, and 3.3% required hospital admission.[6] Most of the injuries in BMX competition were minor, but 6.6% were fractures. BMX competition has a higher risk of injury than road use. During the European BMX Cycling Championship the risk rate was calculated as 1,190 injuries per 1,000 competition hours.[6]

A recent follow-up of 372 children admitted to a hospital after bicycle crashes revealed that 3.2% had died and 1.4% remained institutionalized because of severe impairment from cervical spinal and head injuries. An additional 33% had a persistent disability. Cognitive or behavioral changes were noted in 32%; the most frequent was worsening of school performance.[28] Children riding passively in bicycle-mounted seats are also at risk of injury. The actual number of injuries to children in bicycle carrier seats is unknown, but the US Consumer Product Safety Commission estimates at least 500 such injuries/year. The most frequent age at injury is 2 years, and the most common mechanism of injury is a fall

(80%).[32] The inherent problem of carrying a child in a bicycle-mounted seat is that in a crash the child's body is struck with biomechanic forces resulting from adult-level kinetic energy.[32] The position of the child also raises the cycle's center of gravity and may make falls more likely.

Because alcohol is a significant factor in almost all types of accidents, it is suspected to play a role in bicycle accidents as well. In a recent study in Finland,[30] a breathalyzer was used on cyclists who arrived at the hospital within 6 hours of an accident. The results were compared with a control group of cyclists tested at random on the street. Of those involved in accidents, 24% had a significant alcohol level compared with only 4% of controls. The estimated risk of injury for an inebriated bicyclist was at least tenfold higher at blood alcohol levels above 100 mg/dL compared with a sober bicyclist. Alcohol tended to increase the bicyclist's risk of injury from falls more than from collisions.

The CIBA survey showed that 70% of the respondents had had at least 1 accident or injury during their riding career, and 65% reported at least 1 accident in calendar year 1991. These figures suggest that CIBA members (who are generally experienced riders) average 1 accident for every 94 miles of riding.

CIBA members reported that accidents were due to many factors. The most common were sliding on a turn because of gravel, ice, leaves, or wet pavement (n=29); striking or being struck by another bike (n=22); being hit by or forced off the road by a car or truck (n=22); encounter with a dog (n=21); and getting the wheels caught or losing balance at the road-shoulder interface (n=13). Less common causes included falls while crossing a railroad track (n=6), accidentally hitting the curb (n=4), hitting a pothole (n=4), and falling while making an emergency stop (n=4). Infrequent causes included falls during bicycle mounting, eye injuries during riding, catching the wheel in a storm grate, hitting a speed bump, and falling off the handlebars while riding as a passenger.

CIBA members reported that the following equipment failures produced an accident: broken crank arm, broken front fork, loosened chain, broken derailleur, collapsed front wheel, blow-out of front tire, and broken spoke(s).

Table 4 lists the most common types of fracture injuries suffered by CIBA members from bicycle accidents. Seventeen CIBA mem-

TABLE 4. **Types of Injuries Reported by the 269 CIBA Survey Respondents***

Type	No.
Bruises	24
Fracture of upper extremity	4
Fracture of lower extremity	1
Fracture of spine	1
Other	24

*175 (65%) reported having an accident in calendaryear 1991.

bers had fractures (most commonly in the upper extremities and clavicle); 3 reported being unconscious at the scene of the accident; and 9 had joint injuries, including shoulder separations, shoulder dislocations, and internal derangement of the knee. The pattern of accidents in CIBA riders is fairly similar to that reported in the literature.[12]

Facial and eye injuries are also common. CIBA members reported 7 injuries that required facial sutures, 5 instances of facial abrasions, and 2 instances of fractured teeth. Eye injuries can occur because of falls or running into overhanging objects such as branches or brush. More commonly, eye injuries are due to flying objects, ranging from insects to gravel. Particularly dangerous are small rocks lodged in mud on or between truck tires, which can be thrown backward toward a bicyclist when they dislodge (often when the truck hits a bump in the road). It is important for cyclists to wear protective eyewear. Wraparound styles provide the best protection, but the most important characteristic is that they must be shatter-proof.

The most common bicycle injury is an abrasion of the skin,[4] commonly known as "road rash." Most abrasions are not reported to physicians. They can be graded with the system used for burns: first-degree abrasions are superficial; second-degree, partial thickness; and third-degree, full thickness. Considerable cleansing is necessary to remove road dust, grit, and gravel. Once cleaned, abrasions can be treated as any other open wound. Failure to remove all road grit may leave particles permanently embedded in the skin, perhaps causing a serious cosmetic problem, depending on the location.

The Importance of Visibility

One of the most common reasons for accidents is that bicyclists are struck by drivers who simply do not see them. This type of accident can happen in broad daylight, but it is especially likely at dusk or at night. Being hit by a motor vehicle is perhaps the most dangerous accident that can happen to a bicyclist. Approximately one-half of the hospital admissions that result from cycling accidents involve motor vehicles.[26]

CIBA riders reported 22 accidents due to being hit or forced off the road surface to avoid being hit. In most cases the driver did not see the bicyclist, but in a few cases the bicyclist failed to follow traffic laws. Drivers tend to watch for other autos and trucks, but it is not in their mindset to scan the environment for smaller vehicles.

Bicyclists must endeavor at all times to make themselves as visible as possible. Bicycles should be equipped with reflectors that are visible in all directions. A bright front light and a red tail light are the minimum for use at night. The rider should wear brightly colored clothing for day riding and light or even white clothing at night. Visibility at night can be enhanced by reflective clothing or by adding reflective strips to clothing, helmet, and shoes. A flashing light, especially a strobe light, improves both daytime and nighttime visibility. Additional methods include mounting brightly colored triangular flags on tall stanchions and even using plastic windmill devices to attract attention. All of these measures make the rider more visible to drivers, other bicyclists, and pedestrians.

Bicyclists should ride defensively and assume that others do not see them. When possible, it is advisable for bicyclists to watch the eyes of drivers of oncoming vehicles to make certain that they have been noticed.[26]

Being Heard

One of the major environmental advantages of bicycles is that they are relatively silent vehicles. In some circumstances, however, this can be a major problem. Perhaps the most common example occurs when a bicyclist is trying to pass pedestrians or other bicyclists. Because they cannot hear the bicycle approaching, they are not prepared to stay in their lane of travel or to yield the right of way. A number of tactics have evolved to deal with this problem. The most popular is simply to say something like "passing on your left." A less useful method is to play music that is audible to anyone nearby. Horns mounted on the bicycle or bicyclist, which can now generate a sound volume up to 100 dB, are particularly helpful in dealing with vehicular traffic on busy streets.

Mechanical Bicycle Safety

Defective equipment is a common cause of bicycle accidents. Routine maintenance by either an experienced hobbyist or a professional repairman is essential. It should include an annual tune-up before the start of each year's riding season. Depending on frequency of use, more frequent maintenance may be required. This includes replacement of worn or defective parts such as tires, brakes, and cables. Keeping the bicycle in good operating condition adds not only to safety, but also to the enjoyment of riding. Defective or worn parts can fail and cause an accident at any time. They are particularly likely to cause a problem during a sudden stop or turn, when the bicycle is under maximal stress.

Routine maintenance should also include a brief safety check of the bicycle before each ride to identify loose or malaligned parts. The inspection should include at a minimum a check of the brake pads, seat, headset, derailleurs, and tires.

Bicycle Helmet

A 1-year case-control study at 5 hospitals in Seattle indicated that wearing bike helmets reduced the risk of head and brain injury by at least 85%.[39] A properly fitted helmet can reduce the G-force to the brain in a crash by a factor of 10.[29] An estimated 83% of the mortality and serious morbidity could be prevented by wearing a helmet. The nonuse of helmets is particularly tragic since the death rate from bicycle injuries among children exceeds the death rate from such causes as accidental poisoning, falls, and gunshot wounds.[23]

Spaite, et al. recently did a prospective study of injured bicyclists to determine the potential benefits of using a helmet.[36] Over a 3-year period the investigators assembled 284 cases in which it could be documented whether or not helmets had been worn. The helmet users had a tendency to suffer much less severe head injury. The mortality was much higher for bicyclists who did not use a helmet (6% compared with 0.9%). Another interesting finding was that riders wearing helmets also suffered less severe injuries in body areas other than the head. It was speculated that at least some of the protection was due to safer riding habits in bicyclists who wear helmets.

The CIBA respondents reported that they wore a helmet while riding 94% of the time (range, 0–100%). This tends to indicate that members of organized bicycling clubs have a much higher rate of helmet use than other cyclists. Nineteen CIBA riders reported that they did not use a helmet for the following reasons; discomfort ($n=9$); forgetfulness ($n=7$) uncosmetic appearance ($n=3$), and failure to match their outfit ($n=1$). Of the 63 (31%) CIBA riders who had been in an accident involving a direct blow to the head, 7 were not wearing a helmet at the time; 14 (22%) reported being unconscious at the scene.

Bicycle helmets have some benefit in reducing upper facial injuries but do not provide significant protection to the lower face.[38] In the future helmets may need to be redesigned or a face bar added to improve facial protection. Protection of the lower face is important because repairs of mandibular fractures and periodontal injury are among the most common operations required after bicycle accidents.[25]

Pediatricians and others have attempted to increase the percentage of children wearing helmets for bicycling.[21] A major project to study strategies for increasing use of helmets was undertaken in Seattle, Washington, in 1986.[2] This study found that parents were not aware of the seriousness of bicycle head injuries or of the protection given by helmets. They also found that a major deterrent to helmet use was cost. Another finding was that children were reluctant to wear helmets unless their peers did. The investigators developed a three-pronged strategy of increasing parent awareness, decreasing the cost of the helmets, and providing incentives to children for using them. The awareness campaign included educational materials at doctors' offices as well as a media blitz. The investigators were also able to reduce the price of helmets for children by offering discount coupons. They were successful in overcoming much of the resistance due to peer group pressure by offering prizes and coupons to helmet wearers. The number of children observed wearing helmets while bicycling in the Seattle area rose from 5% at the beginning of the campaign to 16% approximately 1 year later. Appendix A (p. 148) lists excellent educational sources that can be used in campaigns for bicycle safety awareness to increase helmet use.

A recent study of college students who were cyclists showed that only 31% owned a helmet and only about half of these wore the helmet most of the time while cycling. Eighteen percent of the students had been hospitalized in the previous 5 years as a result of a bicycle injury. Helmet ownership was strongly associated with previous injury. Ethnicity was also a factor: helmets were owned by 38% of white non-Hispanic students, but only 4% of all other ethnic groups combined.[16]

Bicycle accidents during races are a major source of injuries. To preserve their strength, bicycle racers lower wind resistance by riding wheel-to-wheel in a tightly packed group called the "pelaton." If one of them falls, the speed at which they are travelling makes likely a chain reaction in which many other riders will fall as well. Because of this danger, the United States Cycling Federation (USCF) mandated helmet use in all sponsored races in 1986.[33] For a detailed discussion of the physics of bicycle helmet design and use, the reader is referred to the article by Mills.[27]

It is critical to purchase a good helmet with a reliable strap-and-buckle system. A wide variety of types and brands are currently available commercially. Cyclists in the United States should buy only helmets certified by the American National Standards Institute (ANSI) or the Snell Memorial Foundation. Excellent articles on the proper selection and use of helmets were published in the popular press in 1990.[3,18]

Dehydration and Sun Injuries

Severe sunburn is frequently reported by Caucasian and other light-skinned riders. Adequate sun block is essential to prevent this painful and unnecessary problem. The long-term effects of the sun on the skin are well known in the medical community, but this knowledge appears to be getting out to the bicycling community only slowly. Cyclists still have a tendency to admire the rider with the darkest tan. Melanoma has been reported in cyclists.[43] One study has suggested that sunblock lotions may impair evaporation from the skin,[42] but the full implications of this finding are not yet known.

Cyclists frequently underestimate their need for fluid replacement, perhaps because the wind causes rapid evaporation of perspiration. Because of the absence of beads of sweat on the skin, the cyclist may fail to notice how much fluid is lost. In addition cyclists sometimes intentionally underdrink on long trips to avoid rest-room stops. Failure to take in adequate fluid can lead to heat exhaustion or heat stroke. A cyclist should drink enough water to prevent overconcentration of the urine. Bicycles can easily be fitted for water bottles, and most cyclists can easily master the technique of safely drinking water while riding. For long rides in hot conditions (over 2 hours), it may be useful to use liquids that replace electrolytes as well.

Safe Riding Techniques

Safe riding practices should be taught as soon as a child is able to ride a bicycle. Because the median age of bicyclists involved in serious accidents is 10 years, one-half of all accidents occur in bicyclists less than 10 years of age.[43] Children should have some ironclad rules, including no riding on busy streets, no riding at night, no playing on the road, obeying all stop signs, and riding on the right with the traffic.[43] An estimated 23% of bicycle/motor vehicle accidents are due to riding on the wrong side of the road, where the bicyclist is much less noticeable to drivers because they expect bicyclists to ride with the traffic. This can be a particular problem at intersections, where a driver may run into a bicyclist riding against traffic if either of them makes a turn.

Safe riding techniques have to be learned, regardless of the age of the cyclist. Children in particular benefit from a safe riding course. One of the best such courses is offered by the League of American Wheelmen (LAW), which has developed a program to train and certify instructors. The instructors offer widely varied courses. Students can qualify for LAW certification by passing the National Effective Cyclist Examination and a road rest. Scouts should endeavor to earn the cycling merit badge.

Appendix B (p. 148) lists resources, recommended by the LAW, that are available on a rental or purchase basis. The excellent booklet "Street Smarts",[1] a relatively detailed book on how to ride bicycles safely in traffic, is available from the LAW.

PREVENTION AND TREATMENT OF OVERUSE INJURIES

Bicycle Sizing

One of the most important means of preventing accidents and overuse injuries is to ensure that the bicycle fits the rider. Where this is important for the occasional, short-distance rider, it is critical for the long- distance rider. The elite rider will benefit from the use of the "Fitkit" system of charts, tables, and measuring devices.[26]

Most riders can fit themselves to a bicycle by using the rules of thumb recently summarized by Mellion.[26] With the rider straddling the bike, there should be 2.5 to 5 cm between the crotch and the top tube. For mountain bikes, this distance should be increased to between 7.5 and 15 cm.

There is no universally accepted way to determine proper seat (saddle) height. According to one method, the seat is raised until the rider has to rock from side to side to pedal, then lowered in small increments until the rocking stops. Another method is to put the seat in the position that places the knee in approximately 15° of flexion at the longest point of the pedal downstroke. Most bicycle seats allow fore and aft adjustment as well. The seat position should be arranged so that when the pedal is in the 9 o'clock position, a line dropped from the tibial tubercle falls through the axle of the pedal.[26] Seat angle should be level, or the front of the seat should be slightly elevated. The reach (distance from the front tip of the seat to the handlebar) should be adjusted so that it is the same distance as the length of the rider's forearm and hand (measured from the tip of the olecranon process to the fingertips).

Slow Progression of Mileage

One of the ways of preventing overuse injuries is to limit the progression of mileage to a rate that can be tolerated as the body adapts to cycling stress. The author's rule of thumb is to increase weekly mileage by no more than 10%, but this guideline has not been formally studied. Due to enthusiasm or sudden changes in the weather, cyclists often suddenly and dramatically increase their mileage and intensity. Cyclists often ask how far they can ride in an organized event compared with their average training distance. In the author's anecdotal experience, cyclists can safely ride twice as far in a *single* nonracing event as they usually ride in training. The key phrase is a single event as opposed to daily routine.

Good Equipment

Although almost any bicycle in good mechanical condition can be used for an occasional trip, serious cyclists need serious equipment. The equipment does not necessarily have to be expensive, but it should be purchased from a dealer who can size the bicycle to the rider and provide training in maintenance and use of the various features. Very good bicycles can now be purchased in the price range of $150 to $500. In fact, spending $2,000 to $3,000 buys only incremental improvements in design, lightness of weight, and cosmetic appearance.

Neck Problems

Neck problems in cyclists vary with the type of bicycle. Symptomatic neck pain develops mainly in cyclists who use racing and touring bicycles and less commonly in riders of mountain or city bikes. Racing and touring bicycles have drop handlebars that permit the rider to get into the classic aerodynamic position in which the hips are flexed and the trunk is almost horizontal over the bike. This position requires the rider to extend the neck to see the road (the so-called head-up position). Chronic neck extension on a long ride can lead to neck symptoms in anyone, but particularly in cyclists with a predisposition to neck pain. Neck muscles may ache in anyone after a ride of 30 minutes or more in the head-up position, but the pain typically resolves in a few hours. Usually due to acute overuse of the neck extensor muscles, it is more common in riders who live in seasonal climates and limit their riding from spring to fall. The tendency for neck muscles to ache during and after cycling is usually worse at the beginning of each riding season and gradually resolves over a few weeks as the neck muscles adjust to extension stress. Riders who advance their training too rapidly at the beginning of the season are the most likely to get acute cervical paraspinal muscle strain.

Neck pain in cyclists with cervical arthritis can be a more serious problem, because extending the neck for long periods of time can activate arthritic symptoms. Cyclists especially at risk for pain after riding are those whose arthritis has reduced cervical range of motion to 50° or less of neck extension.

Cyclists with arthritic and/or disc deterioration also run the risk of developing cervical radiculopathy because the intervertebral foramina are opened by neck flexion and closed by neck extension. Chronic neck extension can trigger irritation of a cervical nerve root and cause radicular pain. The most common levels for involvement in cyclists appear to be C6 and C7 (as in other causes of cervical radiculopathy).

Eliminating neck pain in cyclists can be difficult at times. Most recover by simply slowing down the progression of their riding program at the beginning of each season. Many can alleviate pain by flexing the neck frequently during a ride, sitting as upright as possible during part of the ride, and taking frequent rest breaks. Some cyclists, especially those with arthritis or radiculopathy, simply cannot tolerate riding in the head-up position. Options include changing to a bicycle that allows more upright sitting, such as the mountain or city bike. Sitting up straight on the bicycle helps the neck but may cause more seat pressure problems as well as increasing wind resistance. Upright sitting may be the only way a rider with neck problems can continue the sport.

Neck problems can develop as a result of sudden jolts on any type of bicycle. The most common cause is an unexpected pothole. Mountain bikers often experience a sudden jolt when jumping obstacles on the trail. Jolts can cause cervical strain and/or sprain and are best treated conservatively with ice and rest until symptoms resolve. Most acute cases of neck pain are transient and typically are not reported to physicians. For those with chronic neck pain due to jolts, a number of recent innovations act as shock absorbers to smooth out the ride, including seat post springs, seat post pressure tubes, fork springs, and spring suspension frames.

UPPER-EXTREMITY PROBLEMS

Shoulder Problems

Shoulder problems are relatively rare in cyclists but can occur as a result of trauma or overuse. Shoulder injuries in most sports result from trauma during movement or overuse of a particular shoulder motion. Because the shoulders in cyclists are usually relatively fixed in a position of forward flexion, shoulder problems are not usually due to movement. More commonly, shoulder problems are due to overuse of the shoulder from chronic weight-bearing stress. The shoulders must bear some of the body weight on racing and touring bicycles, especially when the drop handlebars are used to get into the head-up position. Prolonged weight-bearing can lead to capsulitis, bicipital tendinitis, and exacerbations of shoulder osteoarthritis. Cyclists with arthritis of all or any of the shoulder joints (glenohumeral, acromioclavicular, and sternoclavicular) are prone to exacerbate their arthritic symptoms with weight-bearing stress.

Sudden jolts can lead to shoulder problems as well. Mountain bikers must use the shoulders in pulling the bike upward over an obstacle and then in absorbing the shock of landing. Jolts can produce contusions of the shoulder structures as well as muscle strain, sprain, capsulitis, and bicipital tendinitis.

Minor acute shoulder problems usually do not require specific treatment because they spontaneously resolve. If they do not, helpful treatments include rest, ice, and nonsteroidal antiinflammatory drugs (NSAIDs). NSAIDs should be used in most cases only for a short period of time and only if there are no contraindications. Riding only in the upright position on smooth surfaces until symptoms resolve or even temporary cessation of riding may be necessary.

It is critical in any shoulder problem to avoid loss of range of motion due to tightening of the shoulder capsule. This is particularly likely to occur when pain inhibition discourages the normal daily range of motion of the shoulder. The shoulder capsule must be stretched daily, or it begins to shrink around the shoulder joint. Capsular tightness or shoulder capsulitis can become so severe as to be called a "frozen shoulder."

Shoulder pain can also lead to secondary reflex sympathetic dystrophy with shoulder-hand syndrome. In most shoulder problems in cyclists, maintaining full range of motion with passive or active assisted exercise is essential to rapid recovery and prevention of reflex sympathetic dystrophy.

Minor acute shoulder problems in cyclists usually respond to the usual sports medicine principles for acute care, i.e., rest, ice, and maintaining range of motion. NSAIDs may be helpful. In more severe problems, physical therapy, including ultrasound and range of motion exercise, may be necessary. If the shoulder problem becomes chronic or recurrent, riding may have to be limited to smooth surfaces in the upright position to take weight stress off the shoulders.

Elbow Problems

The elbow is a relatively infrequent site of injury, perhaps because the elbow can be flexed or extended during riding, whereas the other joints of the upper extremity are held in a relatively fixed position. Elbow pain is more common in off-road bicyclists using mountain or BMX bikes, probably because of the forces on the elbow during jumps over obstacles or for acrobatics. These elbow problems generally represent acute muscle strains and resolve with relative rest and use of ice.

There are occasional cases of lateral epicondylitis in bicyclists, probably due mainly to lifting the bicycle and bicycle gear rather than to actual riding. Although these cases of lateral epicondylitis are sometimes severe, they typically respond rapidly to icing and relative rest.

Ulnar Nerve Injury

One of the most common overuse injuries in cyclists is ulnar nerve injury. Of CIBA respondents, 52% reported at least one episode, and 11% had sought medical advice. Although it has been reported numerous times in the literature,[7,8,14,20,22,45] it is still not generally recognized by most practitioners and is often mistaken for other conditions. For example, a patient referred to the author with the presumptive diagnosis of amyotrophic lateral sclerosis was found to have ulnar nerve palsy. The rapid onset of intrinsic atrophy of the left hand was due to riding a bicycle 30 mi/day. Sometimes practitioners recognize the ulnar nerve injury but assume that it is due to a ganglion or some cause other than bicycling.

Ulnar nerve injury in bicyclists tends to occur bilaterally or in the left hand, probably because the right hand is frequently used to shift gears; the constant pressure on the ulnar nerve is therefore relieved. Ulnar nerve injury

occurs mainly after long rides over multiple days, but it can occur after a single ride for a few hours. The cause appears to be weight-bearing stress on the ulnar nerve, compounded by road shock and vibration transmitted through the handlebars. It also is made worse by wrist hyperextension, which is required in some handlebar-gripping positions.

The nerve injury, which is almost always a transient type of neurapraxia and rarely if ever requires surgery, may occur as any of the five types cited by Wu et al.[45] The injury site is typically at or near Guyon's canal in the proximal portion of the heel of the hand. Mild cases may have some numbness that resolves in a few hours. Moderate cases have persistent numbness of the little finger and the lateral aspect of ring finger. More severe cases are usually characterized by actual wallerian degeneration of some of the ulnar nerve fibers, the "benediction hand" position, and intrinsic muscle atrophy. Ulnar neuropathy can be prevented in most riders with relatively simple measures. CIBA respondents reported successful prevention with the simple measures listed in Table 5. Thick, padded gloves should be worn, and the handlebars should be padded with foam. The bicycle should have the proper fit and the seat should not be higher than the handlebars. The position of the hands should be changed frequently, particularly of the left hand. Hyperextension of the wrist should be avoided as much as possible. Long-distance riders should avoid staying in the head-up position for long periods of time by alternating with relatively upright postures that remove weight from the upper extremities and hands.

Some riders have a greater tendency than others to develop ulnar nerve irritation or injury. They often have no choice but to adopt a more upright riding style in which the weight of the body is not on the hands. Additional prophylactic measures may be necessary for riders planning to take multiple day-long excursions. In a case personally handled by the author, a rider in the Race Across America was outfitted with custom-made polypropylene forearm trays that shifted body weight to the elbows and forearms rather than the heel of the hand. Despite this intervention, the cyclist developed a relatively severe injury to the left ulnar nerve. He felt that it occurred while "dueling" another cyclist in the West Virginia hills. Although severe, the injury resolved completely in 3 months.

TABLE 5. **Measures Used by CIBA Survey Respondents to Prevent and Treat Hand Numbness**

Measure	No.	%
Change hand position	136	51
Padded gloves	113	42
Less mileage	14	5
Better bike fitting	9	3
Miscellaneous	32	12
Most frequent responses were Aero bars, handlebar angle change, shifting weight, smoother roads		

Wrist Injuries and Carpal Tunnel Syndrome

The wrist is often injured in bicyclists by sudden trauma such as an intentional jump or hitting a pothole. A cyclist typically holds the wrist in a taut position while firmly grasping the handlebars. This position puts the wrist at risk for both sprain and strain injuries. The wrist can also become painful secondary to overuse, particularly with too rapid progression of mileage. In this case the wrist ligaments and bony structures develop generalized tenderness that typically resolves with relative rest, ice, and, in some instances, NSAIDs. It is recommended that the rider change hand positions frequently; persistent wrist hyperextension is particularly likely to cause difficulties.

Carpal tunnel syndrome has been reported in bicyclists, but it is uncertain whether bicycling is the actual cause since the syndrome is common in the general population. When carpal tunnel syndrome occurs in a bicyclist, the issue becomes whether bicycling caused, exacerbated, or had nothing to do with it.

In the author's experience, two types of carpal tunnel syndrome are seen in bicyclists. The first is a transient type seen after a sudden increase in cycling mileage or after a particularly long single event; it is possibly related to stretch or pressure on the median nerve for a prolonged period of time with the wrist in hyperextension and usually resolves in a few days without incident. The only treatment usually required is rest from bicycling. The second type is a persistent, intermittent, and sometimes progressive syndrome that in most ways is similar to that experienced by nonbicyclists. Treatment involves relative rest from bicycling, frequent changes of hand positions, and use of wrist splints to prevent excessive

wrist extension or flexion. NSAIDs may help, and in some cases steroid injections may be necessary to quiet down acutely exacerbated symptoms. Electrodiagnostic studies are important in making certain that the symptoms are due to carpal tunnel syndrome and not to another upper-extremity or neck dysfunction.

Just as in the general population, cyclists from time to time require surgical release of carpal tunnel syndrome. The author recommends early release for most cyclists, because it typically solves the problem and helps to prevent postoperative problems such as causalgic pain. In the author's opinion, in most cases it is inappropriate to wait until the carpal tunnel syndrome has produced significant nerve injury before doing a release; delay can increase the incidence and severity of causalgic symptoms.

PELVIC AND BUTTOCK PROBLEMS

Saddle soreness is quite common in bicyclists. It is particularly likely to occur in cyclists who advance the intensity of their riding too rapidly or who take an unusually long single trip. An inappropriate seat position or angle can also be a cause. If the seat is too high, the cyclist must rock from side to side to pedal. This rocking motion adds sheer force that can create chafing, as noted previously. Chafing can be prevented by proper seat height and by careful selection of undergarments for riding. Inappropriately located or roughened seams in clothing can produce chafing; clothing with chamois lining over the perineal region is recommended.

The more upright the posture on the seat, the greater the weight pressure on the perineum and ischial tuberosities. Pressure over the perineum and ischial tuberosities can produce thickened skin and callus formation, but it is typically not a problem and represents a reaction to overuse. Perspiration has to be carefully controlled to prevent maceration of perineal tissues; thus some cyclists require talcum powder and absorbent undergarments. Because pulling on the hair and subsequent irritation of hair follicles can also be a problem, some cyclists shave as much hair as possible from the perineal region.

Careful personal hygiene is important in cyclists to keep the perineal area free of infection. The most common infections include those due to fungi and candida. Although they can be treated with appropriate topical medications, they can easily ruin an otherwise pleasant cycling experience.

Numerous bicycle seats are currently on the market. The traditional seat is a leather saddle that gradually molds to the shape of the rider over a few hundred miles. Although many cyclists still prefer this seat, more modern materials and designs are now more popular. Seat covers range from lambswool to air-filled, gel-filled, water-filled, and foam-filled types. Some of these materials have recently been built into the seat, particularly the gel type. The rider may need to experiment with different types of seat covers and seats to find the combination best tolerated by the perineum and buttocks. Some will find it necessary to switch to a saddle of a different size or shape. A seat with a broader rear expansion is often helpful for bicycles that require the upright posture, such as the mountain or hybrid bike.

Hemorrhoids can be exacerbated by bicycling because of constant pressure on the perineum. Management usually includes use of topical agents and sitz baths. Individuals with persistent hemorrhoids may require a different type of bicycle seat or surgical hemorrhoidectomy; in rare cases they may even have to discontinue bicycling. Dixon[13] has reported the development of 1–2 cm fibrous masses between the skin and ischial tuberosities. The masses are believed to be due to trauma and pressure in the subcutaneous and fascial tissues; surgical excision may be necessary in some cases.

Too rapid training or too long a trip may also produce a pudendal neuropathy, probably due to compression of the dorsal branch of the pudendal nerve near the pubic symphysis.[5,17,24,26] As a result, the rider experiences numbness of the scrotum and penile shaft. The most important intervention is to ensure that the seat is level or even tilted slightly downward. The rider may have to experiment with different types of seats[40] or even discontinue cycling. Occurrence of pudendal neuropathy in women is likely but has not been reported in the literature.

Impotence has been reported in male cyclists,[9,35] mainly after multiday rides or one long ride. It probably represents another aspect of pudendal neuropathy, but vascular dysfunction also has been suggested.[35] Riding should be stopped until recovery is complete. They should then completely reevaluate the fit of their bicycle and the type of seat[40] they are using before continuing. Some have spec-

ulated that the problem is a common but undiscovered cause of impotence in men and possibly of sexual dysfunction in women.[35] Only careful future studies will determine if this theory is true.

CIBA respondents reported a 5% incidences (10 of 198) of sexual dysfunction due to cycling. The 6% incidence in men (8 of 142) was attributed to genital numbness and/or pain. The men reported that changing seats or lowering the front of the seat, as well as reducing mileage, were the most helpful strategies for relieving symptoms. Women respondents noted a 4% incidence (2 of 56) of sexual problems due to cycling, but the type of problem was not noted.

Problems in urination have also been reported in bicyclists, including the inability to urinate after a long ride.[19] CIBA respondents reported an 11% incidence (22 of 202) of difficulty in urinating after a ride. The incidence was 13% (19 of 147) in men and 5% (3 of 55) in women. Two men with prostate problems reported that riding improved their urination.

Some riders are completely unable to urinate for hours after a long ride. Potential etiologies range from a pressure-and-trauma type of urethritis[31] to pudendal neuritis or preexisting prostatic hypertrophy.[26] All three may be involved in some cases. The treatment is to maintain urination, by intermittent catheterization if necessary. Treatment of secondary infection of the bladder or urethra requires appropriate antibiotics. The cyclist must cease riding until normal urinary flow has resumed. A complete reevaluation of the fit of the bicycle and the type of seat is then appropriate. If the problem persists despite all measures of prevention, the rider may have to cease bicycling completely.

HIP PROBLEMS

Hip problems are relatively rare in cyclists. Cycling can certainly exacerbate problems such as degenerative joint disease of the hip. Tronchanteric bursitis can develop as a result of overuse. Treatment consists of lowering the seat to the appropriate level, using higher cranking cadences instead of higher cranking pressure, ice massage, NSAIDs, and injections with steroid anti-inflammatory medication, if necessary. Most cases are mild and respond to relative rest without the need for further medical treatment.

The iliotibial band friction syndrome can occur in bicyclists but appears to have a lower frequency than in runners and certain other types of athletes. It also usually responds to relative rest, but iliotibial band stretching, NSAIDs, ice massage, and injection may be necessary. A rare individual may require surgery.

KNEE PROBLEMS

Knee pain is common in bicyclists. Patellofemoral pain syndrome, or biker's knee, is perhaps the most common.[15] The most frequent cause is pedaling at too slow a cadence and at too high a pedal resistance. This combination increases the pressure on the patellofemoral interface. Predisposing patellofemoral abnormalities include a high-Q angle and a relatively high or lateral position of the patella.[26] Other predisposing factors can be reduced flexibility of the hamstrings and quadriceps femoral anteversion, external tibial torsion, and pronating feet with calcaneovalgus.[15]

The most critical factor in treating biker's knee is to increase the cadence and to lower pedal resistance. Relative rest may be necessary as well as a reduction in the progression of training rides. Orthotics in the shoes to correct pronation may be helpful. Some patients may require strengthening of the vastus medialis obliquus and stretching of the hamstrings, quadriceps, and iliotibial band. Other patients benefit from an orthotic device for the knee that helps the patella to track in the midline position. Ice massage and NSAIDs may be necessary in some cases. Raising the seat to the proper height is essential. In the author's experience, knee pain can be due to excessive flexion of the knee because the seat is too low or to excessive extension of the knee on the downward stroke because the seat is too high.

FOOT AND ANKLE PROBLEMS

Cyclists with a relatively normal foot and ankle typically have few difficulties. One of the advantages of bicycling as an aerobic form of exercise is that it avoids some of the stresses that occur on the foot and ankle mechanism during running.

One of the most frequent complaints among cyclists is numbness of the feet. Cyclists may complain that their forefeet feel numb and that their toes "buzz" when they walk. The etiology is neurapraxia of the digital nerves between the toes, usually due to an overuse syndrome in which training is progressed too rapidly or cyclists perform a single event that is much longer than they have trained to ride. Excessive pedal pressure is likely to be the basic cause, but the syndrome can also be due to squeezing of the forefoot by toe straps or clips that are too tight or by shoes that are too narrow. Squeezing the forefoot prevents the foot from spreading out completely during the downstroke of pedaling.

The rider should discontinue bicycling until the numbness resolves, typically over a period of a week. Prevention of the problem requires shoes that are wide enough to allow the forefoot to spread out on the pedal downstroke. An in-shoe orthotic device to spread pressure forces may be helpful, and riding at a higher cadence with lower pedal resistance is also advised. Some cyclists find that using various types of pedal-shoe attachment systems helps to prevent the problem. Such a mechanism also improves the mechanical efficiency of pedaling, especially since the rider can use power on the upstroke as well as the downstroke.

Metatarsalgia in cyclists is usually due to a poor foot position on the pedal, which causes too much pressure directly over the metatarsal heads. The condition usually responds to relative rest, orthotics that spread pressure forces over the foot, riding at a higher cadence with lower pedal resistance, and a different type of foot/shoe interface.

SUMMARY

Bicycling is one of nation's most popular activities and extends to all ages. The types of injuries sustained by bicyclists run the gamut from chafing to death; the two most common types, however, are trauma and overuse. The great majority of injuries are minor and are not reported to physicians. Trauma is best prevented by safe riding techniques, sturdy equipment, and clear visibility and audibility when riding on streets. Overuse syndromes are best prevented by slow progression of training intensity, proper fit of the bicycle and shoes, and early treatment of problems that

Chapter 10

ISSUES IN GYMNASTS AND DANCERS

Anthony J. Margherita, MD

Treatment of the dancer or gymnast presents a number of challenges to the sports physician. Dance and gymnastic movements are both aesthetic and explosive, requiring rapid muscular contraction, often beyond normal ranges of motion. These movements demand a strong, supple, and resilient body but also require local muscle and cardiovascular endurance sufficient to maintain a high level of artistry for prolonged periods of time.

Dancers and gymnasts are often younger and therefore less skeletally mature than participants in other sports. The aesthetics of dance and gymnastics mandate a lithe appearance, which predisposes to poor nutrition. Because gymnasts and dancers may begin their artistic/athletic careers prepubertally, the family unit must be incorporated into the rehabilitation team. Coaches and teachers hold special positions of prominence and must also be incorporated into the treatment team, sometimes as surrogate parents. Competitive pressures and grueling practice and performance schedules make the rehabilitation of injuries difficult and often suboptimal. Dancers are likely to seek alternative therapies before incorporating a physician in their treatment. Therefore, they may have already received recommendations and treatment from a chiropractor, naturopath, or herbalist before coming to the sports medicine office. General principles of sports rehabilitation, however, continue to apply.

Although dance and gymnastics are different activities requiring different skills and strengths, they share a common set of disorders related to acute and chronic injuries. The dynamic nature of these activities incorporates explosive acceleration/deceleration motions with strong isometric contractions to maintain stability. Patterns of learned, coordinated movements and agonist/antagonist contraction/cocontraction facilitate the graceful and supple movements and can be "unlearned" during a period of prolonged immobility. For the purposes of this discussion, therefore, dancers and gymnasts are called performer/athletes, and their activities are considered sport.

PRINCIPLES OF EVALUATION

The performing arts physician must have at his or her disposal the full spectrum of skills necessary for treating all disorders of the musculoskeletal system as well as managing and integrating the activities of a health care and rehabilitation team. Injuries of the ankle-foot, knee, and hip account for 60% to 80% of all injuries encountered in the dance population. Therefore, a good understanding of the anatomy and kinesiology of these areas is essential to understanding the pathomechanics of injury in the performer/athlete. Injuries to the low back make up the majority of the remaining injuries and are more common in male dancers. Therefore, the physician must incorporate aspects of industrial medicine and spine rehabilitation into the treatment program. Gymnastic injuries of the upper extremity (primarily the elbow and wrist) can produce significant disability. The physician should therefore be familiar with treating these areas as well.

Injuries can be classified into the following patterns: misuse/abuse, overuse, ill use, disuse, and poor use. Each of these conditions requires a different approach to diagnosis, treatment, and rehabilitation. A diagnostic cascade is described in Figure 1. Injuries in this population most commonly involve acute trauma and chronic or repeated overload. Acute trauma generally involves cartilaginous, ligamentous, or bony structures; chronic overload primarily affects the musculotendinous unit.

Static Evaluation

The static examination of the performer/athlete includes an evaluation of posture, alignment, strength, vasculature, and neurologic function. Muscle balance or imbalance is assessed clinically and, if necessary, through a variety of testing modalities such as isokinetic dynamometry. Dancers and gymnasts are often hypermobile, with lax joints. Therefore, normal considerations of range of motion must be modified according to the needed versus available range for a given activity. The assessment is guided by evaluating static postures in dance movement. As an example, a dancer with inadequate hip flexor mobility will attempt to compensate during barre exercises by increasing the lumbar lordosis and thus predisposing to back disorders (Fig. 2).

Careful neurovascular examination reveals vascular-induced injury or pathology, such as thoracic outlet syndrome in the male dancer who repetitively lifts his 105-lb partner. Careful palpation and percussion distinguishes bony from ligamentous or musculotendinous pain generators. General physical examination provides clues to nutritional status, hydration, and general health.

The general health of the performer–athlete should always be assessed. There is a high propensity toward eating disorders in this population. Amenorrhea, related to poor nutrition and/or high-level training, can result in serious health consequences. The sports physician must be sensitive to the pressures and adaptive behaviors that can result in eating disorders. Often a nutritionist or psychologist makes a valuable contribution to the treatment process.

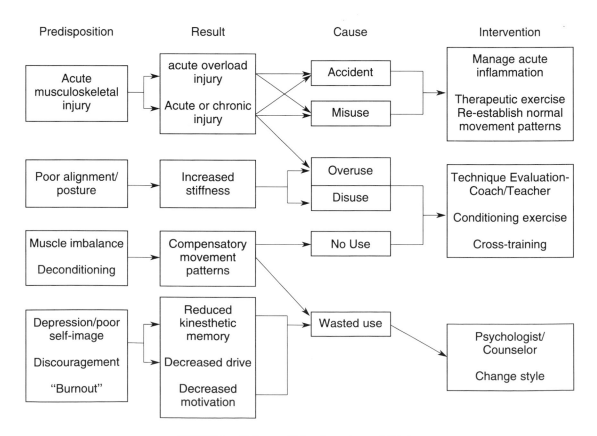

FIGURE 1. Patterns of injury in performer/athletes.

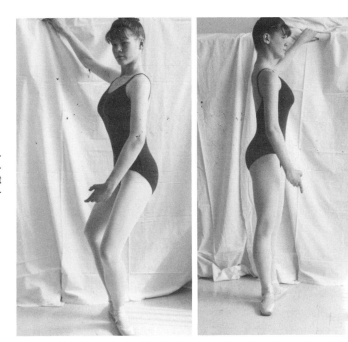

FIGURE 2. Inadequate hip flexor mobility *(left)*, in comparison to proper alignment *(right)*, results in hyperextension at the lumbar spine. Note also other alterations in lower-extremity alignment.

Dynamic Assessment

Dynamic assessment of the performer/athlete is an important aspect of the examination. Errors in technique and form can often be identified only if the patient is allowed to demonstrate the movement pattern in a minimally restrictive environment. Biomechanically inefficient and injurious patterns of movement can be identified. Other methods of dynamic assessment may detect proprioceptive or coordination deficits that predispose to chronic overload. For example, single-legged stance with eyes closed versus open demonstrates excess lateral sway in the dancer with impaired ankle proprioception.

Injury acuity is manifest during this part of the examination. The pattern of movement helps to identify the etiology of disorders. For instance, an acute traumatic injury precludes the patient from performing the desired movement and is associated with pain. Chronic overuse injuries allow the movement to be done, albeit with substitution and inefficient motion. Discouraged or depressed patients exhibit body positions and facial expressions (if not overt emotions) that reveal internal turmoil. Observation of the patient after a long class or period of activity, which accentuates dynamic muscle weakness, is particularly helpful.

Included in the dynamic assessment is an evaluation of the patient's equipment and if appropriate, the environment in which training activity takes place. Because of limited financial resources, the dancer may use footwear well beyond its usable life span.

BIOMECHANICS AND PATHOPHYSIOLOGY OF INJURY

The thin, lithe appearance of the dancer can be both an advantage and a disadvantage. Stress loads imposed by ballistic motions in dance or gymnastics are less when less mass is propelled through the air. However, bony support for muscular activity may be suboptimal, and the ballistic motions may cause fatigue and fracture. Stylistic concerns often require the athlete to assume positions beyond the normal range of anatomic support. Examples of such positions include demi-pointe (Fig. 3) or hyperlordosis on landing from the vault. These maneuvers require strong muscular and bony support to prevent injury. Taping and splinting may be unacceptable, because they restrict the necessary range of motion. Therefore, principles of biomechanics and kinesiology are of great importance in understanding pathology and in designing appropriate treatment.

Anatomic variations can have a dramatic effect on the ability to dance. Long lower

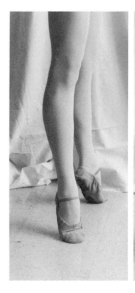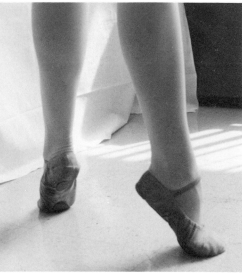

FIGURE 3. Demi-pointe. The ankle becomes destabilized, particularly upon landing or when performing complex tasks on one leg.

extremities relative to torso height (considered "ideal" by some) exert a powerful lever on the lumbosacral spine if range of hip motion is inadequate. Faulty lift technique by the male dancer results in a hyperlordotic posture with increased shear forces in the lumbar spine and lumbosacral junction.

Dancers are more flexible than other athletes[34] and have a higher incidence of joint hypermobility. Structural foot abnormalites such as hallux rigidus, a long second toe (so-called "Greek foot"), and a long first metatarsal or hallux ("Egyptian foot") increase the incidence of significant injury and may preclude the dancer from achieving proficiency in pointe work. In contrast, a "peasant foot," consisting of a squared ankle, strong and sturdy arch, broad forefoot, and equal length of the first three toes, is best for dance activities on pointe. Classical ballet tends to have a Darwinian or "survival-of-the-fittest" effect at increasingly higher levels of skill and training. The anatomically less capable dancers eventually either cannot perform the necessary motions of dance or develop injuries related to anatomic variations. Other forms of dance, such as flamenco, modern, and jazz, though less anatomically extreme, impose their own stresses on the musculoskeletal system.

Biomechanic principles are directly applicable to the study of injuries in dancers and gymnasts. Kinetic chain theory[23,24] can be used to describe many of the potential problems that may occur in performer/athletes. When a limb or body segment is in contact with an immobile object (such as the floor), the chain of motion is described as "closed." Conversely, when there is no direct force against which the muscles work, the chain is "open." Because parts of the body are links in the chain, dysfunction at one level may affect adjacent or distal segments. For example, the hamstring muscles act as a knee flexor. However, when the leg is in contact with the floor, they act as hip extensors. Many such relationships exist throughout the body and are a main reason for muscle overload. Another factor is the contractile properties of muscle. Muscles may be activated either concentrically (i.e., while shortening) or eccentrically (i.e., while lengthening). Thus, when the hamstrings flex the knee, they contract concentrically; with running, however, the hamstrings decelerate the swing leg by firing eccentrically just before the heel hits the ground. Eccentric contractions generate greater force than concentric contractions and therefore are more fatiguing.

"Turnout" is the foundation of ballet movement. Five foot positions, 26 leg positions, 7 trunk, and 7 arm positions performed in foot-flat, demi-pointe or pointe position allow an enormous number of variations (Fig. 4) that must be accommodated through a closed kinetic chain. Many of the forces applied to the lower extremities, pelvis, and lumbar spine are closed-chain in nature and thus require compensation by other segments above or below the region of injury. Open kinetic chain injuries are primarily related to

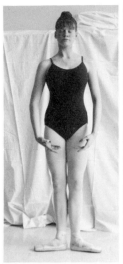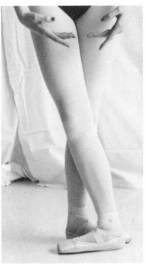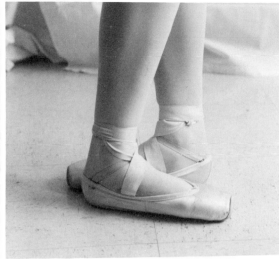

FIGURE 4. Hip external rotation, termed "turnout," forms the basis of movement in dance. Various foot and leg positions are derived from the turned-out position. A reduction in the ability to maintain turnout is a primary cause of injury.

rapid deceleration at floor contact and may be related to faulty technique or fatigue. Studies of gymnasts[26] have suggested a much higher tendency toward injury near the end of a training session.

EPIDEMIOLOGIC CONSIDERATIONS

Musculoskeletal injuries represent approximately 85% of ballet dancers' activity-related diseases.[27] Five anatomic/physiologic factors contribute to the development of these injuries:

(1) muscle imbalance of the hip rotator musculature,
(2) anatomic limitations of hip mobility,
(3) functional gastroc-soleus equinus,
(4) excessive foot plantar flexion, and
(5) hallux rigidus.

Dancers describe eight primary reasons for injuries:

(1) inadequate warm-up,
(2) lack of training specificity,
(3) poor preseason conditioning,
(4) decreased recovery time,
(5) poor instruction in technique,
(6) rehearsal and performance schedules,
(7) starting ballet at too late an age, and
(8) muscle imbalance.

Errors in technique are an additional risk factor for acute injury (more commonly seen in gymnasts).

As one would expect, overuse injuries of the lower extremities predominate. Fractures of the lower extremity tend to be stress fractures, whereas injuries to the wrist and elbow in gymnasts are more commonly acutely traumatic, usually associated with a landing error or faulty technique. Injuries to dancers and gymnasts occur at a rate similar to other athletes engaged in sports with comparable physical demands. Both dance and gymnastics require moderate cardiopulmonary exercise capacity, as demonstrated in comparative studies with other athletic disciplines.[34] They require substantially higher strength-to-weight ratios and strength across a wide range of joint positions. The ankle is the most frequently injured body part in the performer/athlete, as in other sports requiring lower-extremity activity in a closed kinetic chain. The type and character of injuries in the dancer are quite different, owing primarily to the various foot positions required.

GENERAL TREATMENT GUIDELINES

It is helpful to use standard definitions, such as those provided by the World Health Organization, to classify injuries and their treatment. Impairment is defined as an alteration in health status. Disability is the functional deficit that results from impairment. It is clear that some injuries are more disabling than others. What may be a minor injury for other patients seen in the sports medicine office can result in significant disability for the dancer.

Treatment therefore is based on a defined set of rehabilitation goals that are established in consultation with the patient and the treatment team. Acute management of injury incorporates standard treatment modalities such as ice, compression, elevation, immobilization, or rest. Following resolution of the acute phase, reestablishment of normal (or supernormal) range of motion, flexibility, and strength is pursued. During the period of "active rest," the performer/athlete may participate in noninjurious skill activities or movement patterns. When possible, cardiovascular and endurance activities are maintained. Local muscle endurance is developed to prevent fatigue and reinjury, and when possible, sport-specific patterns of dynamic movement are incorporated into treatment. The performer/athlete is progressively returned to active participation in dance or gymnastics but must be reevaluated periodically to gain full clearance to participate in high-level activity or competition. Movement patterns are carefully scrutinized by the coach or teacher during this phase in an effort to identify and correct technique or training faults.

INJURY PATTERNS

Hip and Thigh Disorders

Muscular imbalance about the hip is a frequent cause of dance injuries.[4,5,36,43] Flexibility of the hip is critically important to graceful dance. Strength must be developed through training of large muscles such as the hip extensors, abductors, and flexors, as well as of small rotator muscles. During maturation, the anteversion angle of the femoral neck decreases progressively until the age of 11 years, at which time it reaches its adult value. Children who begin dance between the ages of 6 and 12 years are able to maintain turnout by externally rotating their hips. They can maintain flexibility by frequent and regular stretching of the soft tissues about the hip. After the age of 12 years, the amount of available anatomic external rotation or turnout at the hip becomes fixed from a bony and capsular standpoint. Further increase in external rota-

tion range is limited, even with aggressive flexibility training.[4] Straining the hip in turnout, as sometimes occurs in the male dancer who begins training later in life, can produce tension across the medial capsular attachments and compression of the superior and lateral acetabulum. This results in the formation of osteophytes and predisposes to degenerative arthritis.

In classical ballet there is frequently a highly structured period of warm-up, after which the dancer participates in class or rehearsal. In modern, folk, jazz, or tap dance, the schedule may be less regimented. If the dancer is inadequately warmed-up prior to training, hip and thigh injuries can occur. It is important that all dancers participate in a regular warm-up and stretching program to facilitate turnout and to maximize range of motion to prevent injury. Dancers must understand the specific anatomic limitations of their bodies so that early degenerative arthritis can be avoided.

Stress Fractures

Stress fractures about the hip occur most commonly at the femoral neck. The dancer complains of vague groin pain that is initially relieved by rest. As the condition progresses, the dancer complains of pain earlier during class or rehearsal. During periods of inactivity or rest the pain frequently subsides. Examination may reveal no limitation in range of motion of the hip, even though adduction/ internal rotation and flexion/abduction/ external rotation result in hip or groin pain. Diagnosis by bone scan allows differentiation of stress fractures from early degenerative arthritis or other hip pathology. Treatment of a stress fracture of the hip requires minimal weight-bearing during the healing phase. Crutch ambulation is necessary. If available, barre exercises are performed in a pool with the unaffected limb acting as the weight-bearing structure. To maintain strength, resistive sleeves or air splints can be used to increase hydraulic resistance. Adequate nutrition is critical to maximize the healing process.

Bursitis and Flexibility

Inadequate flexibility or asymmetry of the iliotibial band or tensor fascia lata can result in lateral hip pain and irritation of the subtrochanteric bursa. Acute subtrochanteric bursitis may be treated with ice, friction massage, nonsteroidal anti-inflammatory drugs for pain control, and ultrasound therapy. Tightness of the iliotibial band may occur in the presence of otherwise excellent range of motion and joint mobility. It can be caused by inadequate warm-up and stretching. Occasionally, tightness of the piriformis is identified and must also be treated. Symmetric flexibility and pain-free range of motion must be demonstrated before full return to premorbid activities.

Muscle Strains

Acute muscular tears occur most commonly at the origin of the adductors and in the hamstrings. Acute injuries may result from rapid overload and macroscopic tears of the musculotendinous junction. Less severe injuries are usually associated with fatigue or chronic microinjury (often termed muscle strain). With repetitive microinjury, abnormal or compensatory patterns of movement develop, altering the performer/athlete's kinesthetic awareness and balance. Correction of the anatomic disruption or physiologic event alone is inadequate to return the performer/athlete to participation without a high risk of reinjury. Normal movement patterns and pro-

prioception must be reestablished with proprioceptive neuromuscular facilitory techniques or movement therapies.

Tendinitis

Tendinitis is often caused by overload of the hip rotators or adductors. Some motions (Fig. 5) can produce impingement of the iliopsoas as it inserts on the lesser trochanter. This impingement causes a tendinitis not commonly seen in other athletic populations. Irritation of the short rotators, such as the piriformis, can also occur and may be disabling for the dancer or gymnast who requires extensive hip rotation while performing. Treatment is directed toward reducing inflammation, facilitating pain-free range of motion, and instituting a progressive strengthening program. When evaluating the patient with hip pathology, it is also important to evaluate the lumbar spine, because limitations in lumbar spine mobility result in increased stresses about the hip and vice versa.

Snapping, Popping, and Clicking

Popping, clicking, or snapping of the hip joint is a common complaint. As the iliopsoas

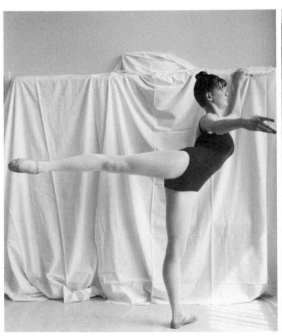
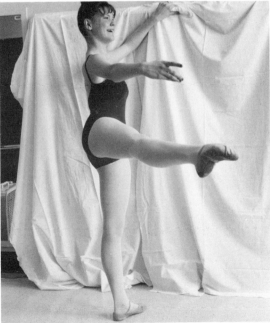

FIGURE 5. Impingement of the iliopsoas, not commonly seen in other activities, can be disabling as the dancer extends and externally rotates the hip from the position shown in the left panel to that in the right.

passes across the anterior hip capsule, a click is felt and occasionally heard.[28] Snapping is described as the dancer lands from a leap or jump. The tensor fascia lata, located posterior to the greater trochanter, snaps forward on landing. This is sometimes described as the hip going "out of place." Clicking or snapping across the hip is usually of no consequence, although snapping of the tensor fascia lata may not be aesthetic. Clicking of the iliopsoas is of no clinical consequence, and simple reassurance is the only treatment necessary. Snapping of the tensor fascia lata can be treated by strengthening the abductor and extensor muscle groups and maintenance or improvement of hip range of motion.

Hip pain may be referred from other sites of pathology. Urinary tract infections as well as thoracolumbar disk lesions may refer pain to the groin. Tumors and other gynecologic disorders may present as hip or groin pain and must be considered in the differential diagnosis. Segmental dysfunction in the lower lumbar spine, particularly at the lumbosacral junction, may radiate primarily to the buttock and posterior hip. Lumbosacral spine abnormalities also increase stress on the hip joint and should be noted and addressed as needed.

Knee Disorders

Performer/athletes have a high incidence of knee disorders, but the nature and type are somewhat different from those in other sports. Injury-causing forces may be applied to the knee from external rotation of the hip in turnout or in dance activities such as the plié or grande plié. The adolescent knee (defined as ages 12 to 17 years) also presents a challenge in diagnosis and treatment. The hypermobility beneficial to the dancer for some movements can result in genu recurvatum and a loss of knee stability. Anatomic variations such as genu varum or genu valgum result in different strengths and weaknesses of the knee relative to dance activities. A dancer with powerful, short muscle bellies, such as the dancer with varus, should not be expected to perform movements that require the flexibility of a dancer with valgus.

Injury patterns of the knee are most often related to the stresses imposed by turnout. Dancers with inadequate external rotation of the hip may compensate for the deficit by rotating the knee to achieve the desired "toe-out" stance. This alters the kinetic chain by applying stresses to the medial collateral ligament and results in medial knee pain.

Major ligamentous injuries, such as those to the anterior cruciate ligament, are rare in dancers. Meniscal injuries also occur relatively infrequently. Musculotendinous injuries tend to result from chronic overload or acute events superimposed on chronic dysfunction.

Collateral Ligament Injury

Strain injuries in the collateral ligaments and patellofemoral problems predominate in dancers and gymnasts. The medial collateral ligament is the primary restraint to medial joint opening. The medial joint capsule acts as an accessory stabilizer of the joint. Traumatic injuries to the medial collateral ligament are generally graded as 1, 2 and 3. Grade 1 injuries consist of a stretch injury to the collateral ligament without significant tear. Grade 2 injuries involve incomplete tears of the medial collateral ligament and grade 3 injuries are complete ligamentous disruptions.

Chronic overload or strain injuries occur frequently in dancers, particularly in those with problems in turnout, as mentioned above. The performer/athlete with acute or chronic injury to the medial collateral ligament may walk, dance, or run with the affected knee in greater flexion that the unaffected knee. This gait pattern is primarily an adaptation to reduce the stress on the ligamentous fibers as the knee reaches full extension. The medial collateral ligament is well vascularized and has a high potential for healing.

Acute treatment of grade 1 injuries consists of standard applications of rest, ice, and anti-inflammatory medications. Grade 2 injuries require the use of a hinged cast-brace initially set at 30° to 90° of knee flexion. Full extension of the affected knee is contraindicated because of the need to prevent increased stress on the healing ligament. Early active and active-assisted range of motion is beneficial. Partial weight-bearing on crutches assists with control of edema and healing. Acute grade 2 or 3 injuries require relative immobilization in the cast-brace for a period of 2 to 6 weeks. Because dancers and gymnasts require significant medial joint stability, caution must be taken not to advance too rapidly and thus risk reinjury.

During the healing phase, cross-training, strengthening, and kinesthetic activities of the unaffected limb are indicated. If a soft-tissue restriction limits turnout, progressive flexibility exercises can maximize hip rotation and minimize stresses on the medial collateral ligament. Hyperpronation is managed as described above. Maintaining aerobic fitness is beneficial to reduce early-onset fatigue when the patient returns to full activities. Isometric exercises can be performed in the cast-brace, and progressive resistive exercises are added as the patient is weaned from brace wear.

Patellofemoral Joint Dysfunction

Syndromes of patellofemoral pain occur commonly in dancers and gymnasts. If one includes patellar tendon and quadriceps tendinitis, these disorders are the most common injuries in performer/athletes.

Rapid deceleration stress is a common cause of injury to the patellofemoral joint. The dancer or gymnast often describes pain with increasing positions of knee flexion, when landing from a jump, or after periods of immobilization, such as while waiting to perform. Examination reveals weakness and easy fatigability of the vastus medialis. Common findings include an increased Q angle in conjunction with lateral patellar tracking and relative inflexibility of the iliotibial band and lateral retinaculum. In most cases plain radiographs are normal.

Treatment of patellar tracking disorders is directed toward stretching the lateral retinaculum and strengthening the vastus medialis, primarily with multi-angle isometrics of the quadriceps and quarter squat lifts for strengthening the closed kinetic chain. Stretching of the iliotibial band and hip musculature provides adequate hip range for turnout and reduces the stress forces across the patella. Balance must be developed in the hip rotator muscles. Myofascial release techniques mobilize the soft tissues about the knee and improve tracking of the patella. McConnell taping may be beneficial in some circumstances to provide kinesthetic feedback and reeducation of the thigh musculature.

Foot and Ankle Disorders

The five basic foot positions in classical ballet require maximal external rotation of the lower extremity (termed "turnout," Fig. 4). Turnout allows the dancer to perform an aesthetic and graceful series of lower-extremity movements. Unfortunately, it also places significant stresses on the joints of the lower extremity.

The female ballet dancer usually begins training at the age of 6 to 8 years.[14,35] Male dancers usually start training between the ages of 12 and 16 years. Dancers first learn barre exercises, then central floor exercises; female dancers progress to "on pointe." According to current recommendations, pointe work should not be permitted before the age of 10 years and should be gradually taught through a series of training exercises between the ages of 10 and 12 years.[35,45] Because the epiphyseal plates are open at this time, compression injury is a risk. Classical ballet involves significant remodeling of the bones in the foot, so that the foot placed on pointe has stable bony support. Ballet may be the only organized physical activity that is actually designed to mold the child's skeletal structure to fit its requirements.

Surveys by Rovere et al.[41] and Quirk[39] found that foot and ankle injuries account for 25% to 42% of all dance injuries. Of these, chronic or overuse injuries tend to predominate. Chronic overload injuries are usually due to repetitive impact-loading of the dancer's foot and ankle on a hard, unyielding dance floor. Often this is exacerbated by using an old or broken-down toe shoe. Overuse injuries are also common in modern dancers but for different reasons. Current footwear for modern dance provides essentially no forefoot structural support. This lack of support renders the mid- and forefoot structures susceptible to repetitive overload injury.

The most common acute injury in dance is an inversion ankle sprain.[13] Grade 1 sprains show primary involvement of the anterior talofibular ligament; grade 2, complete disruption of the anterior talofibular ligament; and grade 3, involvement of both the anterior talofibular and calcaneofibular ligaments. Grade 3 injuries are of great concern in the dancer, because stability in the plantar-flexed position is required to work on pointe. The demi-pointe position renders the ankle intrinsically unstable and requires maximal support from ligamentous and muscular structures. Some authors have suggested that the risk of chronic instability mandates operative intervention for grade 3 inversion injuries. Others, however, note that many injuries recover with good stability and recommend a course of immobilization before consideration of surgical repair.

The term "functional equinus" in dance medicine refers to shortening of the gastrocnemius-soleus complex.[20] This shortening reduces the available dorsiflexion necessary for many dance movements that incorporate plié (Fig. 6). During a plié, the first 10° of dorsiflexion occur with a neutral mid- and forefoot. Shortening of the gastrocnemius causes tightness and reduces the shock-absorbing capacity of the foot. Dancers who lack adequate range of dorsiflexion fail to load the hindfoot during jumping. This predisposes to overuse injuries and stress fractures in the forefoot and ankle. Such stress fractures are particularly common in the second and third metatarsals, but occasionally occur in the distal fibula or sesamoid bones as well. The functional equinus position also predisposes the dancer to the development of Achilles tendinitis or peritendinitis.[12]

Repetitive, forceful dorsiflexion of the weight-bearing foot (as with plié) can result in anterior tibiotalar impingement. With such repetitive activity, exostoses can form at the site at which the tibia impinges on the talus. The result is pain and an inability to push off on the affected foot. Treatment includes the wearing of shoes with elevated heels to unload the impinged structures and to allow healing. The dancer is instructed not to force the foot into the plié position. Nonsteroidal antiinflammatory drugs (NSAIDs) may be of benefit. Surgical intervention can provide short- to intermediate-term relief. However, exostoses often recur several years later in the individual who returns to dance.

Posterior impingement occurs in the pointe or demi-pointe position as the foot is flexed to align the metatarsals with the tibia.[20] In the presence of an os trigonum, total talar flexion is reduced, and proper alignment cannot be obtained. Attempts at forced flexion of such a foot cause posterior impingement. This may repeatedly injure the os trigonum or posterior talar tubercle and cause compression injury to the flexor hallucis longus. The dancer with this anatomic variant may have to be counseled not to perform classical ballet maneuvers that require pointe or demi-pointe positioning. Treatment for impingement of the flexor hallucis longus includes ice, NSAIDs, cross-friction massage, and stretching. Strengthening exercises are added later.

To rise into the demi-pointe position

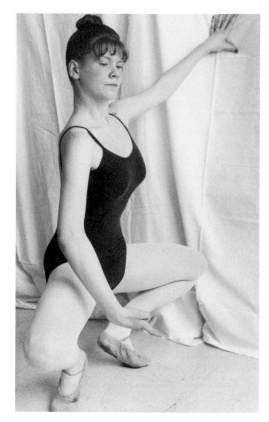

FIGURE 6. Grand plié. Inadequate available gastrocsoleus range will preload the foot and predispose to injury.

(termed relevé), approximately 90° to 100° of dorsiflexion is necessary at the first metatarsophalangeal joint. Inadequate range in this joint can produce degenerative changes and spurring on the dorsal surface of the first metatarsal head. Inadequate dorsiflexion when rising to the ball of the foot produces a phenomenon known as "sickling" (Fig. 6). This phenomenon forces the dancer to shift weight onto the lateral metatarsals, which places excessive forces over the lateral aspect of the foot and increases the risk for injuries to the arch. Initial phases of this disorder are often termed "hallux limitus." In the early stages, NSAIDs, ice, and a toe spacer are indicated. The toe spacer is placed between the first and second digits to maintain first metatarsal alignment with the hallux. Joint mobilization therapy can also relieve symptoms and improve mobility. More advanced cases, called hallux rigidus, may be treated with dorsal debridement and aggressive rehabilitation. Most severe cases of hallux rigidus are disabling and may end the dancer's career.

Resection arthroplasty of the first metatarsophalangeal joint has been recommended[12] in such cases. In the early stages of hallux rigidus, appropriate treatment through joint mobilization, strengthening, and counseling of the dancer may prevent or limit disability.

Cuboid

An often undiagnosed or misdiagnosed condition in the performer/athlete is subluxation of the cuboid.[31,37] The clinical picture includes pain over the lateral midfoot and an inability to propel the foot into plantar flexion without pain or discomfort. The condition may be misdiagnosed as a peroneal tendinitis, because the peroneus longus runs by the cuboid. The astute clinician identifies this condition as separate from tendinitis, because the pain is more localized, not associated with edema or bogginess to palpation in the peroneal tendon, and sensitive to direct palpation of the cuboid. Observing the patient walk or attempt to relevé identifies the limitation. Treatment reduces the subluxation by forceful manipulation of the cuboid. Sometimes termed the "cuboid whip," a forceful downward thrust is applied in a whipping motion, with the patient lying prone on the examination table. When successful, the maneuver is often accompanied by an audible snap or pop. The clinical hallmark for success is at least 50% to 75% reduction in localized pain and improved ability to rise onto the ball of the foot. Supportive arch (Low Dye) taping (Fig. 7) can provide additional support during the acute phase. Chronic or recurrent subluxation may require the use of a foot orthotic in street shoes to prevent the pronation that predisposes to cuboid subluxation. Rarely, surgical intervention with percutaneous pinning of the bone is necessary.

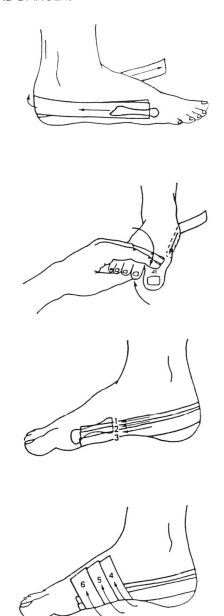

FIGURE 7. Low Dye taping can be used as a diagnostic and therapeutic modality; orthotic inserts cannot be used in dance footwear.

Plantar Fascia

During normal walking, the plantar fascia is loaded during the initial phases of push-off.[4,47] In dance or gymnastics, repetitive loading of the plantar fascia is associated either with landing from a jump on a plantar-flexed foot or toe-running on the dance floor or gymnastics mat. Functional equinus, as mentioned above, can induce a preload phenomenon, because less available range of motion in dorsiflexion of the ankle stresses the plantar fascia earlier in the gait cycle. Treatment is directed toward reducing acute pain through the use of nonsteroidal anti-inflammatory medications and a half-inch heel pad. Such a heel pad reduces the stress loads on the origin of the plantar fascia. The patient is advised not to engage in repetitive loading, such as occurs with dance or gymnastics, for a period of 1 to 2 weeks. Supportive Low Dye taping can reduce the load on the plantar fascia and is often highly beneficial in reducing symptoms in the early treatment phase. Local treatment modalities may include transverse friction massage augmented by ultrasound. Some authors[31] recommend the combination of electrogalvanic stimulation and ultrasound to assist in early local management. The patient is able to augment this treatment with self-administered contrast bath therapy. Following acute treatment, aggressive rehabilitation should include strengthening of the foot intrinsic muscles, stretching of the gastrocsoleus complex, and kinesthetic reeducation with a balance board. Biofeedback may induce more rapid motor learning. The rehabilitation program is completed as the patient progressively returns to premorbid activity. A final review and consultation by the rehabilitation team should precede the performer/athlete's return to full participation.

Flexor Hallucis Longus Tendinitis

Flexor hallucis longus tendinitis is more common in dancers than in other comparable athletic populations. One risk factor for its development is a plantar-flexed first ray, which often occurs in the individual with a cavus foot deformity. Pain is usually felt immediately behind the medial malleolus and can be confused with tendinitis of the tibialis posterior muscle. Stresses are applied to the tendon when the performer/athlete rolls over the ball of the foot in arising to demi-pointe. The tendon is stressed as it crosses the fibro-osseous tunnel directly behind the talus. Repetitive motion, as in relevé or repeated jumps without heel contact, induces microinjury at the level of the tunnel. The tendon may also be irritated under the base of the first metatarsal, where the flexor hallucis longus tendon passes over the flexor digitorum longus.

Treatment of flexor hallucis longus tendinitis consists of acute intervention with ice or contrast therapy, ultrasound, and pain-free range-of-motion exercise. Supportive taping of the arch and padding to allow unweighted first-ray plantar flexion can assist in resolving acute symptomatology. Progressive flexibility and strengthening (particularly eccentric) exercises are added as tolerated.

Achilles Tendon Rupture

Achilles tendinitis, which may be the source of posterior ankle pain, can be caused by repetitive eccentric loading of the dorsiflexors. Such overuse can occur if the dancer fails to reach a foot-flat position when performing dance maneuvers or if the gymnast performs aerial gymnastics with improper talar control on landing. Acute rupture of the Achilles tendon is more common in the gymnast and is often associated with a faulty landing or powerful acceleration during a tumbling run.

Achilles tendinitis is treated with relative rest, ice, or contrast therapy. Ultrasound may be applied to the Achilles tendon to assist in range-of-motion exercises. Rehabilitation is directed toward improving the flexibility of the heel cord and the first metatarsophalangeal joint (a part of the kinetic chain). A heel lift in street shoes is an appropriate short-term measure to reduce the stress on the tendon, but long-term use promotes continued shortening of the tendon. Rarely is surgical repair necessary for Achilles tendinitis. Achilles rupture, on the other hand, should be repaired surgically; it can be a devastating injury and may require a prolonged period of rehabilitation after tendon repair.

"Dancing Pronator"

Forefoot pronation is a normal, physiologic process by which the foot acts as a shock absorber for the lower extremity during gait. Excessive pronation can predispose to significant problems such as flexor hallucis longus tendinitis, cuboid subluxation, patellofemoral dysfunction, and plantar fasciitis. Therefore, control of excessive pronation is important to reduce the risk of injury and to improve the dancer's chances for a long and productive career. Unfortunately, ballet shoes, because of their tight fit, do not allow for the placement of orthotic inserts. The need for total foot mobility makes some forms of taping unacceptable. The physician, therefore, is left with the dilemma of how to provide adequate treatment in a suboptimal situation. All biomechanic factors, such as inadequate hip "turnout" (Fig. 8), must be accurately diagnosed and treated before suggesting a change in dance style or intensity of dance training.

Orthotic inserts may be appropriate for street shoes or when the performer/athlete is not engaged in dance activity. Accommodation of other anatomic abnormalities, such as a plantar-flexed first ray, may be accommodated by padding, orthotics, or supportive taping. The

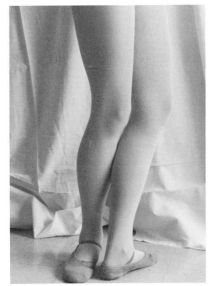
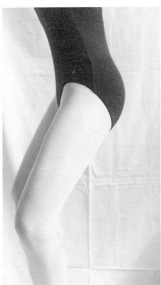

FIGURE 8. Inadequate turnout at the hip resulting in an excessive pronation moment at the foot. This is most evident in the dancer's right foot in the left panel. Note also the stresses placed on the knee in the right panel.

dance teacher, therapist, or trainer must be included in the training and treatment plan to help to correct faulty dance technique.

Fractures

Acute fractures of the foot occur primarily when the dancer "rolls off" the base of support in pointe or demi-pointe (see Figs. 3 and 9). This creates a supination moment and may cause a spiral fracture of the fifth metatarsal. Other acute injuries include acute fibular fracture and lateral malleolar fracture. These injuries can occur in external rotation of the leg on pointe. Medial malleolar fractures may occur with forceful ankle inversion when landing from a jump in the demi-pointe position.

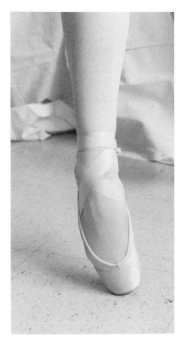
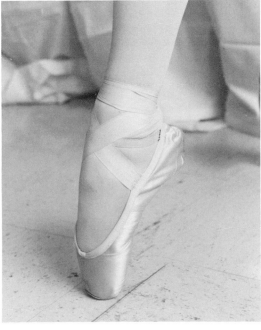

FIGURE 9. A correctly positioned foot on pointe *(left)* compared to a foot that is "rolling off" *(right)*. Fractures of the fifth metatarsal result as the dancer is unable to maintain the position on the right.

The Spine

In gymnastics and ballet the lumbar spine is subjected to repetitive, forceful extension during jumps or dismounts. Spinal motion, which is often extreme in the dancer or gymnast, puts a great deal of strain on the osseous, ligamentous, and muscular structures of the back. Lack of mobility, strength, or endurance can result in significant injury.

In the dancer with complaints of low back pain, a thorough examination of muscular strength and flexibility, segmental spine mechanics, flexibility in the pelvic musculature, and anatomic integrity is needed. Treatment and rehabilitation of the injured performer/athlete with lumbar spine dysfunction must first be directed toward clearly delineating the source of the pathology.

Spondylolysis, a stress fracture of the pars interarticularis, occurs in 10% to 20% of gymnasts and dancers[11] compared with 3% to 5% of the general population.[9] In spondylolysis, pain is localized to the lumbosacral spine; it is exacerbated by extension. During the early phases of spondylolysis, the pain is relieved by rest. Continued activity results in progression of the stress fracture and persistent pain. Treatment includes immobilization with a lumbosacral orthosis (Boston) brace for up to 3 months in the case of spondylolysis, with progressive mobilization thereafter. During the period of immobilization, the dancer is encouraged to maintain a level of aerobic fitness. Certain movement therapies, such as Pilates or Feldenkrais (mentioned below), may prevent the loss of kinesthetic awareness

associated with a prolonged period of down time. Surgical intervention should be considered as a last resort if the performer/athlete is to continue participating at a high level. Immobilization by surgical fusion increases the stress forces and degenerative changes at levels above the fusion. In cases of severe spondylolysis that causes pain and dysfunction, it may be reasonable to counsel the patient to seek an alternative activity.

Biomechanical Factors and Low Back Pain

A number of biomechanical factors may predispose to mechanical low back pain in dancers and gymnasts, including areas of specific muscle weakness or inflexibility. For instance, tightness of the iliopsoas restricts turnout at the hip and increases pelvic tilt, resulting in a hyperlordotic posture. The arabesque (Fig. 10) position results in midline localized pain at the lumbosacral junction as the dancer moves into hyperlordosis in an effort to compensate for poor hip mobility. Segmental dysfunction (hyper- or hypomobility) results in altered coupled motion of the thoracolumbar spine and may also result in injury.

ALTERNATIVE/MOVEMENT THERAPIES

Performer/athletes require a keen kinesthetic sense and ability to perform complicated movement patterns in a skilled and graceful fashion. Standard rehabilitation

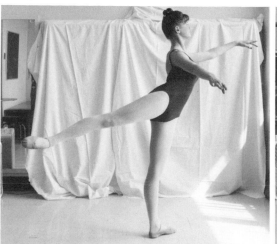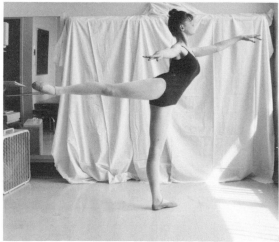

FIGURE 10. Arabesque using incorrect *(left)* and correct *(right)* form. Note the increased lordosis and lower leg position in the right panel.

techniques improve strength, endurance, and functional ability. Dancers frequently employ alternative or movement therapies as an adjunct to standard rehabilitation programs as well as to their dance training. Two primary movement therapies include the Feldenkrais/Alexander technique and the Pilates/Gyrotonics programs to enhance neuromuscular control.

Around the turn of the century (the same time period in which osteopathic and chiropractic techniques were developed), F. Mathias Alexander described numerous musculoskeletal conditions as due to patterns of misuse. Alexander hypothesized that habitual patterns are the product of years of misuse that must be corrected through neuromuscular education, joint mobilization, and postural awareness. The techniques are individualized and therefore difficult to subject to rigorous testing. Different practitioners use different mobilization techniques. Moshe Feldenkrais used some of Alexander's teachings to create a series of exercises he termed "lessons," which are often performed in large groups or classes designed to incorporate mind-and-body activities. He termed the series of activities "awareness through movement" and theorized that muscular activity against gravity makes up the bulk of stimuli to the nervous system. The lessons were designed to isolate movement patterns in the prone or supine position, with gravity eliminated. Once movement patterns were broken down to their most basic level, correct patterns could be developed. The intended result is appropriate kinesthetic feedback and the development of kinesthetic awareness. Principles of joint mobilization are used as necessary to facilitate appropriate muscular contractile patterns.

In the 1920s Joseph Pilates described a series of some 300 exercises performed with and without machines to facilitate muscular isolation and reeducation. Many of the exercises stress stabilization of the lumbar spine and are performed in a neutral spine position. The exercises tend to be exceedingly rigorous and may not be appropriate for the dancer in the initial phases of rehabilitation. As the patient progresses, various movement patterns are incorporated into the exercise program. The machines used in Pilates' training tend to work in a closed kinetic fashion to strengthen the lower or upper body concentrically and eccentrically. The Pilates system is used by many professional dance companies and is available in most metropolitan areas. One of the major benefits of Pilates therapy is balanced strengthening of agonist/antagonist muscle groups in a non–weight-bearing fashion; thus rehabilitation can be facilitated even while full weight bearing cannot be tolerated. Gyrotonics, a variant of the Pilates principle, also uses machines and mat exercises to facilitate neuromuscular patterning.

INJURIES SPECIFIC TO GYMNASTICS

Epidemiologic studies of gymnastics[5,9] suggest a high incidence of both acute and chronic injuries. Garrick and Requa[9] suggest that approximately one-third of gymnasts will sustain a significant injury during the course of a competitive season. Injury patterns tend to be similar to those mentioned above and occur at similar rates. Injuries of the upper extremities, however, occur with greater frequency because of loading of the upper extremities in floor exercise or on various apparatuses. Injuries occur most commonly in floor exercise; this is partially related to the amount of time allotted to floor exercise as well as to the high forces generated with aerial maneuvers. For female gymnasts, the second most common area of injury is the balance beam. Balance beam injuries tend to occur with the wrist in dorsiflexion as the force of body weight is transmitted through the wrist and elbow complexes in a closed kinetic chain. Long training sessions and an extreme number of repetitions of the same movement patterns can lead to physical and/or mental fatigue and may increase the risk of injury.

Some authors have suggested gymnasts have an abnormally high rate of reinjury. Caine[5] felt that the rate of reinjury may be due to underestimation of the severity of the primary injury, inadequate rehabilitation, or premature return to full participation. As with other sports, the ankle and knee tend to be the most frequently injured parts. However, injuries to the upper extremity, trunk, and spine are disproportionately higher in gymnasts. Upper extremity and spine injuries account for approximately 27% and 15% to 20%, respectively.[32]

The Shoulder in Gymnasts

Injuries of the shoulder most commonly involve strain injuries of the scapular stabilizer or glenohumeral muscles. Shoulder injuries occur more frequently in men's than women's gymnastics and may be associated with ring or horizontal bar exercises. Such exercises require high-speed, large-amplitude movements and place significant stress on the shoulder joint, resulting in overuse injury.

Impingement

Findings on examination of shoulder impingement include tenderness to palpation and positive signs of impingement. Treatment is directed toward acute care of the impingement, followed by aggressive training aimed at scapular stabilization. A poor response to therapy may warrant further investigation of other pathology, such as labral injury or partial rotator cuff tear. Acute tears of the rotator cuff are potentially devastating injuries in gymnasts, given the range and strength requirements of the rings and horizontal bar.

Gymnast's Elbow

The biomechanics of performing a back handspring, coupled with the aesthetic requirements of the judges, results in high-peak ground reactive forces.[22] With increasing impact velocity, recreational athletes tend to distribute impact force over a longer time interval through flexion of the hips and knees. As a result, peak impact forces are dissipated. Gymnasts, who are trained to land or dismount without excessive joint motion, do not use a similar strategy and thus are subjected to high-peak impact forces with high-impact velocities. When less competitive or recreational gymnasts perform a hand spring, they increase elbow flexion with increasingly higher loads, thereby dissipating the forces as the hands strike the ground. More competitive, higher-level gymnasts maintain a nearly straight elbow during the double support phase, thereby increasing the peak forces at ground contact. A rigid, partially flexed elbow results in large compression forces, estimated at 2.3 to 2.4 times body weight. Shortly after ground contact, a valgus moment is placed on the elbow.[22] Many gymnasts are young, growing athletes for whom the growth plates have not yet fused.

Elbow injuries in gymnasts can be devastating. Osteochondritis dissecans, a potentially se-

rious affliction of the humeral capitellum, can end a gymnast's career. Jackson et al.[18] described this condition in a series of 7 female gymnasts and reported only 1 athlete who was able to return to competitive gymnastics. The authors postulated that the capitellum is exposed to a combination of factors that cannot be compensated for or avoided in the competitive gymnast. Overuse injuries may also occur at the olecranon.[29] Such injuries cause diffuse, dull elbow pain associated with stiffness and swelling over the olecranon. Recurrent or chronic injuries can result in stress fractures of the epiphysis, especially in growing adolescents.

Gymnast's Wrist

Injuries to the wrist are often attributed to impingement due to disruption of the triangular fibrocartilage and associated instability of the lunate.

Stress fractures of the distal radius or radial growth plate have also been reported.[38] On examination, such instability may reveal pain with mobilization of the lunate. Frank subluxation of the bone may occur. In such cases, bone-scan imaging demonstrates an area of increased uptake at the distal radius. In addition to these conditions, a number of ligamentous injuries may occur at the wrist, especially in activities such as vaulting, pommel horse, or floor exercises. Minor ligamentous injuries can be managed with a dorsal wrist orthosis that limits the amount of wrist extension. More severe injuries may require a period of immobilization.

REFERENCES

1. Alexander E, Kelly DL, Davis CH, et al: Intact arch spondylolisthesis. J Neurosurg 63:840–844, 1985.
2. Bachrach RM: Injury to the dancer's spine. In Stevens RE, Ryan AJ (eds): Dance Medicine: A Comprehensive Guide. Chicago, Plurabus Press, 1987, pp 243–266.
3. Barrett DS: Proprioception and function after anterior cruciate reconstruction. J Bone Joint Surg 73B:833–837, 1991.
4. Bejjani FJ: Occupational Biomechanics of athletes and dancers: A comparative approach. Clin Podiatr Med Surg 4:671–711, 1987.
5. Caine D, Cochrine B, Caine C, Zemper E: Epidemiologic investigation of injuries affecting young competitive female gymnasts. Am J Sports Med 17:811–820, 1989.
6. Chan D, Aldridge MJ, Maffuli N, Davies AM: Chronic stress injuries of the elbow in young gymnasts. Am J Sports Med 64:1113–1118, 1991.

7. Garrick JG, Gillian DM, Whiteside P: The epidemiology of aerobic dance injuries. *Am J Sports Med* 14:67–72, 1986.
8. Garrick JG, Requa RK: Aerobic dance: A review. *Am J Sports Med* 6:169–179, 1988.
9. Garrick RG, Requa RK: Epidemiology of women's gymnastics injuries. *Am J Sports Med* 8:261–264, 1980.
10. Goldstein JD, Burger PE, Windler GE, Jackson DW: Spine injuries in gymnasts and swimmers. *Am J Sports Med* 19:463–468, 1991.
11. Hall SJ: Mechanical contribution to lumbar stress injuries in female gymnasts. *Med Sci Sports Exerc* 18:599–602, 1986.
12. Hamilton WG: Foot and ankle injuries in dancers. *Clin Sports Med* 7:143–173, 1988.
13. Hardaker WT: Foot and ankle injuries in classical ballet dancers. *Orthop Clin North Am* 20:621–627, 1989.
14. Hardaker WT, Erickson LC: Medical considerations in dance training for children. *Am Fam Physician* 35:93–99, 1987.
15. Harris IE, Weinstein SL: Long-term follow-up with patient's with grade III and IV spondylolisthesis. *J Bone Joint Surg* 69A:960–968, 1987.
16. Inglis B, West R: *The Alternative Health Guide.* New York, Alfred A. Knopf, 1983.
17. Irving G: Leisure-aerobics and dance injuries. *Nursing RSA: Verpleging* 5:17–19, 1990.
18. Jackson DW, Sylveno N, Reiman P: Osteochondritis in the female gymnast's elbow. *Arthroscopy* 5:129–136, 1989.
19. Kessler RM, Hertling D: *Management of Common Musculoskeletal Disorders.* New York, Harper & Row, 1983.
20. Kleiger B: Foot and ankle injuries in dancers. In Stevens RE, Ryan AJ (eds): *Dance Medicine: A Comprehensive Guide.* Chicago, Plurabus Press, 1987, pp 115–134.
21. Klemp P, Stevens JE, Isaacs S: Hypermobility study in ballet dancers. *J Rheumatol* 11:692–696, 1984.
22. Koh TJ, Grabiner MD, Weiker GG: Technique and ground reaction forces in the back handspring. *Am J Sports Med* 20:61–66, 1992.
23. Landsmeer JMF: Studies in the anatomy of articulation: II. Patterns of movement of bi-muscular, bi-articular systems. *Acta Morphol Ned Scand* 3:304–321, 1961.
24. Landsmeer JMF, Long C: The mechanism of finger control, based on electromyograms and location analysis. *Acta Anat* 60:330–347, 1965.
25. Letts M, Smallman T, Afansiev R, Gouw G: Fractures of the pars interarticularis in adolescent athletes: A clinical, biomechanical analysis. *J Pediatr Orthop* 6:40–46, 1986.
26. Lindner KJ, Caine DJ: Injury patterns of female competitive club gymnasts. *Can J Sports Sci* 15:254–261, 1989.
27. Loock F, Lorenz M: Berufskrankheiten und Berufsunfahigkeiten in der Theatern and Orchestern der DDR. *Z Gesamte Hyg* 31:716–719, 1985.
28. Lyons LC, Peterson LFA: The snapping iliopsoas tendon. *Mayo Clin Proc* 59:327–329, 1984.
29. Maffuli N, Chan D, Aldridge MJ: Overuse injuries of the olecranon in young gymnasts. *J Bone Joint Surg* 74B:305–309, 1992.
30. Markiewitz AD, Andrish JT: Hand and wrist injuries in the pre-adolescent and adolescent athlete. *Clin Sports Med* 11:203–225, 1992.
31. Marshall P: The rehabilitation of overuse foot injuries in athletes and dancers. *Clin Sports Med* 7:175–191, 1988.
32. Meeusen R, Borms J: Gymnastic injuries. *J Sports Med* 13:337–356, 1992.
33. Micheli, LJ: Back injuries in dancers. *Clinic Sports Med* 2:473–483, 1983.
34. Micheli LJ, Gillespie WJ, Walaszek A: A physiological profile of professional ballerinas. *Clinic Sports Med* 3:199–209, 1984.
35. Micheli LJ, Solomon R: Training the young dancer. In Stevens RE, Ryan AJ (eds): *Dance Medicine: A Comprehensive Guide.* Chicago, Plurabus Press, 1987, pp 51–72.
36. Molnar ME: Rehabilitation of the injured dancer. In Stevens RE, Ryan AJ (eds): *Dance Medicine: A Comprehensive Guide.* Chicago, Plurabus Press, 1987, pp 302–320.
37. Newell SG, Woodle A: Cuboid syndrome. *Physician Sports Med* 9:71–74, 1981.
38. Pettrone FA, Ricciardelli E: Gymnastic injuries: The Virginia experience 1982–1983. *Am J Sports Med* 15:59–62, 1987.
39. Quirk R: Ballet injuries: The Australian experience. *Clin Sports Med* 2:507–514, 1983.
40. Quirk R: The dancer's knee. In Stevens RE, Ryan AJ (eds): *Dance Medicine: A Comprehensive Guide.* Chicago, Plurabus Press, 1987, pp 177–219.
41. Rovere GD, Webb LX, Gristina AG: Musculoskeletal injuries in theatrical dance students. *Am J Sports Med* 11:195–198, 1983.
42. Sammarco GJ: Diagnosis and treatment of dancers. *Clin Orthop* 187:176–187, 1984.
43. Sammarco GJ: The dancer's hip. In Stevens RE, Ryan AJ (eds): *Dance Medicine: A Comprehensive Guide.* Chicago, Plurabus Press, 1987, pp 220–241.
44. Silver JR, Silver DD, Godfried JJ: Injuries of the spine sustained during gymnastic activities. *BMJ* 293:861–863, 1986.
45. Stephens RE: Etiology of injuries in ballet. In Stevens RE, Ryan AJ (eds): *Dance Medicine: A Comprehensive Guide.* Chicago, Plurabus Press, 1987, pp 16–50.
46. Sward L, Hellstrom M, Jacobsson B, et al: Acute injury of the vertebral ring apophysitis and intervertebral disc in adolescent gymnasts. *Spine* 15:144–148, 1990.
47. Taunton JE, McKinzie DC, Clement DV: The role of biomechanics in the epidemiology of injuries. *J Sports Med* 6:107–120, 1988.
48. Thomasen E: *Diseases and Injuries of Ballet Dancers.* Arhus, Denmark, Universitetsforlaget, 1982.
49. Weiker GG: Hand and wrist problems in the gymnast. *Clin Sports Med* 11:189–202, 1992.
50. Weir MR, Smith DS: Stress reaction of the pars interarticularis leading to spondylolysis. *J Adolesc Health Care* 10:573–577, 1989.
51. Zindrick MR, Lorenz MA: The non-reductive treatment of spondylolisthesis. *Semin Spine Surg* 1:116–124, 1989.

Chapter 11

FOOTBALL AND OTHER CONTACT SPORT INJURIES: Diagnosis and Treatment

John C. Pritchard, MD

Football is the most popular contact sport in the United States. An estimated 1.5 million players participate annually and sustain 1.2 million football-related injuries.[29] The overall likelihood of an individual player sustaining an injury varies from 11% to 81%, depending on the level of competition.[27] The significance of these injuries was noted as early as 1905 when President Roosevelt appealed to the Ivy League Schools to improve the safety of the sport after he read an alarming report of 18 deaths and 159 serious injuries during the course of one season.[29]

Overall, lower-extremity injuries account for approximately 50% (knee, 36%) and upper-extremity injuries for 30% of the total, with spine and visceral injuries comprising the remainder. Specific categories include strains and sprains (40%), contusions (25%), dislocations (15%), fractures (10%), and concussions (5%).[29]

Epidemiologic studies since the early 1970s have contributed significantly to our knowledge of football injuries. Changes in coaching techniques, game rules, protective equipment, and playing surfaces have all influenced injury rates.

Anyone participating in the care of athletes must recognize the nature and magnitude of these injuries and understand their diagnosis, treatment, and appropriate rehabilitation (Fig. 1). It is also important to be involved in measures to prevent or reduce the morbidity of injuries in contact sports. This chapter acquaints the practitioner with injuries commonly seen in football and other contact sports that involve high velocity and impact.

BRAIN INJURIES

Brain injury encompasses an area of potentially catastrophic morbidity and mortality in contact sports. It has been recognized as the leading cause of death on the football field.[12] Records indicate that deaths remain fairly constant at 5 to 10/year. This results in a risk ratio of 0.65/100,000 participants.[34]

There are three important considerations for physicians dealing with brain injury in contact sports:

(1) to recognize and to diagnose accurately the presence of a brain injury;
(2) to determine if and when additional diagnostic testing is indicated; and
(3) to counsel the athlete about return to contact activities and future risk of injury.

Brain injuries may be divided into three major categories; mild, moderate, and severe. Moderate and severe brain injuries usually involve a loss of consciousness, whereas mild brain injury may not. The injury may be focal or, more commonly, a diffuse axonal injury. Such diffuse axonal injury can result in loss of consciousness and may cause long-term disability.

Focal injuries include intracranial hemorrhages, cerebral contusions, subdural hemorrhages, and epidural hemorrhages.[34] Intra-

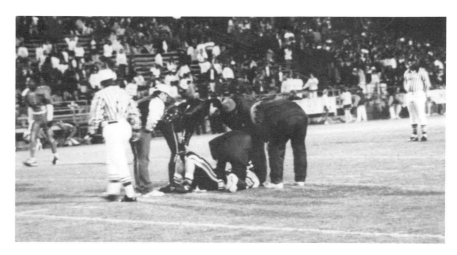

FIGURE 1. Early assessment of the injured athlete helps to reduce morbidity and adds valuable diagnostic information. Caution is required in moving the injured athlete. Suspected neck injuries should be immobilized with cervical spine precautions; the helmet should not be removed. Any injured extremity should be carefully supported to avoid further injury.

cerebral hematoma and cerebral contusion usually cause persistent headaches, periods of confusion, and posttraumatic amnesia. These injuries require computed tomographic (CT) scanning and a complete neurologic evaluation.[2]

Epidural hematomas result from injuries to the meningeal arteries and may involve a rapid deterioration in status, beginning with headaches and progressing to altered mental status, pupillary changes, and decerebrate posturing. These injuries must be approached cautiously because the classic picture may not always be present. Full evaluation and diagnostic studies are required if an epidural hematoma is suspected.[2]

Acute subdural hematoma is a collection of blood in the subdural space. Mortality from subdural hematoma increases to 50% if underlying brain injury is present. Patients often display focal neurologic findings and once again require a full diagnostic evaluation.[2]

In general, severe head injuries present with immediate and prolonged loss of consciousness (>3–5 min). After waking, the athlete may drift back into unconsciousness, an ominous sign that is often seen in subdural or epidural hematomas. When such injury is present, consideration must be given to the possible coexistence of spinal injury and instability.[34]

The initial treatment of severe injuries is directed at maintaining a patent airway, protecting the spine, and initiating appropriate resuscitative procedures with emergent transportation for complete diagnostic evaluation and treatment.[34] Athletes with moderate-to-severe brain injury should not be allowed to return to competitive play.[34]

Concussion

The most common head injury in contact sports is a minor injury or **concussion**.[34] Approximately 250,000 concussions occur annually in football.[4] An estimated 20% of high school football players suffer concussions annually. The likelihood of a repeat, second concussion is increased fourfold in these players.[11] Concussions have been defined as an "immediate and transient impairment of neural function such as alteration of consciousness, disturbance of vision, equilibrium, and other similar symptoms."[6] Theoretic and experimental evidence has implicated rotational acceleration as the primary mechanism of such diffuse brain injury.[2]

Cantu devised a simple on-field grading scheme to aid in diagnosis and initial management of concussions.[4] Grade I, or mild, concussions account for more than 50% of minor injuries. There is no loss of consciousness, impairment of intellectual function is mild, and posttraumatic amnesia lasts less than 30 minutes. Grade I concussions are commonly referred to as "having your bell rung." Treatment requires immediate removal from the game and a short 15 to 30-minute period of observation. Headaches, dizziness, impaired concentration, focal neurologic findings, and full recall of events leading to the injury must be evaluated. Return to contact may be considered if the player is completely asymptomatic.

Grade II, or moderate concussion, involves loss of consciousness for less than 5 minutes or posttraumatic amnesia for longer than 30 minutes. Initial treatment includes removal from participation and full evaluation at a medical facility. Spinal injury must be ruled out.

Grade III, or severe, concussion involves loss of consciousness for more than 5 minutes or posttraumatic amnesia for longer than 24 hours. Grade III concussions must be treated as severe, life-threatening injuries with appropriate life-support measures, spinal injury precautions, and transportation for definitive diagnosis and treatment.

Return to contact sports after multiple concussions has been discussed by several authors.[4,34] A second mild concussion dictates removal from contact activity for a least 2 weeks. All symptoms should resolve prior to return. Consideration for further evaluation may be indicated if the concussions occur close together. A third mild concussion should end the competitive season.

After a grade II, or moderate, concussion the asymptomatic player may return to play in 1 to 2 weeks. A second moderate concussion requires a minimum of 1 month delay with consideration of terminating the season. A third moderate concussion mandates termination of participation.

Athletes with severe, or grade III, concussions may return to activity after 1 month if they are totally asymptomatic and if all studies are normal. A second severe concussion requires termination of the season and consideration of ending the career. High school or college athletes should be counseled that it is safer not to return to contact sports after multiple concussions because of the possibility of permanent damage if they continue to play.

Another important condition, the "second-impact syndrome," involves brain swelling and herniation after a second and possibly minor impact in a patient with preexisting brain injury. The mortality rate, which approaches 50%, underscores the fact that any athlete who is symptomatic from a brain injury must not participate in contact sports until all symptoms have subsided and preferably no sooner than 1 week after injury.[3]

CERVICAL SPINE

Cervical spine injuries encompass a host of pathologic conditions ranging from nerve-root stretch injuries to fractures and dislocations. From 1977 to 1988, 116 permanent cervical cord injuries were recorded in football players. The overwhelming majority (96) occurred in high school football.[24] In 1976, organized football instituted rule changes that eliminated "spearing," or use of the head as an initial point of contact. This change has resulted in a dramatic decrease in the total number and severity of cervical cord injuries.[33] The rate of permanent paralysis for 1990 was approximately 0.72/100,000 players. From 3 to 15 football-related permanent cord injuries still occur each year.[5] Axial loading on the slightly flexed neck has been implicated in the majority of serious cervical injuries.[33]

Any potential cervical spine injury presenting during contact sports must be treated with the utmost respect, and any unconscious athlete must be assumed to have cervical spine injury. Appropriate immobilization of the spine, including in-line traction with the helmet on and a minimum of three persons for log-rolling, is indicated.[12] All steps of basic life support must be addressed as well. Pain in the cervical spine, with or without abnormal neurologic findings, warrants transfer to a medical facility for appropriate diagnostic evaluation. Detailed treatment of all possible injuries is beyond the scope of this text, but in all injuries, the clinician's initial goal is to protect the spinal cord from further injury.

Cervical sprains are frequently seen in contact sports. The diagnosis is one of exclusion and is based on a normal neurologic examination and normal radiographic studies (including flexion and extension views). Treatment may consist of a short period of support with a soft collar and therapeutic modalities to reduce inflammation. Any athlete with less than a full cervical range of motion and normal strength should be prohibited from contact activities.[32]

The most common cervical injuries are the pinch-stretch neurapraxias of the brachial plexus, commonly called "burners" or "stingers." At least one burner episode has been noted in 33% to 67% of college football players (Fig. 2).[14] This injury generally occurs when the shoulder is driven downward and the neck is pushed to the opposite side. The sharp burning pain may be associated with

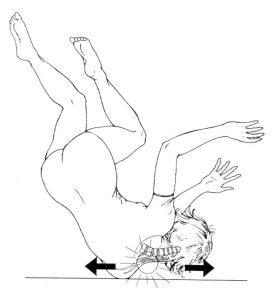

FIGURE 2. The mechanism of brachial plexus stretch injury.

paresthesias and anesthesia of the arm (Fig. 3).[14] The sensation is usually short-lived, and a full pain-free range of cervical motion is present. If the athlete can demonstrate full symmetrical strength of the upper extremities and a full pain-free cervical range of motion, return to play may be considered.[32] Recurrent episodes, persistent neurologic findings, or bilateral symptoms require further diagnostic testing before return to contact activities.[15] This injury has been seen in athletes with stable vertebral fractures.

Several steps are important in preventing cervical spine injuries in contact sports. All coaches, officials, and medical personnel should discourage use of the head as a weapon for tackling or blocking. Protective equipment should fit well and should be inspected often. In adolescents, new equipment is indicated as the athlete grows. Conditioning exercises to strengthen the cervical musculature should be emphasized. Once suspected, cervical injuries need to be assessed rapidly, and the athlete should be protected from further injury during transportation in a safe and efficient manner to a medical facility for definitive evaluation and treatment.[5,24]

BACK INJURIES

The majority of the injuries to the back in contact sports involve the lumbar spine. Up to

30% of college football players have lost playing time secondary to lumbar spine problems.[29] These injuries most commonly include sprains and muscle strains but may also involve bony injuries such as spondylolysis and spondylolisthesis or disc-related problems.

Back sprains and strains typically occur with twisting or bending injuries to the lumbar spine. The pain is localized to the area of the lower back, and radicular symptoms are not present. Osseous injury can be excluded only with radiography. Treatment involves reduction of acute inflammation with rest and application of ice. Standard rehabilitation of the lumbar spine muscles with stretching and strengthening is indicated, and return to full function should be expected within 10 days to 3 weeks.[25] Back pain with sciatica or radicular symptoms may be treated initially in a similar fashion. Persistence of symptoms with or without associated weakness or reflex changes should be further evaluated with diagnostic modalities such as MRI or CT scan to rule out disc disease. Failure of conservative treatment in the face of proven disc pathology may warrant other treatment, such as epidural steroids or surgery.[25]

Repetitive extension and loading of the

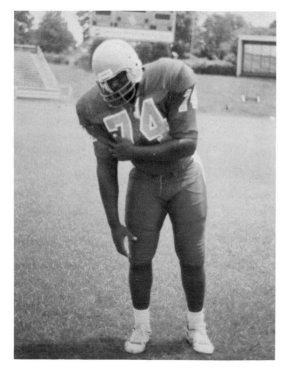

FIGURE 3. An athlete demonstrating the "dead-arm" posturing commonly seen with burner episodes.

posterior elements of the lumbar spine, which occur when linemen rise from their starting stance to blocking posture, may lead to fatigue fracture of the arch of the vertebrae.[29] This spondylolysis occurs in the area of the pars interarticularis and, if not recognized, may lead to spondylolisthesis, particularly in the skeletally immature athlete. Spondylolysis presents with back pain exacerbated by extension. Diagnosis is confirmed by radiographs and bone-scanning in some instances. Treatment involves limiting activities, flexibility and strengthening exercises, and use of a thoracolumbar orthosis.[25] Asymptomatic spondylolysis is not a contraindication to sports participation. Progressive or symptomatic spondylolisthesis may exhibit nerve-root symptoms and may require surgical intervention.

UPPER EXTREMITY

Shoulder Girdle

Some of the most common injuries to the shoulder girdle in contact sports include clavicle fractures, shoulder dislocations, and acromioclavicular injuries.

The most frequently fractured bone around the shoulder in contact sports is the clavicle, which in adolescent athletes is usually due to a direct blow. The middle third of the clavicle breaks and causes obvious swelling and deformity. Diagnosis is confirmed by radiographs. Treatment includes the use of a fig-

ure-of-eight brace to hold the shoulders in a retracted position and of a sling for subsequent comfort. Return to contact sport is generally in 8 weeks if clinical symptoms resolve and radiographs show bony union. Shoulder motion and strength should be regained before return to activity.[18]

Shoulder separations or sprains of the acromioclavicular joint are extremely common in a sport that emphasizes player contact with the shoulders. The mechanism of injury is usually direct contact on the point of the shoulder (acromion) with the arm adducted. Such contact may occur with falling or player impact.[28] Partial separations, grade I and II, involve injury to the acromioclavicular ligament, whereas complete separations, grade III and greater, involve complete tears of the acromioclavicular and coracoclavicular ligaments (Fig. 4).[28] The incomplete injuries occur about twice as often as complete separations.[28] Inspection of the shoulder reveals acute tenderness and a "step-off" at the acromioclavicular joint. Radiographs can readily demonstrate separation of the joint, and stress radiographs with an arm weight can differentiate a grade II, incomplete, from a grade III, complete, separation (Fig. 5).[28]

Treatment includes rest, ice, and possible sling use in grade I and II sprains. Grade III sprains have advocates for either surgical stabilization or closed treatment with slings. Most clinicians recommend surgery if the skin is tented or if significant interposition of the trapezius muscle occurs.[28] Return to contact sports requires full range of motion and strength, with possible additional padding to

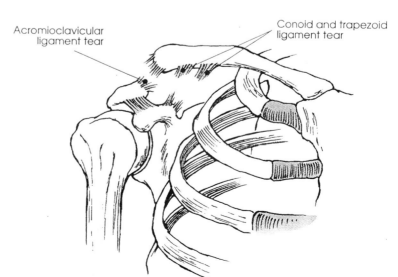

Acromioclavicular ligament tear

Conoid and trapezoid ligament tear

FIGURE 4. A complete disruption of the acromioclavicular and coracoclavicular (conoid and trapezoid) ligaments.

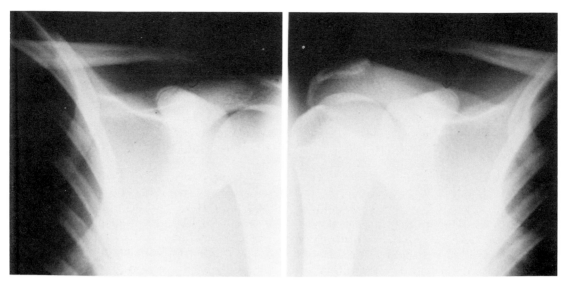

FIGURE 5. Weighted stress radiographs of an athlete's acromioclavicular joints demonstrate increased coracoclavicular distance on the right.

the acromioclavicular joint to protect the athlete. Arthritis of the acromioclavicular joint is a possible delayed complication.

Football is a common cause of shoulder instability; one of the most dramatic and frequent forms is traumatic anterior glenohumeral dislocation.[22] This injury may occur with an anteriorly directed force on the proximal humerus or with forced external rotation and abduction of the arm.[22] The athlete presents with acute pain, flattening of the lateral shoulder contour, and restricted motion. Initial examination must include a careful neurovascular evaluation. Radiographs should include at least anteroposterior views as well as an axillary and scapular lateral view (Fig. 6).[22] It is important not to miss an acute dislocation, and because the dislocation is often not evident on a single radiograph in the anteroposterior plane, the axillary and scapular lateral views are essential. The most common dislocation in the athlete is the subcoracoid type in which the humeral head lies anterior to the glenoid fossa and inferior to the coracoid process.[22]

Initial treatment includes a gentle reduction that may be performed on the playing field by an experienced clinician. In delayed reduction, pain and muscle spasm may necessitate sedation of the athlete to perform the maneuver. The reader is referred to orthopaedic texts for specific techniques. Following reduction and reassessment of neurovascular status, immobilization and symptomatic treat-

FIGURE 6. Axillary lateral radiograph of an anteriorly dislocated shoulder.

ment with modalities such as ice are in order. Redislocation is the most common complication and has been reported by several authors to occur in up to 85% of patients under 30 years of age.[22] After a short period of immobilization, strengthening of the rotator cuff may begin. Before returning to competition, the athlete should be able to perform internal and external rotation exercises against a resistance equal to 20% of body weight.[22] Any athlete with recurrent anterior dislocations despite a vigorous rehabilitation program should be considered for surgical stabilization.

Elbow

Elbow dislocations are not infrequent in contact sports. The mechanism usually involves a compressive load with extension force to the elbow.[16] The coronoid process comes to lie posterior to the distal humerus (Fig. 7). The key to treatment is early reduction, which requires a gentle atraumatic technique with careful attention to the neurovascular status of the extremity. Postreduction radiographs are essential to detect any retained bony fragments. Treatment with early protected range of motion has not been found to jeopardize elbow stability.[16] Return to athletics with protective bracing is generally accomplished within 3 to 6 weeks, depending on range of motion and strength.

Hand and Wrist

Injuries to the hand and wrist are common in football and are probably due to the minimal protective gear and the repeated exposure to trauma.[23]

Wrist injury in football is usually due to macrotraumatic impact, which can cause ligamentous sprain as well as fractures of the carpal bones, the distal radius, or the ulna.[13,23] Diagnosis requires careful examination for tenderness, range of motion, and neurovascular function. Radiographs are essential for any suspected injury. Special carpal views and stress views may be necessary to delineate subtle fractures and instabilities.[13,23]

Treatment is based on individual need, and return to competition does not follow strict guidelines. Distal radius fractures may require 3 months of healing before contact activities are resumed. Some authors have treated various wrist injuries (including stable scaphoid fractures) with early application of a soft splint. These devices have been approved by the National Collegiate Athletic Association (NCAA) and allow earlier return to contact activities.[1]

Injuries to the hand, again the result of exposure to violent impacts in contact sports, may include fractures, dislocations, and ligament sprains. Metacarpal fractures are common and usually result from direct impact (Fig. 8). The thumb metacarpal, however, is usually injured by an abduction force.[13] Most of these fractures can be managed nonsurgically if rotational malalignment and significant shortening of the bones can be controlled.[13] Splints initially incorporate the metacarpophalangeal joint, which is held in 60° to 90° of flexion to help to avoid joint stiffness after healing.[13] Once adequate healing of the fracture is determined by radio-

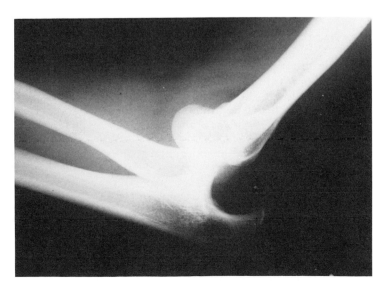

FIGURE 7. Lateral radiograph of a posterior elbow dislocation.

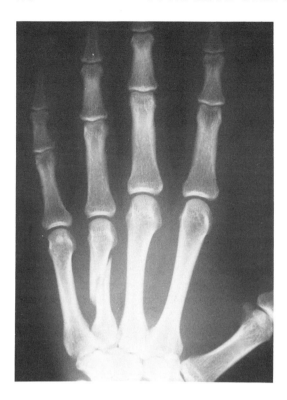

FIGURE 8. Anteroposterior radiograph of a metacarpal fracture, a commonly seen injury in contact sports.

graphs and clinical examination, protective padded splints and buddy taping (Fig. 9) may allow early return to contact sports. Metacarpal fractures with severe angulation, shortening, or displacement may require operative stabilization.

Fractures of the phalanx are also common and are caused by twisting, crushing, and bending forces. Closed reduction and splinting are effective for most of these fractures and also allow early return to sports participation.[13] For stable injuries and injuries with satisfactory healing, buddy taping may allow early controlled motion.[13]

With its prominent position, the thumb metacarpophalangeal joint is quite vulnerable to injuries in contact sports. The radial and ulnar collateral ligaments of the joint are often injured by valgus and varus forces, respectively. If not recognized early, these injuries may lead to functional losses in grip strength.[13,19] If a collateral ligament injury is suspected, manual stress testing of the joint is indicated. In partial injuries (grade I and II), stress testing causes pain and reveals mild or no pathologic joint laxity. In complete inju-

ries (grade III), no firm endpoint is noted on the ulnar or radial stress examination.[8,13] Radiographs may reveal bony avulsions. Stress radiographs may be useful in determining the severity of the injury. Partial ligament tears may be immobilized for 3 to 6 weeks in a spica splint, with subsequent taping to prevent reinjury.[8,13] Complete lesions generally require operative treatment to reestablish stability of the joint.[13,19]

Dislocations of the proximal interphalangeal joint may be seen after direct hyperextension or flexion injuries. Dorsal dislocations are most common and involve some degree of injury to the volar plate of the joint. Volar dislocations involve injury to the central digital extensor tendon.[13,19] Reduction of either dislocation requires exaggerating the deformity in flexion or extension without longitudinal traction and sliding the articular surfaces in the normal anteroposterior plane to a reduced position. Simple longitudinal traction may cause displacement of soft tissues into the joint, thereby blocking further reduction. Following a volar dislocation, the proximal interphalangeal joint is immobilized in extension for 3 to 6 weeks to prevent development of a boutonniere deformity. Dorsal dislocations are best immobilized in 15° to 30° of proximal interphalangeal flexion for 3 to 6 weeks, followed by buddy taping of the digit.[13] Radiographs are recommended to rule out an intraarticular fracture, which may predispose the joint to chronic subluxation. Even after appropriate treatment of proximal interphalangeal dislocations, complete motion may not be achieved. Functional impairment, however, is usually minimal.[13]

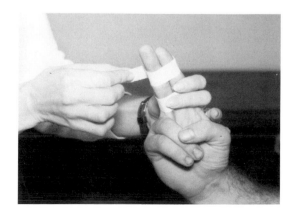

FIGURE 9. Buddy taping of an index and long finger to allow protected motion and early return to competition.

LOWER EXTREMITY

Hip and Pelvis

The area of the iliac crest is highly susceptible to injury in contact sports. Injury along the iliac crest may be in the form of a contusion (hip pointer) or an avulsion of the abdominal muscles attaching to the anterior and inner portions of the iliac wing. The history and physical examination are essential to differentiate between the two lesions. The contusion results from direct trauma and requires simple symptomatic treatment, ice and padding. The avulsion, in contrast, results from forceful contraction of the abdominal muscles with the trunk forced to the contralateral side.[26] The athlete shows great reluctance to straighten the trunk completely because of pain. Complete detachments of the muscles have been treated surgically, but most cases respond to local treatment with ice and compression. Taping of the trunk, which limits motion on the injured side, and gentle stretching exercises, in addition to protective padding, facilitate return to contact.[26]

Adolescent athletes may develop a slipped capital femoral epiphysis. This is a serious condition that needs to be ruled out in any young athlete presenting with a limp and hip or even knee pain.

Thigh

Despite protective padding, quadriceps contusions are ubiquitous injuries in contact sports. The athlete often continues to play, considering the initial injury insignificant. After bleeding into the thigh, however, the muscles become tense, swollen, and quite painful with movement. Compartment syndromes may occur and should be excluded with careful examination and, when clinically indicated, measurements of compartment pressure. For the isolated quadriceps contusion, compression (elastic wrap), immobilization, and icing are important initial treatments to minimize further bleeding (Fig. 10). Rehabilitation is important as early as possible. Gentle stretching and active flexion of the knee are in order.[26] Full symmetrical range of motion of the hip and knee is important before return to contact sports to prevent additional injury to the healing muscle. Chronic irritation of the injured muscle may produce myositis ossificans.[26]

Hamstring

Hamstring strains, which are seen in any running athlete, are common in football. The hamstrings provide a decelerating force as antagonists to the anterior thigh musculature.[25] Sudden changes in force may result in strain or even rupture at the musculotendinous junction. Strains range in severity from mild tearing of a few connective tissue fibers to complete ruptures of the muscle.[25] Treatment is dictated by the severity of the strain. Ice and compression are instituted initially. Rehabilitation is begun as pain diminishes. Slow stretching exercises and moist heat or deep ultrasound then follow. Redevelopment of muscle power begins with isometrics and isokinetics. Gradual return to activity may begin when flexibility, strength, isokinetic power, and endurance are normal.[25] Avoidance of further injury is important and

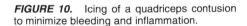
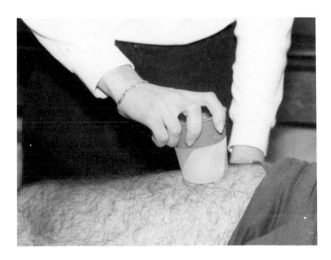

FIGURE 10. Icing of a quadriceps contusion to minimize bleeding and inflammation.

can be facilitated with continued stretching and strengthening exercises, proper technique, and appropriate taping for prevention of knee hyperextension.

Knee

Knee injuries, which are extremely common in football and other contact sports, may present a wide array of morbidity for the athlete. The femur and the tibia offer long lever arms for applied forces, and the joint is poorly controlled by protective equipment. Almost any knee structure can be injured in the athlete, and the causes may range from macrotrauma to overuse injuries. For the purpose of this discussion, only a few of the more common or significant disorders are described.

Injuries to the **medial collateral ligament** are very common and can be seen in athletes participating at any position in football. The classic mechanism of injury to this ligament is a contact-induced valgus stress to the knee while the foot is planted.[25] Physical examination reveals tenderness along the course of the medial collateral ligament and at its femoral and tibial insertions. The knee should be tested in varus and valgus stress, both in full extension and at 30° of flexion. Medial knee laxity at 30° of flexion is indicative of at least partial sprain of the medial collateral ligament, whereas pathologic laxity at full extension is seen with complete sprain and in some cases cruciate ligament injury. A grade I sprain involves 0 to 5 mm of valgus laxity; grade II, 5 to 10 mm; and grade III, > 10 mm without a firm endpoint.[8] Radiographs must be obtained to rule out growth plate injuries in the skeletally immature athlete.

Grade I injuries are treated symptomatically with a short period of immobilization and a subsequent range-of-motion and strengthening program. When symmetrical motion and strength return, the athlete may resume participation. Grade II and III injuries are more serious and can be associated with other ligamentous injuries to be knee.[25] Once cruciate ligament injury has been excluded, conservative treatment is acceptable for grade II and III injuries.[17,25] Once again, initial treatment involves a short period of immobilization. Later, a hinged brace may be beneficial to protect the medial ligaments while allowing range-of-motion exercises. Strengthening exercises begin when the patient is able to perform a straight leg raise. Some rehabilitation programs

limit initial motion to an arc of 30° to 90° but allow strengthening within this range.[17] Even in complete injuries, return to sports may be considered when strength, power, and endurance are symmetrical.[17] Residual laxity of 5 mm in complete tears does not seem to influence the ability to return to contact sports.[17] Prophylactic knee bracing is quite controversial, but protective functional bracing at the time of return to activity seems beneficial.[25,31]

Injuries to the **anterior cruciate ligament** are frequent in contact sports and are significant because of their career-ending potential. The history of injury is important because the player often hears or feels a "pop" with twisting and decelerating activity.[8] This is often a noncontact injury. Effusion usually accumulates within 6 to 12 hours. With immediate tense effusion, osteochondral fracture should be suspected.[10] The most important method of evaluating the integrity of the anterior cruciate ligament is the Lachman test. With the knee flexed to 30°, the examiner pulls the tibia anteriorly on the femur. Increased anterior excursion of the tibia on the femur compared with the uninjured side is pathonomomic of injury to the anterior cruciate ligament.[10] Another similar technique, the anterior drawer test, is done with the knee flexed to 90°. Again, forward movement of the tibia relative to the femur is indicative of injury to the anterior cruciate ligament.[8] Of the two tests, the Lachman test is the most sensitive (Fig. 11). In assessing the injured knee, a careful neurovascular evaluation is also important, as are radiographs to rule out an associated osteochondral fracture or avulsion. Decision algorithms, treatment of injuries to the anterior cruciate ligament, and associated intraarticular pathologies are beyond the scope of this chapter. It is important, however, to establish an early diagnosis, because examination at a later time is often obscured by swelling and secondary muscle spasm.[8] Some patients with isolated injuries to the anterior cruciate ligament may attempt to return to play when they achieve full range of motion and symmetrical strength in the injured extremity. Most, however, require surgical reconstruction of the ligament.

Knee **dislocations** may occur during football. They are a rare injury but are mentioned because of their potentially devastating nature. Dislocations may spontaneously reduce. They allow increased anterior and posterior translation of the tibia on the femur in addition to pathologic varus or valgus laxity.[20,30] If

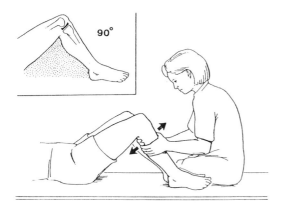

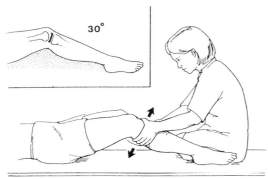

FIGURE 11. **Top,** Anterior drawer testing. **Bottom,** Lachman test. The windows show how the posterior meniscus can act as a wedge to prevent anterior tibial movement. Thus, the anterior drawer test is less sensitive to detecting cruciate ligamentous laxity than the Lachman test. (From Buschbacher RM (ed): *Musculoskeletal Disorders: A Practical Guide for Diagnosis and Rehabilitation.* Stoneham, MA, Butterworth-Heinemann, 1994, with permission.)

gross femoral/tibial displacement is evident, reduction should proceed as soon as possible. Traction is usually sufficient for reduction, but muscle relaxation with sedatives may be necessary.[20] A careful neurovascular evaluation is mandatory because nerve injuries have been reported in up to 35% and popliteal artery injuries in up to 38% of cases.[21] Treatment is controversial, but appropriate initial management of this true orthopedic emergency is essential to avoid limb-threatening sequelae. The athlete should be quickly removed from the field while supporting the injured extremity. The leg needs to avoid a dependent position or any weight-bearing.

Ankle

Ankle injuries are quite frequent in any athletic endeavor, and football is no excep-

tion. The most common cause of ankle injury is inversion stress and plantar flexion, which produce damage primarily to the lateral ligamentous structures.[9] In plantar flexion, the anterior talofibular ligament is taut and most likely to be injured. Further stress to the lateral ligaments may cause injury to the calcaneofibular and, more rarely, the posterior talofibular ligament.

The history is important to determine the mechanism of injury. Physical examination should localize the area of maximal tenderness. Pain in the region of the medial malleolus may indicate involvement of the deltoid ligament. More proximal tenderness may indicate injury to the tibiofibular ligament with interosseous membrane disruption (particularly in rotational injuries.)[9] The anterior drawer test and inversion stress test of the ankle may indicate the severity of the injury (Fig. 12). The anterior drawer test is performed by stabilizing the tibia and grasping the calcaneus while exerting a gentle anterior

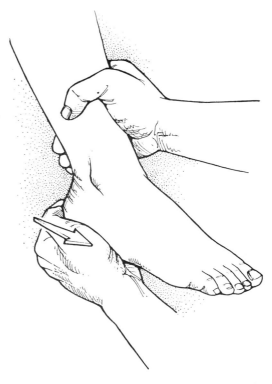

FIGURE 12. The anterior drawer test of the ankle. Excessive laxity is indicative of anterior talofibular ligament rupture. (From Buschbacher RM (ed): *Musculoskeletal Disorders: A Practical Guide for Diagnosis and Rehabilitation.* Stoneham, MA, Butterworth-Heinemann, 1994, with permission.)

force. Increased forward translation of the talus in the ankle mortise (over the noninjured side) indicates damage to the anterior talofibular ligament.[8,9] The inversion stress test is performed while stabilizing the distal tibia and moving the talus and calaneus into inversion. Greater than 10° inversion (a talar tilt) is a sign of an unstable joint.[9] Radiographs are essential to assess any associated fractures of the ankle; stress radiographs may also help to evaluate the severity of the injury (Fig. 13).[9]

The goal of treatment is to minimize disability by reducing pain and swelling and to enable a rapid return to activity. The acronym RICE identifies the elements of treatment in the first 24 to 48 hours, which emphasize pain control and minimization of edema:

*R*est, with weight-bearing as tolerated;

*I*ce, 20 minutes or less 4 times daily;

*C*ompression, by bandage or air splint; and

*E*levation of the affected extremity to control swelling and edema.

Subsequent treatment concentrates on normalizing range of motion, strengthening, and enhancing proprioception.[9] Temperature-contrast baths and electrical muscle stimulation are useful during this period. In addition, surgical tubing exercises are used for strengthening, and stationary bicycling maintains conditioning.

Once the patients have successfully progressed through these treatment modalities, they may begin sport-specific activities with continued motion and strengthening. Return to athletics is permitted on an individual basis and is often based on agility testing.[8] Functional bracing or taping may be beneficial to reduce further injuries during the initial return to athletics.[7] Chronic ankle instability can be very disabling, and in certain cases patients may be candidates for reconstructive procedures.[7,9]

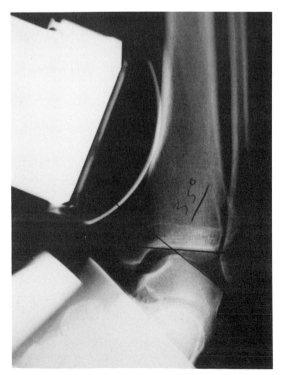

FIGURE 13. Stress lateral radiograph of an ankle demonstrating increased talar tilt and lateral ligament injury.

REFERENCES

1. Bergfeld JA, Weiker GG, Andrish JT, Hall R: Soft playing splint for protection of significant hand and wrist injuries in sports. *Am J Sports Med* 10:293–295, 1982.
2. Bruno LA, Gennarelli TA, Torg JS: Management guidelines for head injuries in athletics. *Clin Sports Med* 6:17–29, 1987.
3. Cantu RC: Second impact syndrome. *Physician Sportsmed* 20(9):55–66, 1992.
4. Cantu RC: Guidelines for return to contact sports after a cerebral concussion. *Physician Sportsmed* 14(10):75–83, 1986.
5. Cantu RC, Mueller FO: Catastrophic football injuries in the U.S.A. *Clin J Sports Med* 2:180–185, 1992.
6. Committee on Head Injury: Nomenclature of the Congress of Neurological Surgeons. *Clin Neurosurg* 12:386–394, 1966.
7. Costello BG: Ligament instability. In Torg JS, Welsh RP, Shephard RJ (eds): *Current Therapy in Sports Medicine,* 2nd ed., Toronto, Decker, 1990, p 229.
8. Crosby LA, Davick JP: Managing common football injuries on the field. *J Musculoskel Med* Nov:62–76, 1990.
9. Drez DJ, Kaveney MF: Ankle ligament injuries. *J Musculoskel Med* Oct:21–36, 1989.
10. Feagin JA: *The Crucial Ligaments,* New York, Churchill-Livingstone, 1988.
11. Gerberich SG, Priest JD, Boen JR, et al: Concussion incidence and severity in secondary school varsity football players. *Am J Public Health* 73:1370–1375, 1983.
12. Halpern BC: Down man on the field. *Pri Care* 10:833–849, 1991.
13. Hankin FM, Peel SM: Sport-related fractures and dislocations in the hand. *Hand Clin* 6:429–453, 1990.
14. Hershman EB: Brachial plexus injuries. *Clin Sports Med* 9:311–329, 1990.
15. Hu R, Burnham R, Reid D, et al: Burners in contact sports. *Clin J Sports Med* 1(4):236–242, 1991.
16. Hurley JA: Complicated elbow fractures in athletics. *Clin Sports Med* 9:39–57, 1990.
17. Indelicato P, Hermansdorfer J, Huegel M: Nonoperative management of complete tears of the

MCL of the knee in intercollegiate football players. *Clin Ortho Rel Res* 256:174–177, 1990.

18. Ireland ML, Andrews JR: Shoulder and elbow injuries in the young athlete. *Clin Sports Med* 7:473–494, 1988.

19. Kahler DM, McCue III FC: Metacarpalphalangeal and proximal interphalangeal joint injuries of the hand, including the thumb. *Clin Sports Med* 11:57–76, 1992.

20. Kremchek TE, Welling RE, Kremchek EJ: Traumatic dislocations of the knee. *Orthop Rev* 18:1051–1057, 1989.

21. Larson RL, Jones DC: Dislocations and ligamentous injuries of the knee. In Rockwood CA, Green DP (eds): *Fractures in Adults,* vol 2. Philadelphia, J. B. Lippincott, 1984.

22. Matsen FA, Zuckerman JD: Anterior glenohumeral instability. *Clin Sports Med* 2:319–338, 1983.

23. Mirabello SC, Loeb PE, Andrews JR: The wrist: Field evaluation and treatment. *Clin Sports Med* 11:1–25, 1992.

24. Mueller FO, Cantu RC: The annual survey of catastrophic football injuries: 1977–1988. *Exerc Sports Sci Rev* 19:261–268.

25. Nicholas JA, Hershman EB: *The Lower Extremity and Spine in Sports Medicine,* vol. 2. St. Louis, C. V. Mosby, 1986.

26. O'Donoghue DH: *Treatment of Injuries to Athletes,* 4th ed. Philadelphia, W. B. Saunders, 1984.

27. Robey JM, Blyth CS, Mueller FO: Athletic injuries: Application of epidemiologic methods. *JAMA* 217:184–189, 1971.

28. Rockwood CA, Young DC: Disorders of the acromioclavicular joint. In Rockwood CA, Matsen FA (eds): *The Shoulder,* vol. 1. Philadelphia, W. B. Saunders, 1990.

29. Saal JA: Common American football injuries. *Sports Med* 12(2):132–147, 1991.

30. Shelbourne KD, Pritchard JC, Rettig A, et al: Knee dislocations with intact PCL. *Orthop Rev* 21:607–611, 1992.

31. Sitler M, Ryan J: The efficacy of a prophylactic knee brace to reduce knee injuries in football. *Am J Sports Med* 18:310–315, 1990.

32. Torg JS: Management guidelines for athletic injuries to the cervical spine. *Clin Sports Med* 6(1):53–60, 1987.

33. Torg JS, Vegso JJ, Oneil M, Bennett B: The epidemiologic, pathologic, biomechanical, and cinematographic analysis of football-induced cervical spine trauma. *Am J Sports Med* 18:50–57, 1990.

34. Wilberger JE, Maroon JC: Head injuries in athletes. *Clin Sports Med* 9:1–9, 1989.

Chapter 12

BODY-BUILDING AND WEIGHT-LIFTING:
Special Issues in Rehabilitation

Robert S. Millard, MD

Thousands of children, adolescents, and young adults in the United States are using weights, either as part of their training regimen or to compete in power-lifting, Olympic-lifting, or body-building contests.[64] Most weight-training programs are based on the premise that if some training is good, then more is better. Injuries result from either training errors (incorrect technique, inadequate supervision, excessively heavy lifts, equipment failure) or overuse (repetitive micro-trauma).[3,10] The most commonly reported injury has been musculotendinous strain, and the most common location has variably been reported to include the lumbosacral spine, patellofemoral joint, shoulder, elbow, or wrist.[10,12,76]

This chapter presents the common injuries associated with weight-training, their presentation, mechanism of injury, and the rehabilitation issues involved. A section on anabolic androgenic steroids is also included because they are commonly used by these athletes.

CATEGORIES OF WEIGHT-TRAINING

The three major types of weight training are body-building, Olympic lifting, and power lifting.

Body-building is a highly competitive aesthetic sport in which athletes are judged on muscle hypertrophy, symmetry, and definition. In an attempt to achieve maximal muscular development, body-builders use free weights (dumbbells and barbells) and weight machines, performing both compound and isolation exercises. They typically train 5 to 7 times a week, with each workout lasting 1.5 to 2 hours. Individual body parts are usually trained twice a week on a rotating basis to allow for adequate recovery. Ten to 20 sets are performed for each body part, and each set contains 6 to 12 repetitions when heavy-to-moderate weights are used.

Olympic lifting involves two techniques: the clean-and-jerk (Fig. 1) and the clean-and-snatch. These lifts require not only strength, but also speed and coordination. Training involves use of heavy weights and low repetitions.[21,64]

Power lifting involves three competitive lifts: bench press (Fig. 2), squat (Fig. 3), and dead lift (Fig. 4). Training sessions involve very heavy weights, multiple sets, and few repetitions.[21,64]

Weight-lifting is also used by athletes to enhance performance in their particular sport. It is especially important for athletes participating in contact sports. Benefits include increases in overall strength and muscle mass, capsular and ligamentous strength, speed, endurance, and coordination.[3]

TYPES OF MUSCLE CONTRACTION

The three basic types of muscle contraction are isotonic, isokinetic, and isometric. Weight-training may incorporate one, two, or all three of them.

Isotonic (which means "same tension") contractions may be concentric (shortening) or eccentric (lengthening). The muscle tension developed during such contractions var-

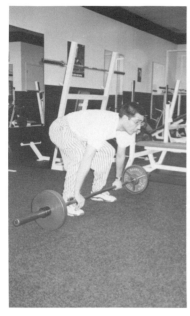
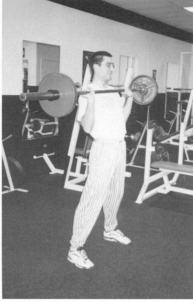
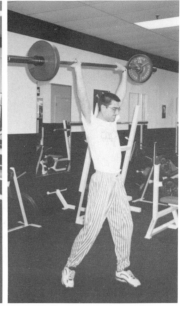

FIGURE 1. The clean-and-jerk lift. The lifter brings the bar to his chest first while squatting (not shown), then stands up and lifts the weight overhead. In the clean-and-snatch, the lift to the chest is bypassed. The lifter brings the bar overhead first while squatting and then stands up.

ies with the applied external force, muscle length, type of contraction, and speed of muscle shortening or lengthening.

With concentric exercise, as speed of contraction increases, the amount of tension in the muscle–tendon unit decreases. During eccentric muscle action, the tension is proportional to the speed of action. At comparable speeds of action against equal external forces, tension during eccentric muscle action is greater than that during concentric contraction.[76] Eccentric work also requires less oxygen, lower consumption of adenosine triphosphate (ATP), and less motor unit activity than a concentric contraction of equal tension and velocity of action.[30] Concentric and eccentric contractions have different effects on adult muscle, with eccentric work causing greater ultrastructural changes in the contractile apparatus, i.e., hypertrophy.[30] Type II (fast twitch) fibers are predominantly affected.[30] Eccentric exercise is important in strength development but also results in significant muscle soreness.[30]

Isokinetic (which means "same velocity") exercise is performed at a constant angular joint velocity, no matter how much force is applied. Resistance and speed of movement

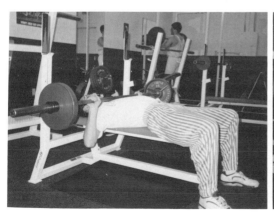
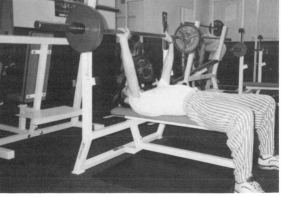

FIGURE 2. Bench press.

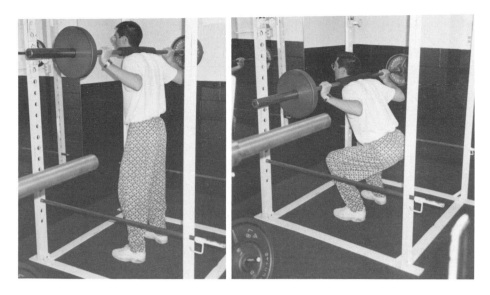

FIGURE 3. Squat.

are controlled electromechanically. No isokinetic device approaches the speeds attained in most athletic competition, and few, if any, natural movements are isokinetic.[76] Most isokinetic machines involve concentric movements. Some of the newer ones offer eccentric tension as well.

During **isometric** muscle action, the muscle–tendon unit length does not change, and no skeletal movement occurs. Consequently, no external mechanical work is accomplished.[22]

PROPHYLAXIS OF WEIGHT-LIFTING INJURIES

Most of the injuries associated with training errors can be avoided if a few guidelines are followed.

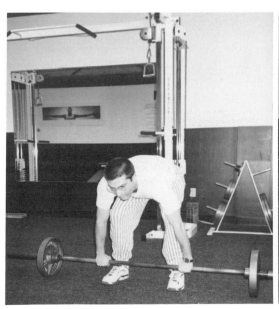
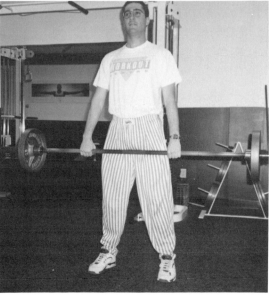

FIGURE 4. Dead lift.

1. *Adequate supervision.* For the beginning weight trainer, the most critical factors in injury prevention are good instruction and knowledgeable supervision. Intensity, duration, and frequency of exercise as well as rate of weight progression should be closely supervised. Recovery from one session before the next is necessary to avoid overtraining. Overtraining, which is signaled by persistent fatigue and muscle soreness, involves no gains in strength or body weight.

2. *Adequate maturity.* The age at which adolescents can safely begin progressive resistance exercise has been thoroughly investigated.[4,10,12,65,70,76] Recent research has revealed that short-term programs in which prepubescent athletes are trained and supervised by knowledgeable adults can increase strength without significant risk of injury.[4] Consideration of physical maturity aids in the selection of appropriate sport-specific exercises. For example, young athletes risk injury during ballistic movements (clean-and-jerk, clean-and-snatch, and the second part of a power clean) because of inadequate strength, coordination, balance, and explosive power.[70]

Generally, adolescents should avoid the maximal lifts incorporated in body-building and power-lifting regimens (dead lifts, power cleans, squats, military press) until they have reached a Tanner stage 5 of development (corresponds to a mean age of 15 years). (*See* chapter 1 on preparticipation examination.) At this point, maximal velocity of height growth has already occurred. Prior to this period, the epiphyses are especially vulnerable to injury.[4] Gumbs et al.[35] presented two cases of bilateral distal radial (epiphyseal—Salter II) and ulnar fractures that occurred in adolescent boys while attempting the clean-and-jerk maneuver. Both lifters were younger than 15 years of age. In both instances, balance was lost during the terminal, or overhead, phase of the lift, resulting in a hyperextension injury to the wrists. In this position, the axial compression force, coupled with the shear force acting on the distal radial epiphysis, can cause a fracture. Skeletally immature individuals are also prone to developing stress fractures of the pars interarticularis, spondylolysis, and spondylolisthesis.[12]

3. *Prehabilitation.* The most common injuries in the beginning weight-lifter involve the shoulder and low back. Many authorities attribute this to a developmental lag of the muscles of the abdomen, trunk (rotational muscles of the abdomen and low back), scap-

ula (stabilizers), and rotator cuff. Therefore, prehabilitation of these muscle groups is recommended, including progressive resistance exercises for anterior, middle, and posterior deltoid muscles, internal and external rotators of the shoulder, and scapular stabilizing muscles (serratus anterior, rhomboids, trapezius); lumbar paraspinous stretching; crunches for the rectus abdominis and obliques; and lumbar extension exercises (*not hyperextension*).[10,73,76]

4. *Proper form.* Proper mechanics during exercise execution is essential.[61] Dumbbell and barbell movements should be slow and deliberate. This is especially important in the eccentric phase of muscle action, during which most muscle strains occur (the highest muscle tendon tension occurs with eccentric muscle action at high velocity).[31] Exercises should be done through a full range of motion to develop strength through the full range and to maintain flexibility.[21] (An exception to this rule is when an injury prevents full, pain-free range of motion; in this case, exercise is performed through the pain-free range).

Development of muscle imbalances can be avoided by strengthening all agonist and antagonist muscle groups equally. This is also important in preventing musculotendinous strains.[33]

5. *Warm-up, stretching, and cardiovascular conditioning.* Inadequate warm-up and stretching predispose the athlete to strain injuries.[68] Light-to-moderate weights should be used for the first set of each exercise.[23]

Soft-tissue flexibility is increased with temperature elevation. Stretching a warmed-up muscle results in an increased musculotendinous unit length at a given load and results in decreased tension along the musculotendinous junction. Subsequently, the incidence of injury to the musculotendinous junction is reduced.[68] Cardiovascular conditioning should be incorporated into the training regimen at least 3 times weekly, because weight-lifting alone provides little benefit in this area.[11,47]

6. *Avoiding a sustained Valsalva maneuver.* *Brief* Valsalva maneuvers may serve an important protective function. The associated elevation in intrathoracic pressure is directly transmitted to the cerebrospinal fluid. This reduces the transmural pressures along the cerebral vasculature, thereby decreasing the risk of vascular injury under the extremes of pressure generated during near-maximal lifts.[52] A *sustained Valsalva* maneuver (straining against a closed glottis during heavy lifting), however, should be avoided because it has been associated with weight-lifter's cephalgia and blackout; brainstem ischemia; subarachnoid hemorrhage; spontaneous pneumopericardium and pneumothorax; ascending aortic dissection; and abdominal hernias.[7,11,16,20,47,52,60,61,71,72,76]

During the concentric phase of heavy lifting, systolic and diastolic pressures may be elevated as much as fourfold.[52] The Valsalva maneuver (increased intrathoracic pressure) contributes greatly to this elevation. Pressures decline rapidly during the eccentric phase of the lift. The pressures rise even if a relatively small muscle mass is exercised, but the greatest elevations occur when the larger muscle groups are used. This is due to the correspondingly higher proportion of vascular mechanical compression by the contracting muscle. Reflex vasoconstriction along the vascular beds of nonexercising muscle also contributes to the observed pressure elevations. Systolic pressures have been shown to increase progressively with each repetition.[52]

7. Weight belts? Several studies have investigated the effectiveness of weight belts in preventing lumbar spine injuries.[9,37,46] Belts purportedly support, stabilize, and attenuate the compressive load applied to the spine during heavy weight training.[9]

The resiliency of the lumbosacral structures under compressive loads is variable. The vertebral endplates are most vulnerable to damage, followed by the muscular and ligamentous structures.[13,46] During heavy lifting, spinal compressive forces have exceeded 10,000 newtons, a force sufficient to cause vertebral structural damage.

A weight belt increases intraabdominal pressure, thereby distributing some of the vertebral compressive load to the abdominal compartment.[23,46,61] With use of a weight belt, lumbar disc compression forces and erector spinae tension are reduced by 2% to 6%, relative to the beltless condition.[9] Because a large portion of the disc compression during lifting has been attributed to the tension developed in the erector spinae muscles,[37] the likelihood of injuring the disc may be reduced.

Based on the above findings, the following recommendations seem appropriate:

1. Weight belts should be worn during heavy lifts, especially squats and dead lifts, or with a history of back pain or injury.

2. Because the abdominal and back muscles are less active when a belt is worn, lighter lifts (< 80% of the maximal lift) should be performed without a belt to strengthen the abdominals, obliques, and back muscle groups.

3. The belt should be loosened between sets, because large elevations in intraabdominal pressure impede venous blood return to the heart.

4. Athletes who typically wear a belt during heavy lifts should exercise caution when attempting lifts without a belt.

8. Spotters. Spotters, as well as sturdy and safe weight racks/safety bars, are especially important when performing near-maximal overhead lifts or simply when exercises are conducted to a fatigue level. Deaths have been reported as a result of crush injuries of the neck or chest during unsupervised barbell bench press.[7,32]

INJURIES

Shoulder Girdle

Shoulder injuries are relatively common among recreational and professional weight lifters. Common shoulder overuse injuries include anterior capsule strain (bench press, behind the neck military press (Fig. 5), or pull-downs (Fig. 6)), acromioclavicular degenerative joint disease (heavy bench press), and rotator cuff tendinitis.[7,76] Weight-lifters are predisposed to developing overuse injuries because of their tendency to continue to train despite pain.

Rotator Cuff Tendinitis

Subacromial bursitis and rotator cuff tendinitis are usually seen in athletes who have trained for at least 4 years.[3] The rotator cuff is placed in an unfavorable position during most overhead lifts, and repetitive exercises place the cuff at risk for injury. The subacromial space is naturally constricted; with overuse and repetitive irritation, the cuff tendons become swollen and inflamed.[59] Pain response in early tendinitis is typically delayed, which allows development of a chronic condition and may lead to impingement.[59] Athletes typically misinterpret the pain to be "muscu-

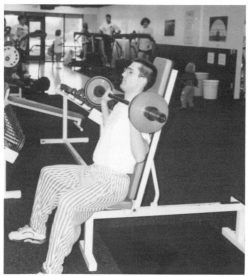
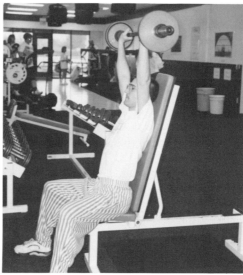

FIGURE 5. Military press. Technique shown is in front of the neck. Similar lifting can be done from behind the neck.

lar soreness," which also contributes to the development of a chronic injury.[59]

Initial treatment consists of relative rest, anti-inflammatory medications, passive stretching, heat, and deep massage. Once full, pain-free, active range of motion is obtained, isolated exercises for rotator cuff strengthening (especially external rotation, internal rotation, and abduction), and gradual return to lifting are allowed.[59] Attention to correcting muscle imbalances and to maintaining flexibility is also critical.

Glenohumeral Instability and Dislocation

The glenohumeral joint is inherently unstable and prone to dislocations, because its stability relies on the integrity of soft-tissue structures.[53] Maximal glenohumeral instability occurs during full abduction.[53] Instability most frequently presents during overhead lifts when the athlete loses control of the weight. Instead of dropping the weight behind, the lifter attempts to pull the weight forward, which results in subluxation or dislo-

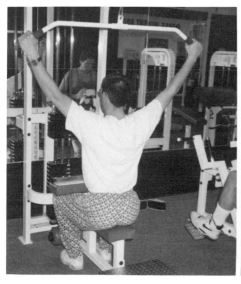
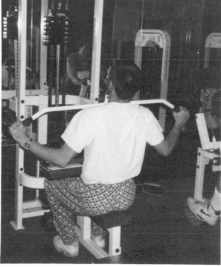

FIGURE 6. Pull downs.

cation.[59] In a high-level competitive athlete with instability, many authorities recommend surgical management, especially if overhead lifts are to be performed.[59] Otherwise, conservative management is pursued first.

Second Rib Fracture

Goeser et al.[34] described a posterior second rib fracture that occurred in a recreational lifter during bench pressing. Fractures of the first three ribs are rare because of their position deep within the shoulder girdle. However, during the bench press, much stress is placed on the shoulder girdle. With the forceful contractions of the scalenus posterior and serratus anterior that accompany the terminal phase of the lift, an opposing traction force is placed on the second rib. If the opposing forces are sufficient, a fracture may result.

Management is conservative, because stability is provided by the intact ribs above and below the fracture. The athlete should be instructed to carry out sustained inspirations to maintain vital capacity and to support the lateral chest wall when coughing. Rib belts and chest-wall taping are not recommended because they merely restrict an already limited ability to inspire.[34]

Midhumerus Stress Fracture

Stress fractures in non–weight-bearing bones are relatively rare but have been reported.[6,17] Under repetitive stress, bones may undergo pathologic changes that lead to stress fractures.

Bartsokas et al.[6] reported the case of a 20-year-old male body-builder who complained of the insidious onset of shoulder and upper-arm pain. The pain was provoked only by certain exercises: bench, incline (Fig. 7), and overhead presses and biceps curls (Fig. 8). He also had been lifting heavier weights than usual. Palpation tenderness coincided with roentgenographic abnormalities (a small lucent line in the anterior cortex of the midhumerus). A bone scan that revealed focal increased activity in the midhumerus confirmed the diagnosis. Relative rest for 6 weeks, followed by gradual return to weight-training, was recommended, and recovery was uneventful.

Acromioclavicular Degenerative Joint Disease

In Cahill's series,[15] 45 of 46 cases of acromioclavicular degenerative joint disease (osteolysis of the distal clavicle) occurred in weight-lifters, and the majority probably resulted from repetitive microtrauma. The onset is insidious, and pain is provoked with bench presses, dips (Fig. 9), or push-ups.[7] Patients present with pain and tenderness at the acromioclavicular joint. Horizontal adduction reproduces the pain. Occasionally, the pain radiates to the deltoid or superior trapezius. Mild swelling of the acromioclavicular joint may be present.

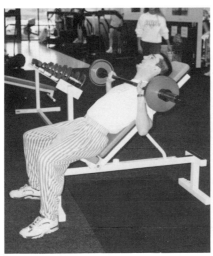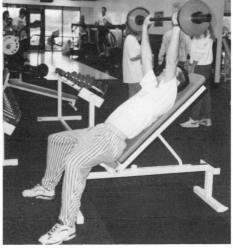

FIGURE 7. Incline press.

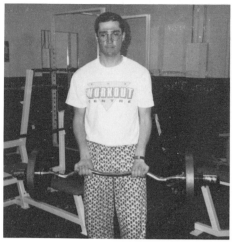
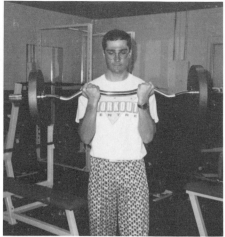

FIGURE 8. Biceps curls.

Roentgenographic findings, present to varying degrees, include osteoporosis, loss of subchondral bone, and cystic changes in the distal clavicle. Joint scintigraphy reveals increased activity in the distal clavicle and occasionally in the adjacent acromion. The findings on joint scintigraphy suggest that the distal clavicle lesion results from microfractures of the subchondral bone and subsequent attempts at repair. During weight-training, stresses are concentrated on the distal clavicle and acromion with resultant subchondral stress fractures.

Conservative management (antiinflamma-tory medication, hydrocortisone injection into the acromioclavicular joint, and avoidance of bench presses, dips, and push-ups) frequently fails in athletes who continue to lift competitively. In such cases, resection of the distal clavicle is required.[7,15]

Forearm and Wrist

Stress Fracture of the Diaphysis of the Ulna

The proposed mechanism of stress fracture of the ulnar diaphysis[17,36] is flexor muscle

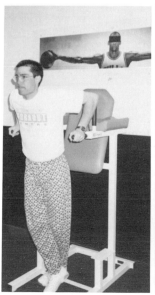
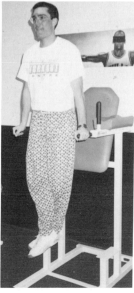

FIGURE 9. Dips.

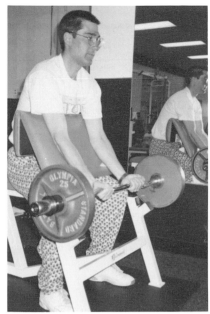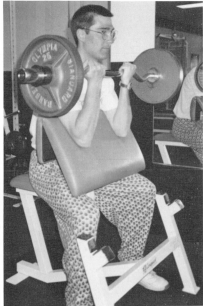

FIGURE 10.   Preacher curls.

overuse during elbow flexion to 90° with the forearm pronated or supinated.[17] Thus, the initial pain typically occurs only when performing preacher-bench biceps curls (Fig. 10) with a barbell. The onset is insidious, and eventually medial forearm pain occurs with any activity. Examination reveals a firm tender mass along the ulnar midshaft. Roentgenographic findings, if present (onset of symptoms precede radiographic findings by approximately 3 weeks), include transverse hairline translucency and reactive periosteal bone formation with sclerosis along the mid-diaphysis. Technetium bone scanning, which may be positive (increased uptake) 1 to 3 weeks before the radiographs, provide an early diagnosis. Some recommend casting for 3 to 5 weeks.[17] Gradual return to weight-training is allowed when serial radiographs demonstrate adequate healing.[36] If there is no evidence of union 4 to 6 months after injury, then excision and bone grafting must be considered.[17]

Volar Forearm Compartment Syndrome

This syndrome has been described in individuals who vigorously exercise with previously untrained arms.[7,8] Forearm pain is progressive and is provoked with finger movement. Physical findings include volar forearm swelling and erythema; tenderness along the flexor tendons; and pain provocation with passive finger extension. Diagnosis is confirmed by measuring compartment pressures. Decompression is accomplished with an extensive midline fasciotomy.[8]

Carpal Dislocations

Wrist degeneration can occur as a result of the repetitive hyperextension that accompanies overhead lifting.[61] For carpal dislocation[26,50,77] to occur, considerable force is required.[50] Lunate or perilunar dislocations and fracture dislocations are considered to be different stages of the same injury pattern. The forces involved in a lunate dislocation are extension (hyperextension), ulnar deviation, and varying degrees of supination.[50] Initially median nerve compressive symptoms are common, but long-term morbidity is rare because symptoms gradually resolve after successful reduction.

Osteochondral Flaps of the Wrist

This condition should be considered in the differential diagnosis of chronic wrist pain. Levy et al.[49] presented a case of a competitive weight-lifter with a 3-year history of wrist pain. Pain was aggravated during movements that involved wrist hyperextension (bench and military press). Intermittent popping and dorsal swelling over the radial aspect of the wrist were also present. Physical examination revealed decreased wrist extension; tenderness over the dorsal radioscapholunate joint; and pain provocation with forced wrist extension. Wrist radiographs and computed tomographic (CT) arthrogram were normal. On wrist arthroscopy, an osteochondral flap was found at the radial ridge between the scaphoid and lunate fossae. With wrist extension, this lesion impinged on the scapholunate ligament. The flap was subsequently debrided to the level of cancellous bone. Two weeks postoperatively, physical therapy was initiated with a gradual return to weight-training.

Lower Extremity

Knee

Meniscal injuries occur most frequently with free-weight exercise (dead lifts), but also with weight machines (leg curls (Fig. 11)).[10,76] The majority of knee injuries, however, are relatively less serious and result from overuse, such as patellofemoral pain, quadriceps strain/tendinitis, and patellar tendinitis.[76]

Open kinetic chain exercises, such as knee extensions, frequently cause patellofemoral pain.[7] During knee extensions, the maximal patellofemoral force occurs at 30° to 40° of knee flexion. Patellar tendon force approaches 8 times body weight simply with performance of deep knee bends. This force obviously increases significantly when weights are employed.[10] Therefore, when patellofem-

oral pain is an issue, closed kinetic chain exercises (leg press, hack-squats, squats), performed to parallel (90° of knee flexion), are preferred.

Injuries due to patellar tendon avulsion may occur during the heavy squat or the clean-and-jerk maneuver. Analyses have shown that the tension on the patellar tendon approaches 15 to 20 times the lifter's total weight.[7]

Collateral ligament sprains, especially involving the medial collateral ligaments, have been reported.[3] The lifter who attempts heavy squats with a broad-based stance and allows the knees to move into relative valgus during weight ascent is particularly vulnerable.

Transchondral Fracture of the Talar Dome

Mannis[54] reported transchondral fracture of the talar dome in an athlete during the performance of squats. Acute ankle pain occurred during descent and prevented completion of the workout. No ecchymosis or swelling occurred, but plantar flexion provoked sharp ankle pain. Radiographs revealed a medial talar dome lesion consistent with osteochondritis dissecans. Increased uptake over the medial talus was evident on a bone scan. The athlete was placed in a short leg cast (non–weight-bearing). Windows were cut anteriorly and posteriorly to allow for daily use of a muscle stimulator unit. The cast was removed 6 weeks later, and calf circumferences were equal. When repeat radiographs showed complete resolution of the osteochondral lesion, a rehabilitation program was initiated for active motion and weight-

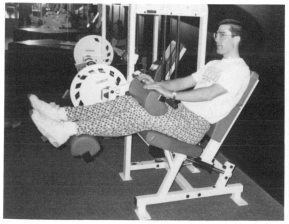
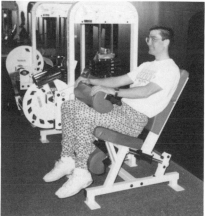

FIGURE 11.   Leg curls.

bearing. Three weeks after cast removal, the athlete resumed his usual activities without incident.

This case is interesting for a number of reasons. First, it reemphasizes the importance of following proper mechanics during the performance of lifts. During the descent phase of the squat, novice lifters tend to incorporate significant trunk forward flexion, which may result in transmission of significant compression forces to the ankle. If a slight lateral rotatory movement of the tibia on the talus also occurs during descent, sufficient shear forces may result and cause a medial lesion of the talar dome. Second, the use of daily electrical stimulation helped the athlete to maintain muscle strength and to return quickly to athletic endeavors.

Musculotendinous Injuries

A strain is an injury to the musculotendinous unit caused by excessive tension.[78] It is not surprising that athletes involved in weight-training are prone to develop musculotendinous injuries. The most frequently reported injuries involve the biceps brachii (barbell or dumbbell curls),[48,78] the pectoralis major (bench press, flies (Fig. 12), overhead lifts),[43,63,79] and the triceps (clean-and-snatch, triceps extensions (Fig. 13), bench press).[5,51,66,71] Other muscles that may be injured are the quadriceps, hamstrings, gastrocnemius, and latissimus dorsi. Risk factors include high level of activity (3 or more sessions/week, session duration $\geq$ 30 min) and demanding repetitive activity.[33] Whether use of anabolic steroid predisposes athletes to muscle tears is controversial. Studies have demonstrated ultrastructural tendon damage associated with anabolic steroids in mice.[56]

As mentioned earlier, strains occur most often during eccentric muscle action. Significantly higher tension is generated on the musculotendinous unit during eccentric contraction compared with isometric or concentric muscle action.[31] The muscles most susceptible to injury are those that span two joints and those with a relatively high percentage of type II (fast twitch) fibers.[33] Fatigued or weakened muscles are also vulnerable to injury because their ability to absorb force is adversely affected.[31]

Normal muscle tendon units fail either at the tendon origin or insertion (avulsion), the muscle belly, or the musculotendinous junction. Failure within the tendon substance proper is rare and is usually preceded by chronic tendinitis.[31,68] Most failures occur at the musculotendinous junction, although the reason is unknown.[31] The triceps most commonly ruptures from its tendo-osseous insertion.[5] In the young athlete, an avulsion fracture through the apophyseal plate is most likely. In youth, the growth plate represents the weakest point in the musculotendinous system.[78] Sartorius avulsion injuries involving the anterior superior iliac spine have been reported in adolescents performing dead lifts and lumbar hyperextension maneuvers.[7,76]

Muscle injuries are graded according to the Ryan scale, which measures extent of damage.[33] Grade I injuries involve the tearing of a

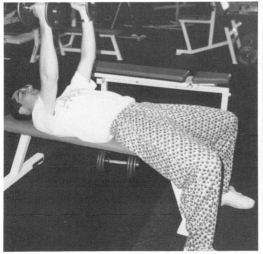
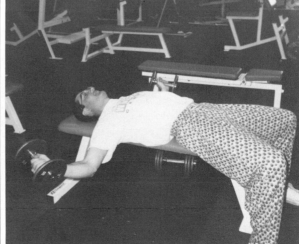

FIGURE 12. Pectoralis flies.

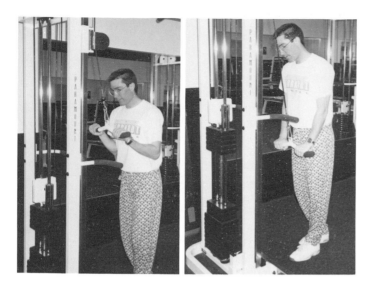

FIGURE 13. Triceps extensions.

few fibers with intact fascia; grade II injuries, the tearing of a moderate number of fibers with localized hematoma and intact fascia; grade III injuries, the tearing of many fibers with diffuse bleeding, ecchymosis, and partial tearing of the fascia; and grade IV injuries, a complete tear of both muscle and fascia.[33]

Partial injuries heal by an initial inflammatory response followed by fibrosis. Because injured muscle fibers do not regenerate, persistent scar formation occurs. Recovery is often slow or incomplete.[33] Although contractile force recovers rapidly (90% complete 7 days after injury), recovery of tensile strength is slower (only 77% normal 7 days after injury). Tensile strength is an indicator of the muscle's ability to withstand reinjury, which therefore remains a distinct possibility even if strength appears near-normal.

When a muscle or musculotendinous injury occurs, athletes typically feel or hear a "pop" that is followed by sudden pain and muscle weakness.[78] Focal pain and swelling are progressive over the first 24 hours. Ecchymosis usually occurs 1 day later.[31] Physical examination usually reveals a visible or palpable defect. Complete muscle ruptures may be misdiagnosed as muscle strains when extensive swelling, in the presence of intact fascia, obscures the discontinuity.[79] Pain is provoked with passive stretching and active contraction of the injured muscle.[31] Weakness of the injured muscle is also present (for example, in pectoralis major injury weakness is felt with internal rotation, flexion, and adduction). The muscle defect can be made more obvious with forceful contraction of the injured mus-

cle against resistance ("clap test" for the pectoralis major).[63]

The **goal of treatment** is to reduce factors that restrict motion: pain, muscle splinting, inflammation, and edema.[33] Ice application, which reduces pain, bleeding, and splinting, is used in conjunction with elevation and compression to reduce swelling.[78] Aspiration of hematoma, followed by compression, may prevent myositis ossificans. This is especially true in muscles closely adherent to bone throughout their course (quadriceps femoris, adductors, biceps, triceps).[33] When a muscle is severely injured or when a minor injury does not respond to treatment, radiographs should be taken to rule out a stress fracture.

For grade I and II injuries, active contraction, stretching, and transverse massage away from the injury site are initiated within the first 24 hours. With a grade III injury, active assisted range-of-motion exercises and stretching begin once swelling is controlled. Weight-bearing is avoided until the muscle can be actively contracted. When active range of motion is restored, gradual return to activity is allowed. The rehabilitation program should include eccentric training and stretching, which represent the maximal stress that can be placed on the musculotendinous unit. Aquatic exercises help to relieve muscle soreness.[33] The risk of reinjury is minimized by proper rehabilitation, including reattainment of full flexibility, strength, and neural control of the muscle.[78]

Grade IV injuries require surgical repair. Most authors recommend early intervention (within the first week after injury) before fibrous adhesions form.[33,43] However, successful delayed repair of a triceps tendon avulsion (6 months after injury) has also been reported.[71]

Nerve Injuries

Long Thoracic Nerve

Injury of the long thoracic nerve has been reported in athletes performing overhead lifts.[69] The mechanism is believed to involve traction because injury typically occurs when the ipsilateral arm is in an outstretched overhead position. Shoulder pain, decreased range of motion, and weakness are the usual presenting complaints. Prominence of the scapula may also be noticeable and can make sitting in a chair uncomfortable. Winging of the inferior angle and medial border of the scapula with forward flexion of the arms is indicative of serratus anterior weakness. This type of winging needs to be differentiated from the scapular winging associated with trapezius weakness, which is most apparent during arm abduction to 90°. The serratus anterior maintains the medial scapular border against the thorax when the arm is thrust forward. Thus, winging can be accentuated by pressing against a wall. Scapulohumeral rhythm during active abduction is abnormal because of impaired scapular rotation. Electromyography and nerve conduction studies are helpful in assessing the severity of the injury.

Treatment includes maintaining range of motion, as tolerated, and instituting a progressive strengthening program. Avoidance of precipitating activity and relative rest are indicated initially. If active range of motion is performed in the supine position, further scapular winging is prevented because the body's weight maintains the scapula close to the thorax. Activities that require forward flexion of the arm are avoided. The latissimus dorsi, levator scapulae, pectoralis minor, and rhomboid muscles must be stretched to avoid their tendency to become painful and contracted. Early serratus anterior and lower trapezius strengthening is accomplished by arm abduction in the supine position. Later, as strength improves, bench press and pushups are helpful.[69]

The prognosis for complete or partial recovery is good. Average recovery time is 9 months. Scapular winging may persist, even when full arm function is regained.[69]

Suprascapular Neuropathy

Repeated, forceful exercises involving shoulder abduction may lead to suprascapular neuropathy.[2,58] The nerve becomes compressed at the level of the suprascapular foramen as a result of the "sling effect."[2,58] Because its plane of origin and plane of termination in the supraspinatus are higher than the plane of the foramen, the nerve forms an angle at the foramen beneath the transverse scapular ligament.[2,58,62] The angulation becomes more pronounced during shoulder depression, retraction, or hyperabduction.[2,58]

The athlete usually presents with complaints of posterior shoulder pain and weakness. The suprascapular nerve contains afferent sensory fibers from the glenohumeral joint and scapula, and posterior shoulder pain is believed to result from compression of these fibers.[2,58] Examination may reveal supraspinatus and infraspinatus atrophy and weakness. EMG helps determine the location (root, plexus, or nerve) and extent of injury (neurapraxic vs axonotmetic).

Ulnar Neuritis

Compression of the nerve as it passes between the two heads of the flexor carpi ulnaris or nerve subluxation across the medial epicondyle on elbow flexion may lead to ulnar neuritis.[7,18] Hypertrophy of the triceps further promotes nerve traction and subluxation.[18]

Other Nerve Injury

Repetitive exercise with associated muscle hypertrophy can result in nerve injury due to compression. The median nerve may be entrapped by the pronator teres, lacertus fibrosis, or flexor digitorum sublimis. Hypertrophy of the forearm may also result in compromise of the posterior interosseous nerve at the supinator muscle or the arcade of Frohse. Involvement of the musculocutaneous and lateral antebrachial cutaneous nerves has also been reported.[40]

Cervical and Lumbar Spine

Cervical radiculitis and radiculopathy of acute onset have been described in weight lifters.[44] Injury results from the combination of axial loading and cervical hyperextension. The compressive forces associated with axial loading may lead to a disc injury. Hyperextension results in decreased neuroforaminal diameter and, in the presence of spondylotic changes, root compression.

Cervical Radiculopathy

The athlete may complain of neck, shoulder, interscapular, or upper-extremity pain. Associated reflex asymmetry, upper-extremity weakness, numbness, or paresthesias may also be present. Cervical range of motion is usually limited by muscle spasm. Signs elicited with the Spurling's and head-compression maneuvers are also useful. Depending on the examination findings, work-up may include a cervical spine series; MRI; or electromyography and nerve conduction studies.

Conservative management includes relative rest, analgesic and anti-inflammatory agents, modalities to relieve muscle spasm, and manual cervical traction. A cervical collar may be helpful initially to limit painful neck motion. Once pain is adequately controlled, passive range of motion and isometric strengthening are initiated. Cervical epidural injections under fluoroscopic guidance are useful in athletes who remain limited by their pain. Stabilization training is important to prevent recurrences after training is resumed.[44]

Lumbar Strain

Repetitive flexion, extension and torsional stresses are placed on the lumbar spine during weight-training.[67] Subsequently, low back injuries are the dominant complaint among weight-lifters. Weight-lifting accounts for proportionately more lumbar injuries than any other sport.[19,74] Risser et al.[65] studied the incidence of weight-training injuries in high school football players. The most common injury was a lumbar strain/sprain. All the athletes who injured their backs were performing one or more of the following lifts: power clean, clean-and-jerk, squat, or dead lift. Many coaches encourage athletes to perform these lifts to allow for the development of explosive, coordinated strength and power in multiple muscle groups.

Disc Injury

Compressive loads on the lumbar spine ranging from 18.8 to 36.4 kN have been recorded in world-champion power lifters.[74] Repetitive torsional loads may cause annular injury that leads to disc degeneration.[67,76] Failure of the annulus fibrosis (linear horizontal tears through all the fibers except the most peripheral) have been demonstrated when rapid, cyclic forward flexion is combined with mild axial compression.[13] Failure of the disc components is associated with low back pain and leads to accelerated degeneration of the lumbar facet joints.[74]

Disc injuries run the gamut from annular tears to herniation of the nucleus pulposus. Transmission of nonuniform forces to the annulus involves the potential for posterolateral rupture.[74] If a nerve root is irritated or compressed, the athlete presents with radicular symptoms or signs, including leg pain, paresthesias, numbness, weakness, and reflex asymmetry. Other physical findings may include limited range of motion in forward flexion, listing away from the side of injury, signs of nerve root tension, and interspace tenderness. MRI is extremely valuable in assessing disc pathology. Electromyography and nerve conduction studies help to document the involved level and extent of injury.

Rest, modalities (ice, electrogalvanic stimulation, ultrasound, transcutaneous electric nerve stimulation), and antiinflammatory medications are implemented initially. Exercise (with a trial of extension exercise), abdominal strengthening, and pelvic tilt follow, once pain is manageable. If pain does not subside, epidural injections play a crucial role in allowing the athlete to participate in therapy.[73] Exercises for flexibility, strengthening, and stabilization training help to prevent reinjury.[67]

Spondylolysis and Stress Reactions of the Pars Interarticularis

Repetitive loading of the posterior elements in hyperextension has been associated with spondylolysis.[1,25,67] With repetitive hyperextension maneuvers, the vertebral isthmus is subjected to excessive stress. This repetitive stress ultimately causes the bone to fail, resulting in a fatigue fracture. Incidence of spondylolysis among weight-lifters is 36% (vs. 5% in the general population) and is most common in athletes who have trained for more than 4 years.[25,74]

Pain is localized to the unilateral paraspinous area and exacerbated by twisting and hyperextension. It is frequently associated with the standing overhead military press.[41] On examination, pain provocation occurs with the standing one-legged hyperextension test on the side ipsilateral to the lesion.[73] There are no associated signs of nerve root tension. Lumbar paraspinous spasm may be present.

Initial roentgenograms are typically negative, but stress reaction is confirmed with a technetium bone scan. If a stress reaction is recognized early, the development of spondylolysis may be prevented.

Treatment includes relative rest, with avoidance of aggravating activities. Form-fitting braces that significantly limit lumbar hyperextension have been used with mixed results. The average time for pain-free return to activities is approximately 7 months, but recovery time correlates with duration of symptoms prior to diagnosis. Of interest, clinical improvement correlates closely with return to normal radioactive uptake on serial bone scans.[41]

Spondylolisthesis

Athletes with spondylolisthesis have pain associated with the hyperlordotic position. Hamstring tightness and decreased overall flexibility are common. Hip and leg extension on the side of the lesion provoke pain. Oblique radiographs may reveal a lytic defect or increased bone density in the pars interarticularis. Spina bifida occulta has a 23% association with spondylolysis.[25]

Most athletes respond to conservative management: antiinflammatory medications; restricted activities; selective antilordotic bracing; flexibility exercises (trunk, hamstrings, hip flexors, hip rotators); strengthening of the back extensor, abdominal, quadriceps, gluteus medius, and quadratus lumborum muscles; and stabilization training.[23,67] Once the athlete is pain-free with full range of motion, training is resumed. Only rarely is surgical stabilization required. In the skeletally im-

mature athlete, close observation for progression of spondylolisthesis is recommended.[25,73] Rapid slip usually occurs between the ages of 9 and 13 years. Later slippage is associated with intervertebral disc and facet degeneration.[73]

Apophyseal fractures of the lumbar ring have been reported in adolescents performing dead lifts. The most common mechanism of injury is axial loading, with or without associated trunk extension. Diagnosis requires clinical suspicion and radiographic (lateral view) confirmation. In cases with concomitant spinal canal narrowing, treatment requires removal of the bony fragment or decompressive laminectomy.[14]

ANABOLIC STEROIDS

Despite legal, legislative, and medical efforts to curtail their use, anabolic androgenic steroids are commonly used among competitive and noncompetitive athletes. Even drug testing by most major sports organizations has failed to eliminate their use. Based on testimonial evidence, anabolic steroids are used by 80% to 100% of male body-builders, weight-lifters, shotputters, and discus, hammer, and javelin throwers of national and international caliber. They are used to a lesser extent by football players and other athletes for whom strength and power are important.[45] Frankle et al.[29] found a 20% incidence of use among people who routinely train with weights.

Anabolic steroids are derivatives of testosterone that were developed in an attempt to minimize androgenic effects while maintaining anabolic potential. They are administered intramuscularly (esters of 19-nortestosterone) or orally (alkyl group at C-17 of the D ring in the basic testosterone nucleus). Most users cycle the drugs: 4 to 18 weeks on steroids, followed by a drug-free period of around 2 to 3 months.[42] The dosages used may be 2 to 40 times greater than those used for medical purposes (hypogonadism, aplastic anemia, debilitated conditions). In an attempt to minimize side effects, combinations of oral and injectable steroids are often used concurrently—a process called "stacking."[27,45]

Anabolic steroids increase strength and lean body mass through their anabolic anticatabolic, and motivational effects.[29,38,42,45] The anticatabolic effects may be the most important, and anabolic steroids have their most profound effects on athletes who have trained to the point that they are in a chronic catabolic state. Haupt et al.[38] found that subjects who had weight-training experience prior to taking anabolic steroids consistently demonstrated increased strength above and beyond that expected from weight-training alone. Novice lifters who took anabolic steroids did not significantly increase their strength.

The anticatabolic effects of anabolic steroids are mediated in two ways: (1) competition for glucocorticoid receptor sites blocks the catabolic effects of glucocorticoids that are released during periods of stress (athletic activity), and (2) improved utilization of protein promotes a positive nitrogen balance. Anabolic steroids induce protein synthesis by binding to skeletal muscle cytoplasmic receptors (anabolic effect).

Athletes using steroids also experience a euphoric state, increased aggressive behavior, and diminished fatigue. They are able to train more intensively and more frequently because of enhanced recovery from exercise.[42] There also appears to be a placebo effect.[38]

Although athletes have been using anabolic steroids since the 1950s, inadequate information exists regarding long-term effects. A thorough presentation of the reported side effects is beyond the scope of this chapter; the reader is referred to any of several excellent reviews.[29,42, 45,79] Most of the known short-term side effects are reversible with cessation of use. In the male, gynecomastia and alopecia may persist. In the female, male-pattern baldness, hirsutism, deepening of the voice, and clitoral hypertrophy are largely irreversible.[75] Premature closure of the epiphyses and resulting short stature may occur when prepubertal adolescents use anabolic steroids.[42] The most frequently reported subjective side effects include changes in libido, increased aggressiveness, muscle spasm, and gynecomastia.[29,38,75]

Orally active steroids are much more hepatotoxic than those administered intramuscularly. The hepatotoxicity appears to be related to duration of usage.[38] Blood levels of the liver isoenzymes, lactate dehydrogenase and alkaline phosphatase, as well as levels of conjugated bilirubin should be monitored. Elevated levels may be indicative of hepatotoxicity. Because muscular stress alone may lead to elevations in AST (aspartate aminotransferase) or ALT (alanine aminotransferase), these levels are not as accurate in identifying steroid-induced toxicity. Cholestatic jaundice may occur but typically resolves several months after discontinuing the offending agents. Peliosis hepatitis and benign and malignant liver tumors have been reported in athletes using oral steroids, but they are rare occurrences.[38,42]

The long-term atherogenic and cardiomyopathic potential of anabolic steroids remains to be elucidated. During steroid use, total cholesterol and LDL-C increase, whereas HDL-C declines. These parameters revert to normal with drug cessation.[3] However, lowered HDL-C has been associated with increased risk of cardiovascular disease; thus anabolic steroids may increase cardiovascular risk.[75] There are case reports of young steroid abusers who, in the absence of the usual predisposing diseases or risk factors, have incurred cerebrovascular accidents, acute myocardial infarction, and cardiomyopathy.[24,28,55,57] Because the precise effects of exogenous androgens on human myocardium are largely unknown, the evidence linking the two is purely anecdotal.[24] Certain oral steroids are associated with increased clotting factors and prothrombin and therefore with a hypercoagulable state. This, coupled with the polycythemia that is induced by most anabolic steroids, could certainly be a factor in the development of vascular disease.[28]

Many athletes who use anabolic steroids develop a dependency. After cycling off, they experience fatigue, depression, anorexia, decreased self-esteem, and body-image dissatisfaction. Subsequently, they have difficulty discontinuing the drugs and have a strong desire to reinitiate use once they have been discontinued.[42]

CONCLUSION

This chapter has presented the most common weight-training injuries reported in the recent literature. Power lifters, body-builders, and other serious weight-trainers are most susceptible to overuse syndromes because they are constantly attempting to progress in terms of strength, power, muscle mass, and definition. Because overuse injuries are basically inevitable, the true genius of these athletes lies in the training modifications that allow continued development, even in the presence of injury. Body-builders have exceptional knowledge in terms of how to isolate, strengthen, and hypertrophy specific muscle groups with a variety of exercises. The carry-over of body-building concepts to rehabilitation appears to be tremendous, including restoration and maintenance of flexibility and strength and correction of muscle imbalances.

REFERENCES

1. Aggrawal ND, Ravinder K, Kumar S, Mather D: A study of changes in the spine in weight lifters and other athletes. *Br J Sports Med* 13:58–61, 1979.
2. Agre JC, Ash N, Cameron C, House J: Suprascapular neuropathy after intensive progressive resistive exercise: Case report. *Arch Phys Med Rehabil* 68:236–238, 1986.
3. Allman FL: Weight lifting—harmful or healthful? *JAMA* 211:2163, 1970.
4. American Academy of Pediatrics Committee on Sports Medicine: Strength training, weight and power lifting and body building by children and adolescents. *Pediatrics* 86:801–803, 1990.
5. Bach BR, Warren RF, Wickiewicz TL: Triceps rupture: A case report and literature review. *Am J Sports Med* 15:285–289, 1987.
6. Bartsokas TW, Palin WD, Collier BD: Case report: An unusual stress fracture site: Midhumerus. *Physician Sportsmed* 20(2):119–122, 1992.
7. Basford JR: Weight lifting, weight training and injuries. *Orthopedics* 8:1051–1056, 1985.
8. Bird CB, McCoy JW: Weight lifting as a cause of compartment syndrome in the forearm: A case report. *J Bone Joint Surg* 65A:406, 1983.
9. Bourne ND, Reilly T: Effect of a weight lifting belt on spinal shrinkage. *Br J Sports Med* 25(4):209–212, 1991.
10. Brady TA, Cahill BR, Bodnar LM: Weight training related injuries in the high school athlete. *Am J Sports Med* 10:1–5, 1982.
11. Breall WB: Risks of weight lifting. *JAMA* 212:2267, 1970.
12. Brown EW, Kimball RG: Medical history associated with adolescent power lifting. *Pediatrics* 72:636–644, 1983.
13. Brown T, Hansen RJ, Yurra AJ: Some mechanical tests on the lumbosacral spine with particular reference to the intervertebral discs. *J Bone Joint Surg* 39A:1135, 1957.
14. Browne TD, Yost RP, McCarron RF: Lumbar ring apophyseal fracture in an adolescent weight lifter. A case report. *Am J Sports Med* 18:533–535, 1990.
15. Cahill BR: Osteolysis of the distal part of the clavicle in male athletes. *J Bone Joint Surg* 64A:1053–1058, 1982.
16. Casamassima AC, Sternberg T, Weiss FH: Spontaneous pneumopericardium: A link with weight lifting? *Physician Sportsmed* 19(6):107–110, 1991.
17. Chen WC, Hsu WY, Wu JJ: Stress fracture of the diaphysis of the ulna. *Int Orthop* 15:197–198, 1991.
18. Dangles CJ, Bilos ZJ: Ulnar nerve neuritis in a world champion weight lifter: A case report. *Am J Sports Med* 8:443–445, 1980.
19. Davies JE: The spine in sports injuries: Prevention and treatment. *Br J Sports Med* 14:18–20, 1980.
20. de Virgilio C, Nelson RJ, Milliken J, et al: Ascending aortic dissection in weight lifters with cystic medial degeneration. *Ann Thorac Surg* 49:638–642, 1990.
21. Dillingham MF: Strength training. *Phys Med Rehabil State Art Rev* 1:555–568, 1987.
22. DiNubile NA: Strength training. *Clin Sports Med* 10:33–62, 1991.
23. Feeler LC: Weight lifting. *Spine State Art Rev* 4:366–376, 1990.
24. Ferenchick GS, Kirlin P, Potts R: Steroids and cardiomyopathy: How strong a connection? *Physician Sportsmed* 19(9):107–110, 1991.
25. Flemming JE: Spondylolysis and spondylolisthesis in the athlete. *Spine State Art Rev* 4:339–345, 1990.
26. Francobandiera C, Mafulli N, Lepore L: Distal radioulnar joint dislocation, ulna volar in a female body builder. *Med Sci Sports Exerc* 22(2):155–158, 1990.
27. Frankle MA, Cicero CJ, Payne J: Use of androgenic anabolic steroids by athletes. *JAMA* 252:482, 1984.
28. Frankle MA, Eichberg R, Zachariah SB: Anabolic androgenic steroids and a stroke in an athlete: Case report. *Arch Phys Med Rehabil* 69:632–633, 1988.
29. Frankle M, Leffers D: Athletes on anabolic androgenic steroids. *Physician Sportsmed* 20(6):75–87, 1992.
30. Friden J, Sjostrom M, Ekblom B: Myofibrillar damage following intense eccentric exercise in man. *Int J Sports Med* 4:170–176, 1983.
31. Garrett WE: Muscle strain injuries: Clinical and basic aspects. *Med Sci Sport Exerc* 22:436–443, 1990.
32. George DH, Stakiw K, Wright CJ: Fatal accident with weight lifting equipment: Implications for safety standards. *Can Med Assoc J* 140:925–926, 1989.
33. Glick JG: Muscle strains: Prevention and treatment. *Physician Sportsmed* 8:73–77, 1980.
34. Goeser CD, Aikenhead JA: Rib fracture due to bench pressing. *J Manip Physiol Ther* 13:26–29, 1990.
35. Gumbs VL, Segal D, Halligan JB, Lower G: Bilateral distal radius and ulnar fractures in adolescent weight lifters. *Am J Sports Med* 10:375–379, 1982.
36. Hamilton HK: Stress fracture of the diaphysis of the ulna in a bodybuilder. *Am J Sports Med* 12:405, 1984.
37. Harman EA, Rosenstein RM, Frykman PN, Nigro GA: Effects of a belt on intra-abdominal pressure during weight lifting. *Med Sci Sports Exerc* 21:186–190, 1989.
38. Haupt HA, Rovere GD: Anabolic steroids: A review of the literature. *Am J Sports Med* 12:469–484, 1984.
39. Herrick RT, Herrick S: Ruptured triceps in a powerlifter presenting as cubital tunnel syndrome: A case report. *Am J Sports Med* 15:514–516, 1987.
40. Herring SA, Nilson KL: Introduction to overuse injuries. *Clin Sports Med* 6:231, 1987.
41. Jackson DW, et al: Stress reactions involving the pars interarticularis in young athletes. *Am J Sports Med* 9:304–312, 1982.
42. Johnson MD: Steroids. *Adolesc Med State Art Rev* 2:79–92, 1991.
43. Jones MW, Matthews JP: Rupture of pectoralis major in weight lifters: A case report and review of the literature. *Br J Accid Surg* 19(3):219, 1988.
44. Jordan BD, Istrico R, Zimmerman RD, et al: Case reports: Acute cervical radiculopathy in weight lifters. *Physician Sportsmed* 18(1):73–76, 1990.

45. Lamb DR: Anabolic steroids in atheltics: How well do they work and how dangerous are they? *Am J Sports Med* 12:31–38, 1984.

46. Lander JE, Simonton RL, Giacobbe JK: The effectiveness of weight belts during the squat exercise. *Med Sci Sports Exerc* 22:117–126, 1990.

47. Langer PH, Mansure FT: Risks of weight lifting. *JAMA* 212:2267, 1970.

48. Leach RE, Schepsis AA: Shoulder pain. *Clin Sports Med* 2:134, 1983.

49. Levy HJ, Gardner RD, Lemak LJ: Bilateral osteochondral flaps of the wrists. *Arthroscopy* 7:118–119, 1991.

50. Lewis DC, Johnson SR: Spontaneous dislocation of the lunate in a weight lifter. *Br J Accid Surg* 21(4):252–254, 1990.

51. Louis DS, Peck O: Triceps avulsion fracture in a weight lifter. *Orthopedics* 15:207–208, 1992.

52. MacDougall JD, Toxen D, Sale DG, et al: Arterial blood pressure response to heavy resistance exercise. *J Appl Physiol* 58:785–790, 1985.

53. Maffulli N, Mikhail HM: Bilateral anterior glenohumeral dislocation in a weight lifter. *Br J Accid Surg* 21(4):254–256, 1990.

54. Mannis CI: Transchondral fracture of the dome of the talus sustained during weight training. *Am J Sports Med* 11:354–356, 1983.

55. McNutt RA, Ferenchick GS, Kirlin PC, Hamlin NJ: Acute myocardial infarction in a 22-year-old world class weight lifter using anabolic steroids. *Am J Cardiol* 62:164, 1988.

56. Michna H: Appearance and ultrastructure of intranuclear crystalloid in tendon fibroblasts induced by anabolic steroid hormone in a mouse. *Acta Anat* (Basel) 133:247–250, 1988.

57. Mochizuki RM, Richter KJ: Cardiomyopathy and cerebrovascular accident associated with anabolic androgenic steroid use: Case report. *Physician Sportsmed* 16(11):108–114, 1988.

58. Montagna P: Suprascapular neuropathy after muscular effort. *Electromyogr Clin Neurophysiol* 23:553–557, 1983.

59. Neviaser TJ: Weight lifting. Risks and injuries to the shoulder. *Clin Sports Med* 10:615–621, 1991.

60. Powell B: Weight lifters cephalgia. *Ann Emerg Med* 11(8):449–451, 1982.

61. Reilly T: Some observations on weight training. *Br J Sports Med* 12:45–47, 1978.

62. Rengachary SS, Neff JP, Singer PA, Brackett CE: Suprascapular entrapment neuropathy: A clinical, anatomical and comparative study. *Neurosurgery* 5:441–455, 1979.

63. Reut RC, Bach BR, Johnson C: Case report: Pectoralis major rupture: Diagnosing and treating a weight training injury. *Physician Sportsmed* 19(3):89–96, 1991.

64. Risser WL: Musculoskeletal injuries caused by weight training. Guidelines for prevention. *Clin Pediatr* 29(6):305–310, 1990.

65. Risser WL, Risser JM, Preston D: Weight training injuries in adolescents. *Am J Dis Child* 144:1015–1017, 1990.

66. Ritchie AJ, Rooke LG: Spontaneous ruptures of the triceps in the presence of a patella cubiti. *Arch Emerg Med* 7(2):114–117, 1990.

67. Saal JA: Rehabilitation of sports-related lumbar spine injuries. *Phys Med Rehabil State Art Rev* 1:613–638, 1987.

68. Safran MR, Garrett WE, Seaber AV, et al: The role of warmup in muscular injury prevention. *Am J Sports Med* 16:123–129, 1988.

69. Schultz JS, Leonard JA: Long thoracic neuropathy from athletic activity. *Arch Phys Med Rehabil* 73:87–90, 1992.

70. Shepherd R: Strength training, weight and power lifting and body building by children and adolescents. *Pediatrics* 88:417–418, 1991.

71. Sherman OH, Snyder SJ, Fox JM: Triceps tendon avulsion in a professional body builder: A case report. *Am J Sports Med* 12:328–329, 1984.

72. Simoneaux SF, Murphy BJ, Tehrahzadeh J: Spontaneous pneumothorax in a weight lifter. A case report. *Am J Sports Med* 18:647–648, 1990.

73. Spencer CW, Jackson DW: Back injuries in the athlete. *Clin Sports Med* 2:191–215, 1983.

74. Stith WJ: Exercise and the intervertebral disc. *Spine State Art Rev* 4:259–266, 1990.

75. Strauss RH, Wright JE, Finerman GA, Catlin DH: Side effects of anabolic steroids in weight-trained men. *Physician Sportsmed* 11:87–96, 1983.

76. Webb DR: Strength training in children and adolescents. *Pediatr Clin North Am* 37:1187–1210, 1990.

77. Wooton JR, Jones DH: An unusual weight lifting injury. *Br J Accid Surg* 19(6):446–447, 1988.

78. Zarins B, Ciullo JV: Acute muscle and tendon injuries in athletes. *Clin Sports Med* 2:167–182, 1983.

79. Zeman SC, Rosenfeld RT, Lipscomb PR: Tears of pectoralis major. *Am J Sports Med* 7:343–347, 1979.

Chapter 13

ALPINE SKIING

Edward R. Laskowski, MD

Skiing is one of the most popular winter-time recreational pursuits. Many ski areas count more than 1 million skier visits each winter. Because of the nature and season of the sport, however, and the need to go to a specific ski hill or facility to participate, one can be especially prone to injuries. In essence, many people will not get in shape in order to ski but will, instead, use skiing as a form of conditioning over the winter months. Thus, being inadequately prepared for the demands of the sport and not having frequent access to practice and training would appear to increase the risk for injury. The following discussion attempts to identify the most common injuries in skiers and explain important aspects of the epidemiology of ski injuries. This information is important to consider when making interventions with respect to technique, equipment, and training/conditioning issues. Specific rehabilitation concerns related to injured skiers will then be addressed.

INJURY PATTERNS

The scope and cost of ski injuries is significant. Approximately 40,000 anterior cruciate ligament (ACL) ruptures occur per year.[27] When analyzing the cost of this injury, one must include aspects such as surgery (including reconstructive graft, anesthesiologist, surgeon, assistants, operating room and inpatient expenses), braces, physical therapy, continued physician follow-up fees, and lost wages and opportunity cost. The impact in terms of monetary expenditure can be significant. About $24 is added to every ski pass sold in the United States to cover insurance and liability.[27]

Accurate analysis and study of skiing injury trends has been difficult due to the inherent difficulty with epidemiologic data related to skiing. Many different populations (children, young adults, middle aged skiers, older adults, males vs. females) are at risk. In addition, terrain and snow condition/environment vary according to the ski area and according to each specific run at the ski area. These conditions may vary during the same day and between days depending on weather conditions. Equipment also varies, including structure of the ski, length of the ski, type of binding and boot, and whether equipment has been adequately inspected for safety. Significantly, skiers have vastly different exposure rates. One person may ski four runs and 12,000 vertical feet in a day while another skier may ski 18 or 19 runs at close to 50,000 vertical feet. Thus, although each visit is counted as one "skier visit," each skier's exposure to injury is much different. There is also significant variation with respect to experience level of the skier. Preliminary data from a large Western ski area indicate that local skiers have a lower incidence of serious injuries. Although residents of one town at the base of the ski hill composed 25% of the skiers at that area, they accounted for only 19% of the injuries.[14] Given all the above, it has been difficult to obtain accurate data regarding ski injury epidemiology.

Johnson et al. have compiled the most complete information on skier injury trends over the past 20 years.[14] Their data cover more than 6,000 patients and 2 million skier visits and have revealed interesting trends over the years. Before 1970, the injury rate was approximately 7 per 1,000 skier days. The current rate ranges between 2 to 3 per 1,000 skier visits.[14,15,29,31] In addition, there has been a 48% decline for all injuries, and the mean number of days between injuries has increased from 214 in 1972 to 408 in 1990.[14]

With respect to patterns of injury, the lower extremities account for approximately 50% of all injuries.[14] A notable decrease has occurred in ankle and tibia fractures, upper body injuries, and lacerations. While the number of knee sprains has remained relatively constant (26% in 1989 to 1990 vs. 20% in 1972 to 1973), the proportion of severe (grade 3, or complete ligament disruption) knee sprains has increased from 15% to 66% in this same time period, with most of these severe sprains involving the ACL. Ski-related ACL injuries have increased approximately 644% over 20 years.[9,11,14,19,25] It is difficult to estimate the amount of ACL injuries that occur in the general population, but Miyasaka et al.[21] have estimated an injury rate of 38 per 100,000 people per year. Among skiers Johnson[15] has estimated an injury rate of 50 per 100,000 skiers per day.

In Johnson's study,[14] shoulder injuries accounted for approximately 8% of total injuries. Fifty-two percent of these injuries were dislocations, and 18% were acromioclavicular sprains, the majority being grade 1. Of the total shoulder injuries, 1.5% were clavicular fractures. The ever-present "skier's thumb," or ulnar collateral ligament injury, accounted for up to 75% of upper-extremity injuries, 20% of which required surgical repair.

With respect to competitive skiers, McConkey surveyed the Canadian Women's National Team from 1984 to 1992.[20] He found that the risk of a knee injury per year per skier was 50%. Specifically, the risk of an injury to the anterior cruciate ligament and to the medial collateral ligament were both 17% per year; the risk of lower extremity fracture was 11% per year, and the risk of needing an operative procedure on the knee was 29% per year. Worldwide, approximately 6% of World Cup skiers sustain season-ending injuries each year. Injuries can be severe and can include comminuted fractures of the lower leg bones, tibial plateau fractures, compression fractures of the spine, and patellar tendon ruptures.

EPIDEMIOLOGIC ASPECTS OF SKI INJURIES

Optimally, causative and contributing factors of ski injuries should be identified to permit intervention, either with respect to external factors (terrain, snow conditions), internal factors (experience of skier, technique, training), and equipment-related issues.

Forces encountered in downhill skiing can be impressive; it has been reported that the lower extremities are exposed to 2G (where G = the force of gravity) during a sliding "hockey stop" of 15 feet, 15G during a shorter 2-foot drop, and 139G during an instantaneous stop or "edge catch."[7]

Optimal ski length has been debated, as a longer ski means a longer lever arm, which can decrease the force necessary to break a bone or tear a ligament. Conversely, longer skis mean greater stability, especially at higher speeds. With respect to bindings, Eriksson[7] reports that a 1973 survey indicated that only 3.6% of skiers had their bindings "correctly tuned" (Fig. 1). This has improved, but only to the point at which a similar survey in 1992 indicated that 50% of bindings were appropriately maintained. The issue of ski boot design also has been discussed. Greenwald[13] reports that 68% of all skiers in one sample population used rear entry boots. In the same population, 77% of all females who were injured used rear entry boots (Fig. 2), and 88% of tibial plateau fractures occurred with rear entry boots. The latter survey raises the possibility of equipment design modification, such as a break-away back on the boot to prevent high loading forces.

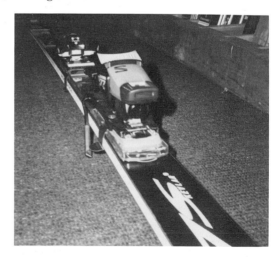

FIGURE 1. Ski binding. Arrows point to a screw that is used to adjust the tension of the binding. Too low a tension allows the ski to detach from the boot during ordinary skiing. Too high a tension keeps the ski attached even during a fall. The long lever arm of the ski can cause injury.

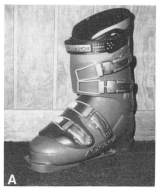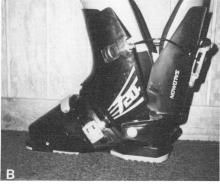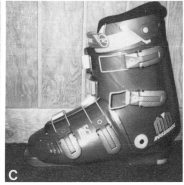

FIGURE 2. Three commonly used ski boots: **A,** front entry design; **B,** rear entry design; and **C,** hybrid "mid" entry type.

With the recent growth of instructional ski programs for the physically challenged, it is interesting to note that Ferrara et al.[8] and Laskowski and Murtaugh[17] have examined the injury experience of physically challenged skiers in competitive and instructional programs, respectively. Both studies suggested that the rate and severity of injury in physically challenged skiers are similar to those in the able-bodied population. Locations of injuries were similar in both groups, and injury patterns were determined primarily by the adaptive equipment and mode of skiing used by the physically challenged skiers. Thus, upright skiers tended to have more lower-extremity injuries and sit skiers or mono skiers (wheelchair bound) had more upper-extremity and shoulder injuries. Physically challenged skiers appeared to incur approximately the same proportion of injuries as skiers without a disability, and, in some cases, seemed to have fewer severe bony injuries and lacerations and more (but less severe) soft-tissue injuries.

With respect to the individual skier, factors such as experience and ski technique may play a role. There is no definitive study on the injury rate of those who have been instructed in the basics of proper ski technique vs. those who have learned on their own, but variation in technique is a possible contributing factor to injury. In addition, fatigue plays a great role, especially during ski vacations that last up to one week. Surveys have shown that rates of injury increase at the end of a ski day. In addition, Nygaard et al.[24] have shown that, after biopsy of the vastus lateralis muscle, there is an average 50% decrement of glycogen on the fifth vs. the first day of consecutive

skiing. The importance of appropriate diet and carbohydrate loading to replenish lost glycogen is essential in helping skiers to avoid fatigue and possible injury. The inherent risk of skiing in general is also a factor that is hard to estimate. Skiers skiing on slopes that are beyond their ability can be a problem, and collision-related injuries can occur when skiers are unable to control their skiing. In addition, the paradox of young children not being allowed to drive but being allowed to ski at 40 to 50 miles per hour is intriguing.

Of note, the increasing popularity and dramatic growth of the related sport of snowboarding have stimulated interest in injury patterns specific to this sport (Fig. 3). Preliminary data by Johnson[14] suggest that snowboarders predominantly sustain upper-extremity injuries, especially to the hand and wrist. The incidence of serious ligamentous (including ACL) knee injury appears to be markedly lower, possibly due in part to equipment differences, such as nonrigid boots, and less confining binding interfaces.

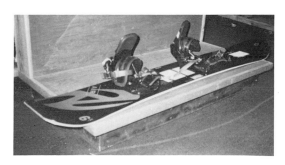

FIGURE 3. Snowboard, similar to water-ski or surfboard.

BIOMECHANICAL FACTORS IN ACL INJURY

Current biomechanical explanations for ACL injury include a passive and an active model. The "active" ACL injury, or "quadriceps-induced" ACL injury, occurs during recovery from falling backwards. This usually occurs in expert skiers who are trying to recover from a fall. During the attempted recovery, the accelerating upper body and active quadriceps contraction create increased force, directing the tibia anteriorly. This occurs in combination with a rigid high-backed ski boot that creates a longer lever arm and moves the "fulcrum" of movement to the knee. This combination of factors provides more force to be directed anteriorly. During this injury, both eccentric and concentric muscle contractions of the quadriceps may occur. Bindings may not release, and the skier may not fall (the classic "injury that caused the accident").

The passive biomechanical explanation for ACL injury includes the "phantom foot" phenomenon. This usually occurs in beginning and lower-level skier and entails hyperflexion and internal rotation of the knee. Again, this biomechanical position, combined with a rigid high-backed boot, produces increased anteriorly directed force on the tibia and the potential for an ACL tear. Both of these explanations are probably generalizations, and multiple other variables are probably involved that contribute to the force needed to rupture the ligament.

REHABILITATION ISSUES IN SKIERS

Prevention

Specific exercise parameters for ski injury prevention have yet to be clearly delineated and objectively proved, but interesting data have been presented by Greenwald[13] regarding a knee injury prevention program for skiers. A program was designed at a large Western ski area to prevent knee injuries in ski area employees through flexibility, strength, stability, and muscle endurance assessment and treatment. Testing included isokinetic measurements of quadriceps/hamstring ratios and KT-1000 measurements. In two consecutive years, 18.9% and 16.0% of individuals diagnosed with a problem in one of the assessed areas were subsequently injured during that season. Only 0.8% and 4.6% of those with no identified problem sustained subsequent injury. In addition, individuals who complied with an exercise program designed to correct their area of deficiency had fewer injuries. As discussed previously, many other epidemiologic variables likely influence these findings. Nonetheless, attempting to identify problem areas in physical status that can be improved by a ski-specific exercise program may be a key aspect of injury prevention.

Training

Many factors are involved in a comprehensive rehabilitation program for the injured skier. In addition to specific rehabilitation concerns, it is important to remember that prevention of recurrent injury, as well as prevention of initial injury, are affected by the skier's particular conditioning and training program.

Education is an important aspect of training and rehabilitation and should include information about appropriate pre-season conditioning and ski-specific conditioning in hopes of preventing injury or re-injury. Pre-season conditioning should begin with cross training off the slope after the ski season ends. The conditioning can be a continuum of the skier's regular recreation, sport, or physical fitness pattern, with an emphasis on cross-training activities and exercises that contribute to optimal musculoskeletal health of ski-specific muscle groups along with aerobic and power bases. In general, physical preparation should include strength training, power training, and sports-specific endurance. Performance will likely be limited by a weak link in any one of these three aspects. In addition, ski-specific training includes preparation with respect to psychological status (focus, imagery, relaxation), tactical education, and technical education.

Appropriate cardiovascular training is essential for optimal skiing performance and also should be maintained and enhanced in any rehabilitation program. Though skiing may be considered anaerobic by many, it is important to train all three energy systems: ATP-phosphocreatine, anaerobic, and aerobic. The ATP-phosphocreatine system, which provides for explosive power, is extremely short-lived (5-10 seconds). Training in this system helps to improve speed and quickness. This system can be enhanced through plyometric-type activities, which stress muscle power. Lower weight, higher repetition weight training emphasizing speed and explosiveness of movement in "skiing specific" patterns (i.e., squat, lateral lunge) also contribute to enhancing this system.

Intermediate duration (60-90 seconds) power comes from the anaerobic system (glycolysis). Training of this system improves speed endurance. Exercises that enhance this system include 220- and 440-yard sprints, stair runs, and interval training on a bicycle or in-line skates. This type of training enables high-speed, high-intensity types of activity to be sustained over short segments of time.

Finally, endurance training is important for an optimal aerobic base and fat and carbohydrate metabolism. Aerobic training enables sustained intervals, allows quicker recovery, and helps in sustaining aggressive skiing and maintaining a high tempo. An aerobically fit individual also has more efficient transport of oxygen through the tissues and muscles and recovers more quickly from a strenuous day or week of skiing. Aerobic endurance must be improved during the off season, as routine skiing and even training is not sufficient to raise the oxygen uptake ($\dot{V}O_2$ max) to the level required for aggressive skiing. The aerobic exercise prescription is well known and will not be reviewed in detail. Of importance in rehabilitation, however, is the principle of "relative rest" after injury. The principle of relative rest dictates that the injured body part be "rested" and protected from further trauma or injury while the remaining muscle mass is utilized to provide appropriate stress to the cardiovascular system for maintenance of optimal aerobic conditioning. A 50% reduction in aerobic capacity has been shown after just 4–12 weeks of detraining.[10,16,28] In addition, strength training should continue in uninvolved body parts, and it is documented that "crossover" training effects occur in the rested limb when the contralateral limb is exercised.[22]

INJURY REHABILITATION

Pain control remains an essential first step in the rehabilitation of an injured skier. Pain can be a great inhibitor, and muscle co-contraction and substitution are just two of the suboptimal biomechanical and neuromuscular effects that can result from "going through the pain."

Once pain control is established, it is essential to ensure that range of motion and flexibility are optimal. Symmetrical flexibility may be the most important aspect, rather than "perfect geometry," especially after an injury. In essence, it is not as important that the popliteal angle of the hamstring muscle group is $0°$ rather than $20°$, but that it is equal compared to the uninjured side. Tight muscles can act like an effusion and have an inhibitory effect on antagonist muscle groups. Stretching may decrease facilitation of muscle spindle afferents and assist the facilitation of Golgi tendon organs.[6] In addition, stretching may increase temperature, which may have a protective effect.[23] Stretching techniques should be reviewed in detail with the skier, as poor body positioning may make the stretch worthless or even harmful. In addition, an insufficient duration of hold when stretching may fail to provide proper benefit. Ideally, one should stretch before and after an exercise session; if compliance is a problem, stretching after exercise is probably the best option. At that time, muscle blood flow has warmed the muscle to the point that collagen and elastin are more extensible and, it is hoped, greater long-term benefits can be obtained from the stretch. Muscle co-contraction and substitution patterns should be avoided during stretching.

Important muscle groups for the skier to stretch include the heel cord (Achilles tendon), hamstrings, hip group muscles (hip flexors, hip extensors, hip abductors and adductors), iliotibial band, lumbar spine, and shoulder groups. The latter should include the rotator cuff groups and the scapular stabilizers (trapezius, rhomboids, latissimus dorsi, serratus anterior, levator scapulae). In addition, if a bicycle is used for off-season conditioning, the skier should be careful to avoid hip flexor tightness and should pay special attention to stretching this muscle group.

Early range of motion and gentle stretching after injury are important for the skier to obtain maximal strength of the healing tissue. If collagen is left to heal without any force applied, cross-linkage patterns will be random and disorganized. With a stretching force applied, the collagen will heal in linear bundles and will provide the greatest tensile strength.[1,2]

STRENGTHENING

Prerequisites to successful strengthening include pain-free range of motion (which is almost full) and acceptable flexibility. During rehabilitation, therapeutic exercise in the lower extremity will naturally focus on ski-specific muscle groups. It has been postulated that hamstring dominance is important in an anterior cruciate ligament-deficient knee and may be prophylactic in helping to prevent ACL injury.[30] Open kinetic chain hamstring exercise done in the prone position safely provides an effective form of strengthening to this muscle group without causing an undue amount of shear force to the knee joint. Other lower extremity muscle groups that need to be optimally strengthened include the quadriceps, gluteus maximus, and hip group musculature, especially the hip abductors and adductors. Eccentric quadriceps strengthening should be included as part of an exercise routine because this is the manner in which the muscle will be used most during the sports-specific skiing position.

Abdominal exercise is also essential for optimal kinetic chain muscle function. A strong abdomen will serve to protect the back muscles and also will help with upper body stabilization. Some skiers have advocated use of an elastic support or wrap for episodes of back pain and to assist in preventing fatigue in this area. The efficacy of this device has not been proven conclusively, and a dynamic lumbar stabilization program stressing coordinated strengthening of the back and abdominal musculature may be preferable.

Upper body strengthening helps balance during skiing and also aids the skier's ability to withstand turning forces without unwanted body rotation. Triceps strengthening, such as with triceps pull-downs, can aid with propulsion during race starts and also when using ski poles during turns. Closed kinetic chain upper extremity exercises, such as push-ups and pull-ups, provide coordinated triarticular strengthening for most of the major upper extremity muscle groups. In general, the posterior shoulder groups and upper back musculature are neglected during strengthening in favor of the more popular anterior group strengthening exercises (bench press, pectoral strengthening). To ensure balanced shoulder strengthening and good function, scapular stabilization exercises should be included. These can include strengthening for the latissimus dorsi via pull-downs (Fig. 4), serratus anterior via push-up "plusses" (pushing up into even more torso elevation after a push-up [Fig. 5]), rhomboid strengthening via pull-backs and reverse flies, trapezius strengthening via shoulder shrugs, and also levator scapulae strengthening.

Closed kinetic chain exercises should be

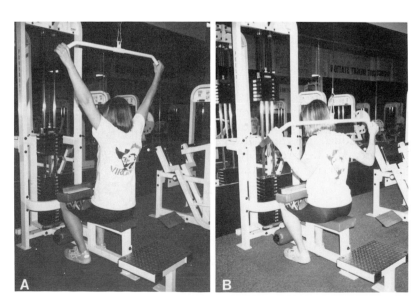

FIGURE 4.   Latissimus pull-downs for upper back and posterior shoulder strengthening. **A,** upward; and **B,** downward positions.

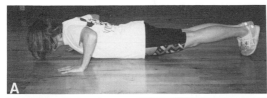

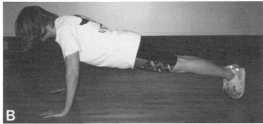

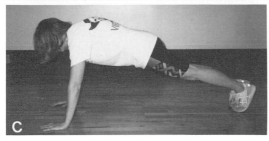

FIGURE 5. Push-up "plusses:" After fully extending the arms during push-up, the body is raised further, stressing the serratus anterior. **A,** bottom; **B,** top; **C,** "plus."

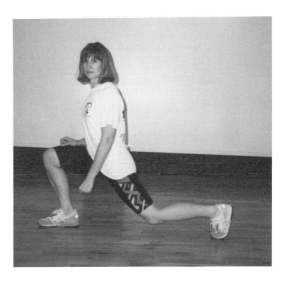

FIGURE 6. Closed kinetic chain exercise: a lunge.

the foundation of lower extremity muscle strengthening. These exercises entail triarticular movement (ankle, knee, and hip) with the distal portion (foot) in a fixed position. As muscle co-contraction is a stabilizing factor, shear force and compression force at the knee are diminished as compared to open kinetic chain exercises.[18] Closed-chain exercises are particularly essential in strengthening the knee after anterior cruciate ligament reconstructive surgery and also for general lower extremity conditioning. These exercises can be ski specific and functional. They may include squats, lunges, step-ups, leg press, bicycling with toe clips, and variations of the above (Figs. 6 & 7).

Speed and power are especially important for full rehabilitation after a ski injury. Power is essential for rapid weight transfer during skiing, especially during suboptimal snow conditions and for aggressive edging. In essence, power is the amount of work done over a unit of time and can be thought of as a dynamic measure of strength. Plyometric exercise is basically the power component of a comprehensive program. These exercises en-

tail a rebound muscle contraction after a stretch (i.e., jumping down off a box and immediately jumping back up). Concentric and eccentric muscle activity are combined during the exercise, loading the elastic and contractile elements of the muscle. It is thought that an element of neuromuscular facilitation occurs that provides for increased muscle contraction and power after the prestretch.[3] Higher level plyometrics must be monitored closely, as the high impact nature of the exercise increases the risk of injury. Low level plyometrics, however, can be safely

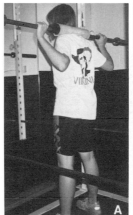

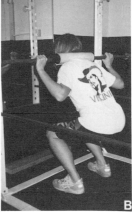

FIGURE 7. Closed kinetic chain exercise: a squat. **A,** top; **B,** bottom.

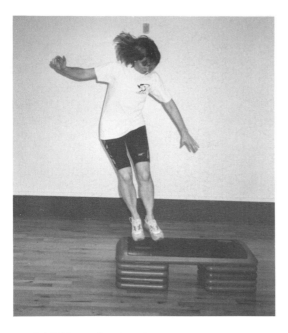

FIGURE 8. "Box jumping" plyometric exercise.

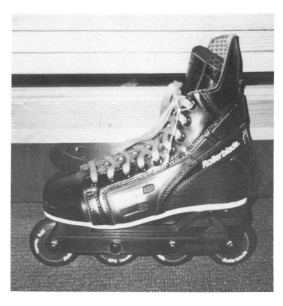

FIGURE 9. In-line skate. When used with poles, it can be an effective simulation exercise for skiing to be used in the off-season.

begun after a sufficient strength base is established. Ski-specific plyometric exercises may include bounding, box jumps (Fig. 8) and hops, high stepping, hopscotch exercises, skipping, and tuck jumps. All these help to create a more explosive power component for the exercise program.

Resistance band exercise, such as use of a theraband or sport cord, provides for multiple plane strengthening in diagonal/spiral and sport-specific patterns. The advantages of this type of exercise are that equipment needs are minimal and the resistance bands are easily transported. In addition, they enable the muscles to be worked in a sport-specific fashion. Some of the sport-specific ski simulators (i.e., Fitter, Skier's Edge) use resistance bands in a lateral plane to enable the lateral muscle groups to be worked in a ski-specific side-to-side fashion.

Before returning to the slopes, a base strength program maximizing muscle strength and symmetry should be undertaken. Work on muscle endurance (low weight, high repetitions) should be followed by a gradual progression to resistance training. Once this is accomplished, the remaining aspects of rehabilitation include ski-specific strengthening and the development of quickness and agility.

PROPRIOCEPTION AND SPORTS-SPECIFIC SKILLS

Rehabilitation is not complete unless proprioception and sports-specific skills have been optimized. Proprioception, which can be thought of as the body's ability to vary contractile forces of muscles in immediate response to outside forces, may be the most important factor in returning functional stability to joints and in limiting the occurrence (recurrence) of injury.[6,26] In addition to the mechanical and anatomical disruption that soft tissue injury may entail, the disruption of muscle spindles, Golgi tendon organs, and joint receptors has an impact on joint stability and function. These functions must be "retrained" to ensure optimal stability. With respect to sports-specific training, exercise gains are specific to the type and pattern of movement training, velocity of training, and the range of motion and angle at which training occurs.[5,12,32]

Skiing specific exercises include running or in-line skating (Fig. 9) through a slalom course, using a sliding board for lateral and medial hip group strengthening, using a wobble board to challenge the balance (Fig. 10) and proprioceptive system, and using plyometrics to aid in explosive rebound move-

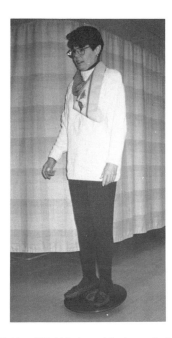

FIGURE 10. "Wobble board," also called BAPS (biomechanical ankle proprioceptive system) board, is used for proprioceptive exercise.

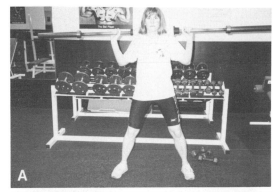

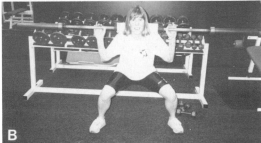

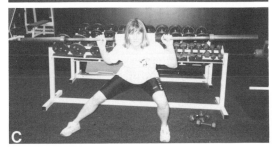

FIGURE 11. Ski-specific exercise. Lateral squats with a weight bar. **A,** top; **B,** bottom; **C,** lateral.

ments. As mentioned, use of a ski simulator exercises the hip adductors and abductors. Similar benefits can also be accomplished by performing lateral squats with a weight bar. (Fig. 11) In-line skating and tight rope walking help to enhance ski specific muscle strength and balance. Foot quickness and agility can be enhanced by participation in tennis and racquet sports, touch football, basketball, soccer, fencing, and aerobic dance.

BRACING

There has been much controversy in the literature regarding the use of functional bracing after an anterior cruciate ligament injury (see also chapter on knee bracing). Some skiers question whether they should wear a brace to protect themselves from injury. There is no evidence to support that the wearing of a functional knee brace will protect the skier from an ACL injury. After ACL rupture, functional braces are often prescribed both for post-reconstruction and rehabilitative treatments. While these braces, during static testing, do not seem to control anterior tibial translation, they do seem to provide proprioceptive help. Patients who are ACL-deficient and who have worn functional braces report fewer episodes of "giving way" and instability.[4] This likely is a result of an enhancement of dynamic muscle activity, perhaps entailing earlier activation of the hamstring muscle groups because of the custom-fit nature of most of these braces. Definitive studies in this realm have yet to be completed. The author's opinion is that after an ACL rupture, skiing can safely be resumed when deemed appropriate after surgical reconstruction and rehabilitation or after an aggressive rehabilitation alone. The risk of ACL disruption, as previously mentioned, is increasingly present in skiing; however, once the ACL is torn, it is not essential for participation in the sport. Skiing is done in a functional stance with a flexed knee position, a position in which the ACL can be compensated for by aggressive closed-chain, sport-specific, and proprioceptive exercise. In essence, "you can tear your ACL skiing, but you can ski without your ACL."

SUMMARY

There are many inherent difficulties in the collection of epidemiologic ski data, but important trends have been identified. Further investigation into equipment design is currently in progress in an attempt to reduce injury incidence, along with prophylactic strength training and conditioning programs. A comprehensive rehabilitation program entailing training of all three energy systems, flexibility, and sport-specific strengthening, power, and coordination/agility exercise are essential to ensure the optimal performance and safety of the skier.

REFERENCES

1. Akeson WH: An experimental study of joint stiffness. *J Bone Joint Surg* 43A:1022–1034, 1961.
2. Akeson WH, et al: The connective tissue response to immobility: A study of chondroitin-4 and 6-sulphate and dermatan sulphate changes in periarticular connective tissue of control and immobilized knees of dogs. *Clin Orthop* 51:183–197, 1967.
3. Chu DA: Understanding plyometrics. In Jumping Into Plyometrics. Champaign, IL, Leisure Press, 1992, pp 1–4.
4. Colville MR, Lee CO, Ciullo, JV: The Lenox Hill brace: An evaluation of effectiveness in treating knee ligamentous instability. *Am J Sports Med* 14:257–61, 1986.
5. Coyle EF, Feiring DC, Rotkis TC, et al: Specificity of power improvements through slow and fast isokinetic training. *J Appl Physiol* 51:1437–1442, 1981.
6. Day RW, Wildermuth BP: Proprioceptive training in the rehabilitation of lower extremity injuries. *Adv Sports Med Fitness* 1:241–257, 1988.
7. Eriksson E: Recent Trends in European Skiing Injuries. The Utah Symposium for Skier Safety, April 2, 1993, Salt Lake City.
8. Ferrara MS, Buckley WE, Messner DG, Benedict J: The injury experience and training history of the competititve skier with a disability. *Am J Sports Med* 20:55–60, 1992.
9. Freeman JR, Weaver JK, Oden RR, et al: Changing patterns in tibial fractures resulting from skiing. *Clin Orthop* 216:19–23, 1987.
10. Fringer MN, Stull GA: Changes in cardiorespiratory parameters during periods of training and detraining in young adult females. *Med Sci Sports Exerc* 6:20–25, 1974.
11. Garrick JG, Requa RK: Injury patterns in children and adolescent skiers. *Am J Sports Med* 7:245–248, 1979.
12. Graves JE, Pollock ML, Jones AE, et al: Specificity of limited range of motion variable resistance training. *Med Sci Sports Exerc* 21:84–89, 1989.
13. Greenwald R: Retrospective Analysis of Skiing Injury Trends in Utah. The Utah Symposium for Skier Safety, April 2, 1993, Salt Lake City.
14. Johnson R: Skiing Injury Research. The Utah Symposium for Skier Safety, April 2, 1993, Salt Lake City.
15. Johnson RJ, Ettinger CF, Shealy JE: Skier Injury Trends. In Johnson RJ, Mote CJ, Binet MH (eds): Skiing Trauma and Safety: 7th International Symposium. Philadelphia, American Society for Testing and Materials, 1989, pp 25–31.
16. Kendrick ZB, Pollock ML, Hickman TN, Miller HS: Effects of training and detraining on cardiovascular efficiency. *Am Corrective Ther J* 25:79–83, 1971.
17. Laskowski ER, Murtaugh PA: Snow skiing injuries in physically disabled skiers. *Am J Sports Med* 20:553–557, 1992.
18. Lutz GE, et al: Comparison of tibiofemoral joint forces during open kinetic chain and closed kinetic chain exercises. *J Bone Joint Surg* 75A:732–739, 1993.
19. Mather P, Ziegler WJ, Holzach P: Skiing accidents in the past 15 years. *J Sports Sci* 5:319–326, 1987.
20. McConkey P: Canadian Team Ski-Injuries. The Utah Symposium for Skier Safety, April 2, 1993, Salt Lake City.
21. Miyasaka K, Daniel D, Stone M, Hirshman P: The incidence of knee ligament injuries in the general population. *Am J Knee Surg* 4:3–8, 1991.
22. Moritani T, deVries HA: Neural factors vs hypertrophy in the time course of muscle strength gain. *Am J Phys Med* 58:115–130, 1979.
23. Noonan TJ, et al: Thermal effects on skeletal muscle tensile behavior. *Am J Sports Med* 21:517–522, 1993.
24. Nygaard E, Andersen P, Nilsson P, et al: Glycogen depletion pattern and lactate accumulation in leg muscles during recreational downhill skiing. *Europ J Appl Physiol* 38:261–269, 1978.
25. Pope MH, Johnson RJ: Skiing injuries. *Artif Organs* 9:1–13, 1981.
26. Root ML, Orien WP, Reed JH: The mechanics for motion and stability of joints in the foot. In Normal and Abnormal Function of the Foot. Los Angeles, Clinical Biomechanical Corp. 1977, 5–37.
27. Rosenberg T: Skiing Injury Research: Current Status. The Utah Symposium for Skier Safety, April 2, 1993, Salt Lake City.
28. Roskamm H: Optimum patterns of exercise for healthy adults. *Can Med Assoc J* 96:845–899, 1967.
29. Sherry E: Skiing injuries in Australia. *Med J Aust* 140:530–531, 1984.
30. Steadman, JR: Rehabilitation of skiing injuries. *Clin Sports Med* 1:289–294, 1982.
31. Stoddard C: Alpine Skiing Accidents Fact Sheet. Springfield, MA, National Ski Areas Association, 1987.
32. Thorstensson A, Sjodin B, Karlsson J: Enzyme activities and muscle strength after "sprint training" in man. *Acta Physiol Scand* 94:313–318, 1975.

Chapter 14

KNEE BRACING

Wilhelm A. Zuelzer, MD

Sprains and strains are the most frequent musculoskeletal injuries, resulting in 14.5 million physician visits/year.[32] The knee is a common site for significant injury. Teitz et al.[40] reported that Division I football players had a mean knee-injury rate of about 8%. Hewson et al.[20] found that football players in high-risk positions (e.g., linemen, linebackers, and tight ends) have a 23% chance of a knee injury per season and a 64% chance of a knee injury during a 4-year career. He also found that season-ending knee injuries averaged 8/year in one NCAA football team over an 8-year period. Among patients in a health maintenance organization (HMO), Miyasaka et al[28] found that ligament disorders were the leading reason for referral of patients with significant knee injuries. The anterior cruciate and medial collateral ligaments were the most commonly involved. Extrapolation of their data to the entire population of the United States reveals the extent of the national problem (Table 1).

A brace can be defined as a device that clasps objects together to resist deforming forces and to support weakened structures.[13] External bracing is used for prevention of knee injuries, enhancement of performance, and prevention of giving way in an injured knee. It is also used for protection during postoperative rehabilitation. A classification scheme devised by the American Academy of Orthopaedic Surgeons[14] divides knee braces into three categories:

1. Prophylactic knee braces are designed to reduce the likelihood or severity of knee ligament injuries in a relatively normal knee.
2. Rehabilitation knee braces are designed to allow protected motion of an injured knee treated operatively or nonoperatively early after the injury.
3. Functional knee braces are designed to improve stability for an unstable or postoperative knee in activities of daily living and sports.

OVERVIEW

Knee braces grip bone indirectly through soft tissue. Pressure applied to skin is transmitted to the underlying fat, muscle, blood vessel, and nerve. This external compression from the brace increases intramuscular pressure.[27] The efficacy problems of brace construct are demonstrated, to a somewhat exaggerated degree, by Figures 1, 2, and 3. In Figure 1 the brace is aligned with the model knee, and in Figure 2 the brace is strapped to the soft tissue. Because of soft-tissue deformation and brace pistoning (sliding of the femur proximally on the strap), the brace protection is compromised (Fig. 3). Even long leg casts, applied tightly to cadaver legs, allow significant anterior-posterior translation, varus-valgus, and rotatory motion.[24] In vivo muscle contractions, however, stiffen and enlarge the underlying soft tissue and may improve the protection provided by braces or casts.

Experimental studies of brace efficacy use cadaver knees, knee models, and the in vivo knee. However, no ideal way exists to evaluate knee braces. We lack knowledge about speed, amount, and direction of forces that result in knee injuries; moreover, mechanisms of knee injuries vary greatly. A well-controlled study of

TABLE 1. Acute Knee Injuries Per Year in theUnited States with Pathologic Motion*

Isolated anterior cruciate ligament	61,000
Isolated medial collateral ligament	37,000
Anterior cruciate ligament/medial collateral ligament	16,500

*Extrapolation of data from Miyasaka et al.[28]

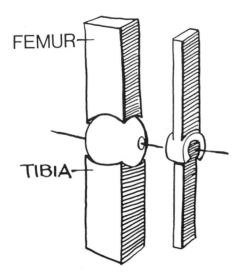

FIGURE 1. Brace lined up to knee.

brace efficacy faces formidable barriers, including variation in playing surfaces, shoes, conditioning, prior knee injuries, tackling technique, and normal fluctuations in yearly injuries among teams.

PROPHYLACTIC BRACES

Prophylactic braces attempt to prevent or to reduce severity of knee injuries, typically for a normal knee. There are two basic designs[43]: (1) a lateral bar with various hinge designs strapped to soft tissue (Fig. 2) and (2) medial and lateral bars with plastic cuffs or straps as well as various hinges. Prophylactic braces are off-the-shelf (not custom-made) with a retail cost between $35 and $60 per brace. Many colleges and professional teams use them extensively.

In Vitro Assessment

Baker et al.[2] used one cadaver with fixed foot, suspended femur, and lateral impact

loads on the knee with and without a prophylactic brace. The brace, they concluded, had limited capacity to protect the medial collateral ligament. The small number of cadavers, intrinsic biologic variability among cadavers, low-impact load (because significant loads would damage the ligaments), and low speed make cadaveric studies inconclusive. Because

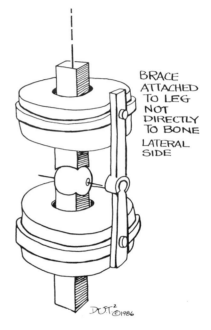

FIGURE 2. Brace strapped to soft tissue.

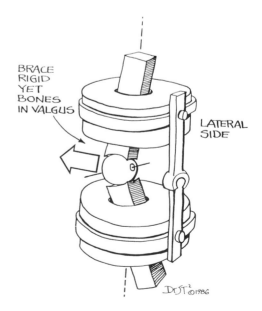

FIGURE 3. Angulation because of soft tissue deformation.

of this, Brown et al.[8] devised a mechanical knee to simulate a cadaver knee. They found that prophylactic braces, with the knee in full extension and high-impact lateral loads, offered modest protection, at best, to the medial collateral ligaments. They recommended design changes to improve prophylactic braces.

Paulos et al.[31] and France et al.[15,16] evaluated prophylactic knee braces for both cadaver and mechanical knee models. They used higher speeds and loads to approximate the in vivo situation. They found that a majority of prophylactic braces are biomechanically inadequate to protect the medial collateral ligament from direct lateral impact. They reported some protection for direct lateral hits but could not comment on the degree of protection if the hit came from another direction. They recommended that prophylactic knee braces be used voluntarily, but only if applied properly and maintained in good condition. They concluded that improvement in brace design was needed. Finally, Daniel,[12] using KT1000, demonstrated that fresh taping was superior to all prophylactic knee braces in limiting laxity during the Lachman maneuver (anterior drawer at 20° flexion).

In Vivo Assessment

Clinical studies are not conclusive. Hewson et al.[20] studied university football players and found no reduction in severity, number, or type of knee injuries with use of prophylactic braces. At another university, Taft et al.[38] reported a decrease in knee injuries with prophylactic knee braces. Grace et al.[19] followed 580 high school football players and found an increase in knee, ankle, and foot injuries with use of prophylactic knee brace. Teitz et al.[40] collected data from about 50% of all Division I NCAA colleges over 2 years and found a higher injury rate among football players who used prophylactic braces than among those who did not (10.2% vs 6.2%). Garrick and Requa[17] noted significant methodologic problems in the above studies and found no persuasive support for or against knee bracing.

More recently, Sitler et al.[35] reported on the efficacy of prophylactic braces in reducing knee injuries for intramural tackle football players at West Point. In their prospective, randomized study, the total number of knee injuries was reduced with the use of a unilateral biaxial (double-hinge) knee brace, but reduction in severity of injuries to the anterior cruciate and medial collateral ligaments was not statistically significant. Ankle injuries were not affected by wearing a prophylactic knee brace. The brace-related reduction in injury was found in defensive but not offensive players. They believed that the biaxial hinge was instrumental in the beneficial outcome. Finally, they found that the most frequent mechanism of knee injuries was direct lateral hit (47%), at the site where the brace is located.

REHABILITATION BRACES

Rehabilitation braces are designed to provide early protection of an injured knee joint treated with or without surgery.[14,43] They protect the healing structures from excessive elongation and load. Historically rehabilitation braces replaced casts and cast braces because of their light weight and adjustability for swelling or atrophy. They are off-the-shelf (not custom-made) with a typical retail cost between $80 and $200. Few data are available regarding their efficacy. They are commonly used for a 6- to 12-week period. Rehabilitation braces often have hinges that can be locked in one position or dialed to limit range of motion. Typically they consist of circumferential wraps and straps attached to medial and lateral sidebars with hinge attachment at the level of knee joint line. They usually cover most of the calf and thigh (Fig 4, Table 2).

In Vitro Assessment

Hofmann et al.[21] tested six rehabilitation braces with fresh cadavers, measuring anterior, valgus, and rotational stability. There were significant differences among braces in the ability to stabilize the cadaver knee after sectioning the anterior cruciate and medial collateral ligaments. Lateral and medial molded supports and increased sidebar rigidity appeared to result in greater stability. Cawley et al.[9] compared eight commercial rehabilitation braces using the mechanical knee model described previously. Most of the knee braces significantly reduced both translation and rotation relative to the unbraced limb. However, low loads were used. The au-

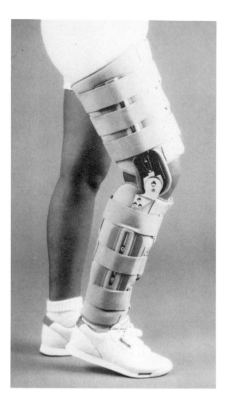

FIGURE 4. Representative rehabilitation brace. (Reproduced with permission of Medical Design, Inc.)

thors reached two conclusions: (1) joint line contact was the key to controlling varus-valgus and rotation and (2) the stiffness of the assembled brace improved the degree of knee control. The presence of shells, the design of the hinge bars, and the number of brace straps influenced the stiffness.

Clinical Assessment

No clinical data support or deny the efficacy of rehabilitation braces. Reported clinical problems include brace migration, pressure sores, excessive bulk, and heat. Stevenson et al.[36] showed that a walking subject wearing a rehabilitation brace had an extension of some 20° more than the setting on the hinge.

We need to know the ideal loads and motion to enhance and protect healing of cartilage, bone, and ligaments. Only then can rehabilitation braces be appropriately designed and assessed. Early motion with some significant loads on ligaments appears desirable,[34] but the degree is unknown.

FUNCTIONAL BRACES

Functional braces are designed to reduce laxity and disability in a person with a chronically unstable knee during activities of daily living and/or sports.[14,43] They are also used to protect a repaired ligament after rehabilitation is completed and athletic activity is resumed. Functional braces allow significant motion and speed, yet they must be durable and resist brace migration. They typically have medial and lateral bars and are differentiated by hinge and strap design. There are two general types of braces: strap dominant (Fig. 5) and shell dominant (Fig. 6). These are not as adjustable as rehabilitation braces to changes in swelling and muscle size. Off-the-shelf functional braces are cheaper and more readily available than custom-made braces. Selection of size for an off-the-shelf is determined by measurements of leg length and/or thigh circumference. Custom functional braces are made from cast molds or leg measurements. Functional braces weigh from 12 oz to 2 lbs and usually retail between $200 and $600 (Table 3).

TABLE 2.   Rehabilitation Braces*

Manufacturer (telephone)	Brace	Retail Cost† ($)
Anodyne 800-446-6236	1030	98.00
Bauerfeind 800-423-3405	Mos Gen U Long	459.00
Bledsoe 800-527-3666	Postop I	99.75–137.50
Deroyal 800-251-9864	3 Way	161.16
	2 Way	150.34
Donjoy 800-336-6569	IROM	109.00
Innovation Sports 800-222-4284	Century	150.00
	Dual Stage	155.00
	KMD Postop	95.00
Med Design Inc. 800-433-5179	Universal leg brace	150.00
OMNI Scientific 800-448-6664	OS5 Rehab	288.50
	OS5 Postop	315.25
Orthotech 800-227-1554	Rehab 3	99.00
Spademan Sports 800-442-2996	Postop	175.00
Zinco 818-405-0660	Soft Lehman Rehab	130.00

*Information provided by manufacturers.

†Cost may vary. This is the cost to the physician for ordering a brace for a patient.

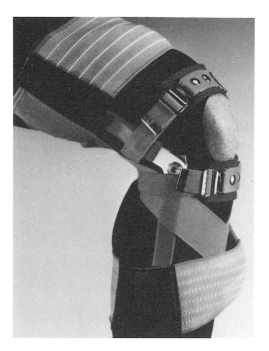

FIGURE 5. Functional brace, predominant strap design. (Reproduced with permission of Lennox Hill Brace Company.)

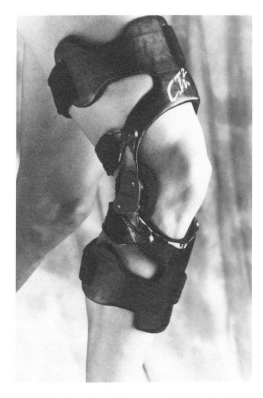

FIGURE 6. Functional brace, predominant shell design. (Reproduced with permission of Innovation Sports, Inc.)

In Vitro Assessment

Baker et al.[1] evaluated functional braces for their effect on abduction and external rotation forces applied to one cadaver with or without disruption of anterior cruciate and/or medial collateral ligaments. Most functional braces demonstrated some protective effect; however, low loads were used on one cadaver knee. Using a lateral impact mechanical knee model, Baker et al.[2] found functional bracing provided some protection to tibial rotation and abduction. Mortensen et al.[29] also evaluated the effect of functional braces on anterior-posterior translation and rotation in cadavers with the anterior cruciate ligament intact and disrupted. In general, the braces diminished anterior tibial translation at low loads but not at higher loads. Again, loads were lower than anticipated for activities of daily living. Noyes et al.[30] hypothesized that the anterior cruciate ligament is subjected to loads ranging from 0 to 454 newtons (N) during most activities of daily living. Wojtys et al.[44] tested the relative restraints of 14 functional braces using 125 N (28 lbs) of anterior-posterior forces and 12 N-m (8.8 ft-lbs) of internal-external rotation on cadavers at 30°

and 60° flexion. The braces limited abnormal anterior-posterior tibiofemoral displacement by 10% to 75%. Application of the braces controlled rotational displacement to a greater degree than anterior-posterior translation. The strap tension was standardized to 6.8 kg (15 lbs). The authors found that some braces were better than others. Although the test loads were low compared with loads probably occurring in vivo, they concluded that functional braces can be helpful.

In Vivo Assessment

After placing a strain gauge arthroscopically on the anterior cruciate ligament, Beynnon et al.[6] studied the effects on strain of seven functional braces under four different loading activities. The braces provided no strain-shielding effect at the higher anterior shear loads expected for athletic activity. Custom braces showed no advantage over off-the-shelf braces. This unique study was performed on subjects with normal anterior cruciate liga-

TABLE 3. Functional Braces*

Manufacturer (telephone)	Brace	Retail Cost†† ($)	Off-Shelf/ Custom	Shell or Strap	Hinge‡	Weight§ (oz)
Bauerfeind 800-423-3405	Mos Gen U Short	379.00 459.00	Off-shelf	Shell	Simple	22
Bledsoe 800-527-3666	Force 1	225.00	Off-shelf	Shell	Polyaxial	35
	Force 2	225.00	Off-shelf	Shell	Polyaxial	35
	Force 3	275.00	Off-shelf	Shell	Polyaxial	42
	Proshifter ACL	275.00	Off-shelf	Shell	Polyaxial	28
	Proshifter Contact	300.00	Off-shelf	Shell	Polyaxial	34
	Custom available″	475.00				14
Deroyal 800-251-9864	Three-D	237.95	Off-shelf	Shell	Polyaxial	
Donjoy 800-336-6569	Gold Point	335.00	Off-shelf	Strap	Polyaxial	48
	4 point Supersport	309.00	Off-shelf	Strap	Polyaxial	64
	CE 2000	439.00	Custom	Strap	Polyaxial	25
	Defiance	500.00	Custom	Strap	Polyaxial	15
Generation II USA. Inc. 800-462-7252	GII Sports Brace	489.00	Custom	Shell	Polyaxial	26
Innovation Sports 800-222-4284	MVP	280.00	Off-shelf	Shell	Polyaxial	24
	CTI Classic	400.00	Custom	Shell	Polyaxial	15
	CTII Superlight	430.00	Custom	Shell	Polyaxial	14
	CTI Standard	440.00	Custom	Shell	Polyaxial	15
	CTI Pro Sport	450.00	Custom	Shell	Polyaxial	17
Lennox Hill Brace Co. 800-222-8837	Regular	420.00	Custom	Strap	Single	27
	Light	420.00	Custom	Strap	Single	24
	Spectralite	420.00	Custom	Strap	Single	22
Medical Designs Inc 800-433-5179	Lorus	225.00	Off-shelf	Shell	Multiplanar	23
Med Techna 800-225-2610	Can Am	340.00	Custom	Shell	Polyaxial	40
Mueller Sports Medicine Inc 800-356-9522	Magnum Lite Pre-fit	295.00	Off-shelf	Shell	Triaxial	16
	Magnum Competition	460.00	Custom	Shell	Triaxial	16
Omni Scientific 800-448-6664	Spectrum	295.00	Off-shelf	Strap	Biaxial	26
	OS-5	260.00	Off-shelf	Strap	Biaxial	
	Elite	425.00	Custom	Strap	Biaxial	
	TS-7	415.00	Custom	Strap	Biaxial	30
Orthotech 800-227-1554	Contender	145.00	Off-shelf	Shell	Single	16
	Oti Performer	424.00	Custom	Shell	Single	19
Orthomedics 800-733-6999	Ecko II	195.00	Off-shelf	Shell	Single	19
Spademan 800-422-2996	Custom	485.00	Custom	Strap	Dynamic fitting system	22
	ACL sport	345.00	Off-shelf	Strap		
Townsend Design 800-432-3466	Off-shelf	245.00	Off-shelf	Strap	4 Bar linkage	16–32
	Air Custom	425.00	Custom	Shell	Cam bearing	
	Original	425.00	Custom	Shell	Cam bearing	
Vixie Enterprise 800-255-1700	MKS2 OTS	295.00	Off-shelf	Shell	Polyaxial	18
	MKS2 Custom	455.00	Custom	Shell	Polyaxial	18
	MKS2 PCL	455.00	Custom	Shell	Polyaxial	18
Zinco 818-405-0660	Lerman Multilig	240.00	Off-shelf	Strap	Single	
	MSO	175.00	Off-shelf	Strap	Single	
Zimmer 800-348-2759	Sports Caster I	545.00	Custom	Shell	Biaxial	33
	Sports Caster II	570.00	Custom	Shell	Biaxial	

*Information provided by manufacturers.
†Cost may vary. This is the cost to the physician for ordering a brace for a patient.
‡Polyaxial includes biaxial, triaxial, etc.
§Weight may vary with patient size.
″Also, light models are available at reduced prices.

ments. The authors believed that brace performance depends somewhat on design and technique of application; soft tissue to which the brace attaches may be the limiting factor. They noted that even with active muscle contraction and small magnitudes of force, simply pushing a thumb perpendicular to the limb axis results in significant displacement of soft tissue. Many other studies measured anterotibial displacement in subjects with deficient anterior cruciate ligaments, with and without functional braces. Beck,[5] for example, found that at low loads some braces were more effective than others in controlling anterior-posterior displacement. Jonsson and Karrholm[23] found that some braces reduce anterior-posterior instability, but not to normal levels, with loads up to 150 N. Liu et al.[25] found that 10 different functional knee braces were ineffective in controlling anterotibial displacement at forces over 150 N (34 lbs).

The straps of functional braces clearly compress muscle,[27] and external compression of the lower limbs can impede muscle blood flow.[37] Because of the weight of the braces, increased energy consumption and early fatigue can be anticipated. Zetterlund et al.[45] found a 4.58% increase in energy expenditure when subjects wore a Lenox-Hill brace while running on a treadmill. Houston and Goemans[22] found increased energy expenditure and reduced velocity with the use of a functional brace in prolonged exercise. Cook et al.[11] evaluated the effect of one type of functional knee brace on running and cutting maneuvers in 14 athletes with arthroscopically proven absence of the anterior cruciate ligament. They found that the brace improved exercise performance, especially in patients with a quadriceps deficiency. Of note, they found that the braced knee had increased forces compared with the unbraced knee during cutting maneuvers. Subjectively, 40% of tested athletes performed to preinjury level with the brace. All athletes reported fewer episodes of subluxation.

Proprioception is defined as position sense. Loss of the anterior cruciate ligament has been associated with a proprioceptive deficit measured by lost ability to detect joint motion.[3] With injuries to the anterior cruciate ligament, normal efferent pathways are disrupted, and it has been conjectured that bracing can substitute for this lost pathway. This theory could explain the positive subjective response to bracing. Branch et al.[7] used surface electrodes to compare muscle firing and timing with or without a functional brace in subjects with anterior cruciate deficiency during a step-step cut. Subjects with deficient limbs showed a decrease in quadriceps and gastrocnemius activity and an increase in hamstring activity compared with normal subjects. Bracing decreased slightly the muscle amplitudes and had no effect on muscle timing patterns. This decrease in cofiring of quadriceps and hamstrings may indicate that bracing reduced the need for muscular contraction; thus, less muscular stability is required. Vailas et al.[41] compared a placebo brace with a functional brace during a run-and-cross cut using a forceplate and photography. The functional brace reduced torque produced by the limb compared with the normal limb. The placebo knee brace had no effect on torque. Thus, although bracing alters muscle amplitude and limb torque, no conclusive evidence supports its role in proprioception.

Regalbuto et al.[33] applied functional braces on normal subjects and measured the forces and moments at the hinges. This technique was believed to measure the mismatch between knee and brace motion. Hinge design was not as critical a factor as hinge placement. Forces on the hinge were increased with anterior placement of the hinge and decreased with posterior placement. The hinge design may not be as critical because any mismatch in motion between hinge and joint can, to some degree, be taken up by soft-tissue deformation and cuff-to-skin slippage.[42] However, abnormal patterns of ligament lengthening may also occur.

Bassett et al.[4] evaluated the Lenox-Hill functional brace by manual testing with low forces. They found that in 70% of patients with significant laxity, giving way continued in spite of the brace. Gerber et al.[18] evaluated anterior-posterior translation in patients with anterior cruciate reconstruction. Of interest, they found that the long leg cast decreased the anterior-posterior translation by 70%, the Lenox-Hill brace by 53%, and a cast brace by 14%. Colville et al.[10] studied 45 patients with anterior cruciate deficiency. Of the patients who received the brace, 91% felt better. Objective improvement in the amount of laxity, however, was slight. This interesting dichotomy of mild objective and significant subjective improvement has not been explained. Research needs to be done in this area.

TABLE 4.   Denegerative Joint Disease Braces*

Manufacturer (telephone)	Brace	Retail Cost† ($)	Off-Shelf/ Custom	Shell or Strap	Hinge	Weight (oz)
Generation II USA Inc 800-462-7252	GII Unloader	589.00	Custom	Shell	Polyaxial	26
Orthotech 800-255-1700	Performer	424.00	Custom	Shell	Single	18
Vixie Enterprises Inc 800-255-1700	MKSIII	250.00	Custom	Shell	Single	12

*Information provided by manufacturers.
†Cost may vary. This is the cost to the physician for ordering a brace for a patient.

Psychological benefits of wearing a brace may account for its subjective success.

FUNCTIONAL BRACE SELECTION

There are numerous functional knee braces. The manufacturer must accept responsibility for demonstrating brace efficacy. Studies must be designed to approximate the in vivo situation. Previously described studies show that some braces are better than others in restraining specific motions. Because of testing conditions, however, no conclusions can be made. Further research is essential.

The clinician must choose the orthotic by being a critical consumer. The manufacturer must be asked to verify claims and to provide documentation of efficacy. The clinician must realize that the brace is only one part of the treatment of a ligament-injured knee. Neuromuscular rehabilitation and activity modification may be far more important. Tegner and Lorentzon[39] found serious knee injuries in elite ice hockey players even when functional knee braces were worn.

To select a brace, the following features should be considered:
1. Documented efficacy testing with speeds and loads anticipated in vivo.
2. Pattern of instability targeted for control. Some braces may work better for varus-valgus and others may work better for anterior-posterior control.
3. Durability. The braces should hold up for at least 1 year; straps should be easily replaceable by the manufacturer.
4. Brace slippage. Repetitive slipping in the brace decreases efficacy and may increase injuries elsewhere. Manufacturers' claims about slippage resistance should be verified.

5. Comfort and ease of application.
6. Reasonable price.

OSTEOARTHRITIS BRACING

One well-designed study has looked at the efficacy of valgus knee bracing for osteoarthritic knees (Table 4, Fig. 7).[26] In a double crossover study of 79 patients, all patients had medial compartment osteoarthritis

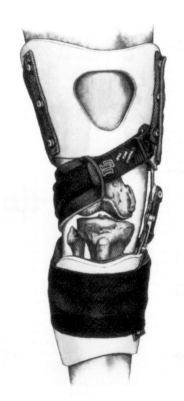

FIGURE 7.   Degenerative joint disease brace. (Reproduced with permission of Generation II USA, Inc.)

of the knee. Two braces were compared, one with a medial hinge and one with a lateral hinge. With the medial hinge, 19 of 21 elderly patients and 19 of 19 athletic patients reported significant relief of pain. The overall success rate for relief of pain with the brace forcing with valgus strap was 82% and with the brace in neutral, 72%. There was no improvement in function and no radiographic evidence of any change in the femorotibial angle. Of the patients with a medial hinge brace, 93% were still wearing their brace at 20-month follow-up. Thus, bracing appears to be a useful modality for patients with medial compartment arthritis of the knee. However, the rationale for success is unknown.

SUMMARY

Braces can be categorized into three general categories: prophylactic, rehabilitation, and functional. They protect the joint mechanically to different degrees at low loads and have some effect on muscular activity. However, the subjective benefits have not been objectively supported by high-load teting. Psychological support may be the greatest benefit. Further research for improved design, tailored to patient's build, specific laxity, and individual demands, is needed before recommending any currently marketed brace.

REFERENCES

1. Baker B, VanHanswtk E, Bogosian S, et al: A biomechanical study of the static stabilizing effect of knee braces on medial stability. *Am J Sports Med* 15:566–570, 1987.
2. Baker B, VanHanswyk E, Bogosian S, et al: The effect of knee braces on lateral impact loading of the knee. *Am J Sports Med* 17:182–186, 1989.
3. Barrack R, Skinner H, Buckley S: Proprioception in the anterior cruciate deficient knee. *Am J Sports Med* 17:1–6, 1989.
4. Bassett G, Fleming B: The Lennox Hill Brace in anterolateral rotatory instability. *Am J Sports Med* 11:345–348, 1983.
5. Beck C, Drez D, Young J, et al: Instrumented testing of functional knee braces. *Am J Sports Med* 14:253–258, 1986.
6. Beynnon B, Pope M, Wertheimer C, et al: The effect of functional knee-braces on strain on the anterior cruciate ligament in vivo. *J Bone Joint Surg* 74A:1298–1311, 1992.
7. Branch T, Hunter R, Donath M: Dynamic EMG analysis of anterior cruciate deficient legs with and without bracing during cutting. *Am J Sports Med* 17:35–41, 1989.
8. Brown T, Van Hoeck J, Brand R: Laboratory evaluation of prophylactic knee brace performance under dynamic valgus loading using a surrogate leg model. *Clin Sports Med* 9:751–762, 1990.
9. Cawley P, France E, Paulos L: Comparison of rehabilitative knee braces. *Am J Sports Med* 17:141–146, 1989.
10. Colville M, Lee C, Ciullo J: The Lennox Hill brace. An evaluation of effectiveness in treating knee instability. *Am J Sports Med* 14:257–261, 1986.
11. Cook F, Tibone J, Redfern F: A dynamic analysis of a functional brace for anterior cruciate insufficiency. *Am J Sports Med* 17:519–524, 1989.
12. Daniel D: Quoted in *Knee Braces Seminar Report*. Chicago, American Academy of Orthopaedic Surgeons, 1984, p 11.
13. Drez D: Knee braces. In Jackson D, Drez D (eds): *The Anterior Cruciate Deficient Knee*. St. Louis, Mosby, 1987, pp 286–289.
14. Drez D, DeHaven K, D'Ambrosia R, et al: *Knee Braces Seminar Report*. Chicago, American Academy of Orthopedic Surgeons, 1985, pp 1–90.
15. France E, Paulos L, et al: The biomechanics of lateral knee bracing: P II. Impact response of the braced knee. *Am J Sports Med* 15:430–438, 1987.
16. France E, Paulos L: In vitro assessment of prophylactic knee brace function. *Clin Sports Med* 9:823–840, 1990.
17. Garrick J, Requa R: Prophylactic knee bracing. *Am J Sports Med* 15:471–476, 1987.
18. Gerber C, Jakob R, Ganz R: Observations concerning the limiting mobilization cast after anterior cruciate ligament surgery. *Arch Orthop Trauma Surg* 101:291–296, 1983.
19. Grace T, Skipper B, Newberry J, et al: Prophylactic knee braces and injury to the lower extremity. *J Bone Joint Surg* 70A:422–427, 1988.
20. Hewson G, Mendini R, Wang J: Prophylactic knee bracing in college football. *Am J Sports Med* 14:262–265, 1986.
21. Hofmann A, Wyatt R, Buorne M, Daniel A: Knee stability in orthotic knee braces. *Am J Sports Med* 12:371–374, 1984.
22. Houston M, Goemans P: Leg muscle performance of athletes with and without knee support braces. *Arch Phys Med Rehabil* 63:431–432, 1982.
23. Jonsson H, Karrholm J: Brace effects on the unstable knee in 21 cases. A roentgen stereophotogrammetric comparison of three designs. *Acta Orthop Scand* 61:313–318, 1990.
24. Krackow K, Vetter W: Knee motion in a long leg cast. *Am J Sports Med* 9:233–239, 1981.
25. Liu S, Lunsford T, Vangsness T: Comparison of functional knee braces for control of anterior tibial displacement. Presented at the American Academy of Orthopaedic Surgeons, Washington, DC, February 1992.
26. Loomer R, Horlick S: Valgus knee bracing for osteoarthritic knee. Presented at the International Society of the Knee, Toronto, Canada, May 1991.
27. Lundin O, Styf J: Intramuscular pressure varies with the tensile force used at knee brace application. *Trans Orthop Res Soc* 310, 1993.
28. Miyasaka K, Daniel D, Stone M, Hirshman P: The incidence of knee ligament injuries in the general population. *Am J Knee Surg* 4:3–8, 1991.
29. Mortensen W, Foreman K, Focht L, Daniel D: An in

vitro study of functional orthoses in the ACL disrupted knee. *Trans Orthop Res Soc* 520, 1988.

30. Noyes F, Butler D, Grood E, et al: Biomechanical analysis of human ligament grafts used in knee-ligament repairs and reconstruction. *J Bone Joint Surg* 66A:344–352, 1984.

31. Paulos L, France E, Rosenberg T, et al: The biomechanics of lateral knee bracing: Pt I. Response of the valgus restraints to loading. *Am J Sports Med* 15:419–429, 1987.

32. Praemer M, Furner S, Rice D: *Musculoskeletal Conditions in the United States.* Park Ridge, IL, American Academy of Orthopaedic Surgeons, 1992, p 118.

33. Regalbuto M, Rovick J, Walker P: The forces in a knee brace as a function of hinge design and placement. *Am J Sports Med* 17:535–542, 1989.

34. Shelbourne K, Whitaker J, McCarroll J, et al: Anterior cruciate ligament injury: Evaluation of intraarticular reconstruction of acute tears without repair. *Am J Sports Med* 18:484–489, 1990.

35. Sitler M, Ryan J, Hopkinson W, et al: The efficacy of a prophylactic knee brace to reduce injuries in football. *Am J Sports Med* 18:310–315, 1990.

36. Stevenson DV, Shields C, Perry J, et al: Rehabilitative knee braces. Control of terminal knee extension in the ambulatory patient. *Trans Orthop Res Soc* 517, 1988.

37. Styf J: The influence of external compression on muscle blood flow during exercise. *Am J Sports Med* 18:92–95, 1990.

38. Taft T, Hunter S, Fundurbeck C: Unpublished data. Presented at American Orthopaedic Society for Sports Medicine, Nashville, TN, July 1985.

39. Tegner Y, Lorentzon R: Evaluation of knee braces in Swedish ice hockey players. *Br J Sports Med* 25:159–161, 1991.

40. Teitz C, Hermanson B, Kronmal R, Diehr P: Evaluation of the use of braces to prevent injury to the knee in collegiate football players. *J Bone Joint Surg* 69A:2–9, 1987.

41. Vailas J, Tibone J, Perry J, et al: Dynamic biomechanical effects of functional bracing. *Med Sci Sports Exer* (suppl):S82, 1989.

42. Walker P, Rovick J, Robertson D: The effects of knee brace hinge design and placement on joint mechanics. *J Biomech* 21:965–974, 1988.

43. Wirth M, Delee J: The history and classifications of knee braces. *Clin Sports Med* 9:731–736, 1990.

44. Wojtys E, Loubert P, Samson S, Viviano D: Use of a knee brace for control of tibial translation and rotation. *J Bone Joint Surg* 72A:1323–1329, 1990.

45. Zetterlund A, Serfass R, Hunter R: The effect of wearing the complete Lenox-Hill derotation brace on energy consumption during horizontal treadmill running at 161 meters per minute. *Am J Sports Med* 14:73–76, 1986.

Chapter 15

ANKLE SPRAIN EVALUATION AND BRACING

Ralph M. Buschbacher, MD

The use of ankle bracing, taping, and wrapping for athletic injuries is both overused and underused. The overuse occurs in patients who do not need ankle support or who no longer need it. Underuse occurs in patients who could potentially return to activity sooner with the extra support.

It is now well established that prolonged immobilization of a body part can cause a number of deleterious effects. Immobilized animals have been shown to have decreased strength of muscles, bones, tendons, and ligaments.[1,65,66] Immobility adversely affects the healing process in rats and has been shown to decrease ligamentous tissue DNA, collagen synthesis, and tensile strength compared with ligaments in mobilized rats.[70] Similar effects are seen in humans.

Proprioception can be impaired after immobilization of the ankle,[18–20,37] and atrophy of the leg muscles may occur.[52] Weak muscles and poor proprioception predispose the athlete to further injury. Thus it is clear that immobilizing joints as a part of treatment brings its own morbidity. That is not to say that immobilization is never necessary and useful. Certainly an unstable joint needs to be stabilized, but in recent years the emphasis has shifted from complete immobilization to providing support in only the unstable planes, allowing functional activity to occur in the stable planes. Bracing, taping, and wrapping are increasingly used to provide such support.

This chapter was adapted from Buschbacher RM: The use and abuse of ankle supports in sports injuries. *J Back Musculoskel Rehabil* 3:(3):57–69, 1993; with permission of Butterworth-Heinemann Publishers.

ANATOMY

Bones

The bones of the lower leg (Fig. 1), the tibia medially and the fibula laterally, form a dome for the articulation of the talus bone of the foot, in what is usually considered to be the ankle joint proper. The tibia contributes the medial and upper portion of this dome, whereas the fibula contributes to the lateral portion. Above the ankle, the tibia and fibula are connected by a tough fibrous membrane called the interosseous membrane or syndesmosis. Distally the fibula extends further downward than the tibia. The prominent palpable portions of these bones are called medial and lateral malleoli.

Articulating with the tibia and fibula is the talus, which is the most superior foot bone. The talus is somewhat wedge-shaped, i.e., wider in the anterior than in the posterior portion. Thus, when the foot is dorsiflexed, the talus becomes wedged into the talocrural joint and becomes more stable. When the foot is plantarflexed, the talus sits in the joint more loosely and allows the foot to move more freely.

Inferiorly, the talus articulates with the calcaneus, which is the bone that forms the heel of the foot. Distally, the talus and calcaneus articulate with the navicular and cuboid. Beyond this lie the rest of the tarsal bones: the cuneiform bones, metatarsals, and phalanges.

Joints

The primary ankle joint as described above is the talocrural joint, which is an articulation

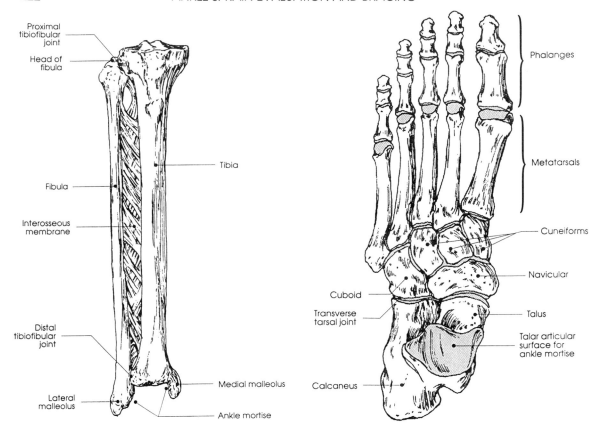

FIGURE 1. Bones of the lower leg and foot (superior view). (From Buschbacher RM (ed): *Musculoskeletal Disorders: A Practical Guide for Diagnosis and Rehabilitation*. Stoneham, MA, Butterworth-Heinemann, 1994, with permission.)

of the dome created by the tibia and fibula with the talus below (Fig. 2). Below this joint is the subtalar joint, which connects the calcaneus and the talus. More distally lies the transverse tarsal joint, which is actually a combination of the talonavicular and calcaneocuboid joints.

Muscles

The primary muscles that are important to understanding ankle motion are the lower leg muscles, which can be divided into three groups: anterior, lateral, and posterior (Fig. 3). The anterior muscles of the lower leg include the tibialis anterior, extensor digitorum longus, extensor hallucis longus, and peroneus tertius. These muscles are the dorsiflexors of the foot and help to absorb shock during gait by gently lowering the foot to the ground on heel impact. The medial tibialis anterior is also an ankle invertor, whereas the lateral peroneus tertius contributes to eversion. The tendons of the anterior muscles are

held in place by the superior and inferior extensor reticulae, which are fascial bands that hold down the tendons.

The primary evertors of the foot are the lateral muscles, the peroneus longus and peroneus brevis. The ligaments of these muscles pass behind the lateral malleolus to insert on the bones of the foot. The peroneus brevis inserts on the base of the fifth metatarsal, whereas the peroneus longus runs under the foot to attach to the underside of the base of the first metatarsal and the medial cuneiform bone. As they pass behind the lateral malleolus, the ligaments of the lateral muscles are held in place by the superior and inferior peroneal retinaculae.

The posterior muscles of the lower leg are divided into superficial and deep groups. The gastrocnemius and soleus, which attach to the calcaneus and are the primary plantarflexors of the ankle, make up the superficial group (along with the small plantaris muscle). The deep muscles include the tibialis posterior, flexor digitorum longus, and flexor hallucis longus. The tendons of these ligaments pass

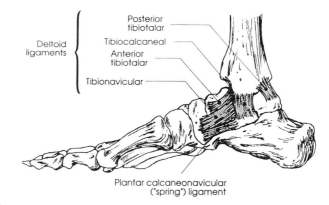

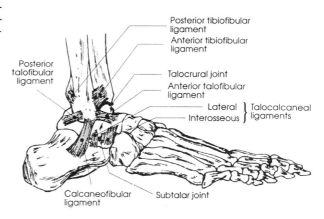

FIGURE 2. Joints and ligaments of the ankle, medial (top) and lateral (bottom) views. (From Buschbacher RM (ed): *Musculoskeletal Disorders: A Practical Guide for Diagnosis and Rehabilitation.* Stoneham, MA, Butterworth-Heinemann, 1994, with permission.)

behind the medial malleolus to insert on the bones of the foot. The flexor hallucis longus and flexor digitorum longus insert on the phalanges and flex the toes in addition to contributing to ankle plantarflexion. The tibialis posterior attaches to the navicular bone and contributes to ankle inversion along with the tibialis anterior, described above. The posterior deep lower leg muscles are held in place behind the medial malleolus by the flexor reticulum.

Nerves

The sciatic nerve branches near the knee into the medial tibial nerve and the lateral common peroneal nerve. From the common peroneal nerve originate the deep peroneal nerve, which supplies the anterior muscles of the leg, and the superficial peroneal nerve, which innervates the lateral muscles. The tibial nerve supplies innervation to the posterior muscles of the lower leg and passes with the flexor tendons behind the medial malleolus to innervate some of the foot muscles and to

provide sensation to the plantar surface of the foot.

Ligaments

The bones of the foot and ankle are held together by numerous interosseous ligaments (Fig. 2). For a discussion of ankle sprains and injuries, it is essential to understand the medial and lateral stabilizing ankle ligaments.

The medial ligaments are often grouped together and called the deltoid ligament. They are divided into a superficial tibiocalcaneal ligament and a deeper portion that includes the anterior tibiotalar, the tibionavicular, and the posterior tibiotalar ligaments. The deltoid is a broad, strong ligament that effectively restricts ankle eversion.

Laterally, the stabilizing ligaments of the ankle include the anterior talofibular, the calcaneofibular, and the posterior talofibular ligaments. These ligaments are more distinct than on the medial side and are more easily damaged. When the foot is dorsiflexed, the anterior talofibular ligament is somewhat lax.

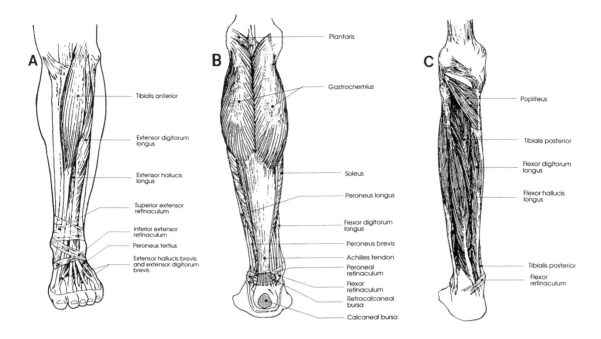

FIGURE 3. Muscles of the lower leg: **A,** anterior view; **B,** posterior view, superficial muscles; **C,** posterior view, deep muscles. (From Buschbacher RM (ed): *Musculoskeletal Disorders: A Practical Guide for Diagnosis and Rehabilitation.* Stoneham, MA, Butterworth-Heinemann, 1994, with permission.)

When the foot is plantar-flexed, the anterior talofibular ligament becomes taut, whereas the calcaneofibular ligament becomes somewhat more relaxed.

Other important ligaments of the foot include the calcaneonavicular ligament, also known as the "spring ligament," which helps to maintain the medial longitudinal arch of the foot. The bifurcated ligament, which runs between the calcaneus, navicular, and cuboid, is sometimes injured in inversion sprains.

Ankle Movement

The talocrural joint primarily allows dorsiflexion and plantarflexion. The talus has some ability to tilt medially and laterally within this joint, and such movement occurs primarily when the foot is in a plantar-flexed position. When dorsiflexed, as described above, the wider portion of the talus wedges into the joint and prevents motion. The subtalar joint allows a degree of inversion and eversion and also, in a more general sense, pronation and supination.

When the foot is pronated, it becomes loose and allows shock absorption during ambulation. As the foot contacts the ground, it pronates and accommodates to the surface. During push-off the foot supinates, which stiffens its integrity. This allows the foot to act as a rigid lever during the push-off phase of gait.

INJURIES

Ankle sprains are the most common injuries in sports.[23,25,37,41] Most (85% to 95%) involve the lateral ankle ligaments, and 5% to 15% involve the medial ligaments.[4–6,24,44] Two-thirds of ankle sprains are isolated to the anterior talofibular ligament, whereas one-fifth to one-fourth involve both the anterior talofibular ligament and the calcaneofibular ligament.[4–6,37] Lateral ankle sprains may be associated with peroneal nerve damage[53] and peroneal muscle weakness,[43] which can lead to deficits in proprioception and strength. Inversion ankle sprains are more likely to occur than eversion sprains because the medial malleolus extends distally to a lesser extent than the lateral malleolus. Thus, inversion of the talus is less restricted than eversion. The inversion sprain is also more likely to occur because the ligamentous support on the lateral side is not as continuous and strong as the medial deltoid ligament. An additional factor is probably biomechanical and associated with the way we walk, run, and participate in sports. Syndesmotic injuries are rare.

Injuries to the medial ligament are often severe and have a high rate of associated fractures and disruptions of the ankle mortise,[4–6,31] which must be looked for carefully. If such extensive damage has occurred, a surgical opinion is warranted. Most patients with ankle sprains, especially lateral sprains, recover without medical assistance. Those who go to a physician also in general do well as long as they have ligamentous damage not associated with fractures, tendon subluxation, or gross deformities.

There are three grades of ankle ligamentous injury. Grade I (mild) involves a stretch of the ligament with no macroscopic tearing or functional loss and little swelling, tenderness, or instability of the joint. Grade II (moderate) injuries involve partial tearing of the ligament associated with moderate pain, swelling, tenderness, and some ligamentous laxity (but with a firm endpoint) and functional loss. Grade III (severe) injuries involve complete ligament ruptures with no endpoint on stability testing.[12,37]

EVALUATION

Evaluation of the injured ankle must detect conditions such as fractures, ligamentous sprains, or nerve damage. It should identify which ligaments, if any, were sprained and should distinguish between stable and unstable ankle injury.

History

The history should focus on the type of injury sustained and the position of the body during injury. Most often the diagnosis of a sprain can be made by history alone; in fact, for minor sprains most people make a self-diagnosis. The overwhelming majority of sprains are of the inversion type, and people usually feel the ankle give way in an inversion direction.

It is also important to note whether the injury involved a rotational component and where the pain was located. Such information may help to localize the specific ligaments that were injured. It is also helpful to know whether or not the patient heard a popping sound, whether he or she was able to walk after the injury, whether swelling occurred immediately or slowly, and whether such an injury has been sustained previously.

Observation

It is, of course, optimal to examine the ankle as soon as possible after injury. Once swelling has developed, it is sometimes difficult to perform a full examination and to determine exactly which structures were injured. Observation should include looking for swelling, areas of ecchymosis, and gross deformities of the ankles.

Palpation

Palpation, in general, should proceed from the structure least likely to be damaged to the structures most likely to be damaged. This strategy avoids excessive pain early in the examination. Such pain makes the patient resistent to continued examination.

The fibula should be palpated carefully. Squeezing the fibula and tibia together often reveals a fracture of the fibula if in fact it has occurred. The area between the tibia and fibula should be palpated to assess the syndesmosis. The medial deltoid ligament should be palpated in all its components, along with lateral ligaments. Special attention should be paid to the anterior talofibular and the calcaneofibular ligaments. Often a mild sprain affects only the anterior talofibular ligament, whereas more severe sprains also involve the calcaneofibular ligament. As described above, these ligaments are lax in different positions of dorsiflexion or plantarflexion; thus sprains of one or both ligaments may give an indication of foot position when the sprain occurred. In addition, the bones and malleoli of the foot and ankle should be palpated to assess whether associated avulsions or fractures are present.

Range of Motion

Range of motion should be assessed, but assessment is often difficult, especially with associated swelling. In general, however, a decrease in dorsiflexion may indicate the presence of effusion of the talocrural joint or injury to the ankle mortise.

Stability Testing

Because the talocrural joint mainly moves in dorsiflexion or plantarflexion, stability testing is used mainly to assess the lateral and medial ligament complexes. A number of specific tests can be used.

Talar Tilt

The calcaneus and talus are tilted medially and laterally in an attempt to invert and evert the ankle joint. These motions involve normal joint "play," and the injured ankle should always be compared with the noninjured ankle to assess whether or not range of motion is excessive. The ankle can be tested for passive eversion to stress the deltoid ligament. It can also be pushed into inversion. If pushed into inversion with the foot plantarflexed, it primarily assesses the anterior talofibular ligament. Stressing the ankle in neutral is a test of the anterior talofibular as well as the calcanofibular ligaments.

Pain on these maneuvers is common and often makes it difficult to perform a proper examination. In such cases, history and palpation usually indicate what structures were injured. In some cases, however, the affected areas may be injected with a local anesthetic to facilitate the stability testing.

Anterior Drawer Test

The anterior drawer test (Fig. 4) assesses mainly the anterior talofibular ligament, which is nearly horizontal in its orientation (with the foot in neutral). Stabilizing the lower leg with one hand and pulling the heel forward stresses the ligament, and excessive forward movement indicates rupture. Again, side-to-side differences help to validate the determination.

Side-to-Side Movement of the Talus

Holding the ankle without tilting it and moving the heel side to side reveals whether

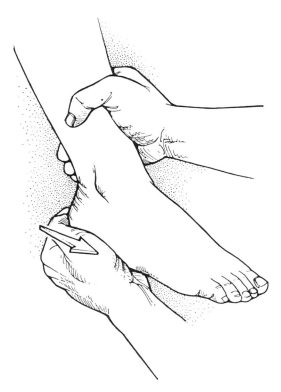

FIGURE 4. The ankle drawer test. While the foot is in 20° of plantarflexion, the examiner pulls the foot anteriorly to stress the anterior talofibular ligament.

the ankle mortise is widened. A widened mortise indicates a syndesmotic injury, in which the tibia and fibula have been allowed to separate.

Radiographic Stress Testing

Occasionally it is useful to obtain radiographs while performing the inversion and eversion tilting maneuvers. This technique allows the direct visualization of bony alignment and helps to make the diagnosis of instability. The talar tilt test is performed with an anteroposterior view. A lateral view can be obtained during the anterior drawer test.

Plain Radiographs

Radiographs without stress testing can also be useful in determining whether or not fractures have occurred. Such evaluation is not necessary in every case of simple ankle sprain. In more severe cases, however, a radiograph can help to detect the presence of an associated fracture, which of course would change the treatment.

Arthrography

Arthography is rarely needed; however, injecting radiopaque dye either into the peroneal sheath or into the talocrural joint can facilitate the diagnosis of ligamentous rupture. Leakage of dye from the peroneal sheath may indicate that the calcaneofibular ligament has been torn, and leakage of dye upward from the talocrural joint may indicate that the syndesmotic membrane and tibiofibular ligaments have been injured.

Electromyography

Electromyography is also rarely required, especially in acute management. However, it can aid in the diagnosis of nerve damage sometimes associated with ankle sprains.

TREATMENT

Patients with isolated grade I and II sprains heal well with nonoperative treatment. Grade I and II sprains are best treated with early functional mobilization and rehabilitation.[14,31,37]

A recent review[37] of prospective randomized treatments of grade III lateral ligament sprains compared surgery followed by cast immobilization, cast immobilization alone, and functional treatment with bracing, taping, or wrapping. All forms of treatment gave good or excellent long-term results, but the functionally treated groups recovered sooner and with less cost and morbidity. Rates of functional instability (a feeling of the ankle "giving way"), pain, swelling, stiffness, long-term loss of range of motion, atrophy, reinjury, mechanical instability, and return to preinjury level of activity were not appreciably different among the different forms of treatment. Furthermore, in the case of an unsatisfactory conservative outcome, a delayed operative repair can be performed with results comparable to primary repair.[2,4–6,37] Clearly, conservative functional treatment of all grades of lateral ankle sprains is the initial choice, even in cases of clinically unstable

ankles.[50] Exceptions may be patients with associated large bone avulsions, simultaneous medial and lateral ligament damage, or osteochondral fractures; young athletes who need a return to perfect ankle function; and patients with severe recurrent injury or chronic instability.

The following sections describe the rationale, technique, and uses of taping, wrapping, and bracing for functional injury treatment as well as specific items available to the clinician for use about the ankle.

ANKLE SUPPORTS

Taping

In 1973 Garrick[22] reported on the use of prophylactic ankle taping and shoe type in basketball players. He divided the players into four groups: one group was treated with high-topped shoes and tape; one with high-topped shoes and no tape; one with low-topped shoes and tape; and one with low-topped shoes and no tape. Both high-top shoes and tape appeared to have a protective effect on the ankle; both were associated with a lower rate of sprain, although the protective effect of the shoes was relatively small. Prophylactic taping reduced the reinjury rate in players with previous sprain by about two-thirds. Other studies also support the use of tape to help in stabilizing the ankle, and it is believed that taping reduces the incidence of sprains.[2,7,17,26,33,56]

The goal of taping is to prevent the ankle ligaments from being stressed to the point of injury. The taping method should be designed to limit ankle inversion and eversion but to allow functional dorsiflexion and plantarflexion. Some evidence suggests that by stimulating proprioceptive afferent nerve fibers, taping may cause the peroneus brevis muscle to be activated just before heel strike. This may help to prevent injury independent of any mechanical effect of the tape on the joint itself.[19,20,31,67]

There are four potential uses for taping: treatment of acute injury, prevention of reinjury, prophylaxis, and treatment of chronic instability (Table 1). For an acute injury, taping may be used to provide support and to help reduce edema. The open Gibney wrap, used in conjunction with rest, ice, and elevation,[23] is preferred in this stage (Fig. 5). It involves application of 1-inch-wide tape to the

TABLE 1.   Overview of the Use of Tape in Ankle Sprains

	Technique	Advantage	Disadvantage	Recommendation
Acute injury	Open Gibney basketweave	Good support Compression Can be left in place for up to 3 days	Requires skill in application	Recommended—may use with a lace-up support
Prevent reinjury	Closed Gibney basketweave with stirrup and double-heel lock	Proprioceptive feedback Good initial support	Cost Loses support rapidly May slightly decrease performance	Recommended for early stages of rehabilitation only
Prophylaxis	Closed Gibney basketweave with stirrup and double-heel lock	Proprioceptive feedback Good initial support	Cost Loses support rapidly May slightly decrease performance	Not recommended for routine use, may consider if athlete prefers it
Chronic instability	Closed Gibney basketweave with stirrup and double-heel lock	Proprioceptive feedback Good initial support	Cost Loses support rapidly May slightly decrease performance	Not recommended for routine use, may consider if athlete prefers it

anterior foot and lower leg. The strips are not applied completely around the leg to avoid the circulatory compromise that may ensue from circumferential taping. Felt or foam pads applied under the tape may help to reduce edema.

After swelling subsides, the closed Gibney basketweave technique may be used (see Fig. 5). This technique, which helps to decrease the risk of reinjury,[2] involves application of circumferential strips of tape. It should not be used if circulatory compromise is a potential problem. The final tape application involves stirrup and figure-of-8 straps around the ankle to give a "heel lock" (see Fig. 5) and to prevent inversion/eversion. This method has been shown, both on a prosthetic foot and in humans, to provide more support than simple basketweave taping,[54,56] although other techniques may be functionally equivalent in athletics.[47]

Using taping to prevent reinjury is a costly and time-consuming procedure. Taping an ankle costs about $1.75, and it is estimated that most of the $16,000/year in tape typically used by an NCAA division I football team goes toward ankle taping. Added to this is the cost of countless hours spent by trainers in taping ankles; thus it is easy to appreciate the mounting costs of ankle taping.[8,49,57,58] Tape may be applied for the first few weeks after return to activity or during rehabilitation of ankle injuries, but it is probably not the treatment of choice indefinitely. This principle applies

also to the prophylactic use of ankle taping. Although taping probably reduces the rate of ankle injuries, it is not a cost- and time-effective option compared with the alternatives described below.

Taping has also been recommended as a possible treatment for chronic instability.[2,40] Again, this approach is probably not as cost-effective as the alternatives described below.

When the option of taping an ankle is selected, a number of guidelines should be followed to ensure the best possible outcome. The anatomy of the joint and the mechanism of injury must be understood to ensure that the tape is applied in a manner that provides protection in the weakened plane. The skin should be cleaned and shaved prior to tape application; cuts must be covered; and areas sensitive to blistering must be protected with lubricated gauze sponges. Special adherent spray may be applied under the tape. If tape is to be reapplied often, an underwrap should be used to prevent chronic skin irritation. Tape should always be applied in strips. Using one long, continuous wrap may cause pressure inequalities and compromise blood flow. Tape should overlap one-half to three-fourths of the underlying strip to prevent "gapping" where the strips separate. Proper tape width must also be selected to avoid gapping (for the foot, 1 in; for the ankle, $1^1/_2$ in).

It is also important to understand the limi-

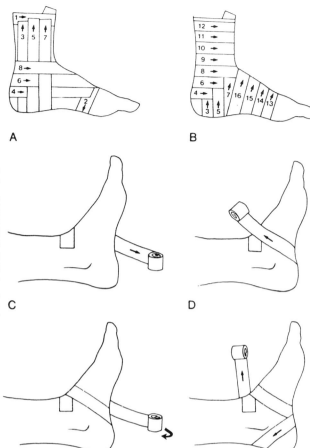

FIGURE 5. **A** and **B, The basketweave technique.** A, Application of the basketweave; B, After the basketweave, circular strips are applied; **C–F, The medial heel lock.** For clarity the underlying basketweave is not shown. After the medial heel lock is finished, a lateral heel lock (not shown) is applied. In the open basketweave technique, the tape strips are not applied all the way around the limb. This technique is preferred in cases of acute injury or fluctuating edema where circulatory compromise is a potential problem. (From Miller EA, Hergenroeder AC: Prophylactic ankle bracing. *Pediatr Clin* 37:1175–1185, 1990; with permission.)

tations of taping. Tape initially offers good support, with as much as 30% to 50% decrease in ankle range of motion immediately after application, but with movement and sweating tape rapidly loses its effect.[25,40,45,51,56] After 10 minutes of exercise, up to 40% of limitation of range of motion is lost,[16,21,40,51,56] and toward the end of exercise it may have little or no effect at all other than perhaps to improve proprioceptive feedback. This decline in effect is probably not a factor in the treatment of acute sprains, in which the tape is not stressed so much, and such a decline has not been documented in all studies.[42]

Elastic tape has also been studied,[51] and although it provides more compression than nonelastic tape,[9] it loses its restriction of range of motion even more than standard tape. Elastic tape may continue to offer benefits of proprioceptive feedback, but it rapidly loses its elasticity[47] and has been shown to provide little support to the ankle.[69]

Tape may impair athletic performance. It has been shown to decrease vertical leap, to slow down a sprint, and to limit the standing broad jump.[8,36,46] These effects tend to be fairly mild (< 4%) and may not cause functional differences in many sports (especially since the effects wear off so quickly), but they need to be kept in mind. Ankle taping does not appear to increase the incidence of knee injuries.[22]

Elastic Wrapping and Sleeves

Wrapping with elastic bandages is useful in the early stages of ankle sprain to provide compression that reduces swelling. It is used as an adjunct to ice and elevation. Care must be taken not to overtighten the wrap, and it should be changed often to monitor the skin. Wrapping provides little or no support during activity, and because of its bulk may even impair proper function (Table 2).

Similarly, elastic ankle sleeves (Fig. 6) that

TABLE 2.   **Overview of the Use of Elastic Wrap or Bandages in Ankle Sprains**

	Technique	Advantage	Disadvantage	Recommendation
Acute injury	Ankle wrap, changed often	Reduce edema	Excess compression Poor support	Recommended
Prevent reinjury	Ankle wrap, changed often	Inexpensive Reusable Possible proprioceptive feedback	Unproven Poor support	Not recommended
Prophylaxis	Ankle wrap, changed often	Inexpensive Reusable Possible proprioceptive feedback	Unproven Poor support	Not recommended
Chronic instability	Ankle wrap, changed often	Inexpensive Reusable Possible proprioceptive feedback	Unproven Poor support	Not recommended

are pulled over the foot like open-ended socks offer no value as supports.[51] If they have a beneficial effect at all, it is due to enhanced proprioception. They may also provide compression to reduce edema, but they are not recommended for support.

Bracing

Like taping, bracing can be used to prevent injury, to treat an acute injury, to prevent reinjury, or to treat chronic instability. Braces come in three main types: casts, lace-up

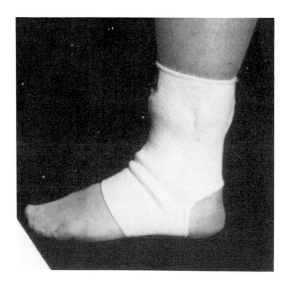

FIGURE 6.   Elastic ankle sleeve. (From Miller EA, Hergenroeder AC: Prophylactic ankle bracing. *Pediatr Clin* 37:1175–1185, 1990; with permission.)

wraps, and plastic orthoses. Other braces are basically variations of these types. Casts can be either semirigid or rigid; lace-up braces and plastic orthoses are considered semirigid.

Casting

Rigid plaster casting, once a common treatment for acute ankle sprains, has now been generally abandoned (Table 3). Compared with taping, it has been shown to increase the time to return to activity and has not been shown to produce a better outcome, even in grade III sprains.[5,6,34,37] Still, rigid casting is an option to consider for the early postoperative phase or in cases of gross ankle instability. It should be replaced with semirigid bracing as soon as possible, usually within 1 to 2 weeks. Its potential advantage over semirigid bracing is that it may facilitate healing by holding the ends of the ruptured anterior talofibular ligament in opposition. It is available in either a weight-bearing, short-leg walking cast[15] or in non–weight-bearing casts. Weight and discomfort are relative contraindications to its use, as is fluctuating edema. When acute swelling subsides, the cast must be replaced with a better fitting one. A sugar-tong splint may be considered if circumferential casting is not used.[30]

Semirigid, or soft, casting is done with a wrap that hardens somewhat after application but does not become rigid. The Una (Unna's) boot (Graham Field, Inc., Hauppage, NY), which is commonly used for this purpose, consists of a gauze bandage that contains glyc-

TABLE 3. Overview of the Use of Casting in Ankle Sprains

	Technique	Advantage	Disadvantage	Recommendation
Acute injury	Semirigid	Compressive effect	Cost Not much support Not proven more effective than tape	Not routinely recommended but may be considered
	Rigid	Best support	Side effects of immobility Unable to accommodate fluctuating swelling Cost Not proven to be better than tape	Not recommended
Prevent reinjury	Not applicable			
Prophylaxis	Not applicable			
Chronic instability	Not applicable			

erin and gelatin and is applied over a felt pad around the malleolus.[59] In an acute sprain it provides some support and compression. Ice is commonly applied around the boot, but no studies have demonstrated adequate tissue cooling with this technique. Soft casting does not give enough support to be used during the rehabilitative phase of ankle injury or for sports participation.

Lace-Up Braces

Lace-up braces are in common use in athletics (Table 4), and a number of brands are available. They have been proved to be as effective as tape at restricting ankle range of motion, and they tend not to lose their supportive ability during exercise.[7,24] One study

TABLE 4. Overview of the Use of Lace-up Ankle Supports in Sprains

	Technique	Advantage	Disadvantage	Recommendation
Acute injury	Lace-up support worn under shoe	Inexpensive Can be used with tape Good support	May be uncomfortable Nonuniform compression	Not recommended alone but may be useful if used in conjunction with tape, pads or elastic wrap to give uniform compression
Prevent reinjury	Lace-up support worn under shoe	Maintained support throughout exercise Can be retightened Can be reused Possible proprioceptive feedback	May become psychologically dependent	Recommended
Prophylaxis	Lace-up support worn under shoe	Maintained support throughout exercise Can be retightened Can be reused Possible proprioceptive feedback	May become psychologically dependent	Recommended if prophylaxis is chosen
Chronic instability	Lace-up support worn under shoe	Maintained support throughout exercise Can be retightened Can be reused Possible proprioceptive feedback	May become psychologically dependent	Recommended

found that lace-up braces may decrease rates of ankle injury and reinjury when used prophylactically.[57] This noncontrolled retrospective survey showed that the best results occurred when lace-up braces are used in conjunction with low-topped rather than high- topped shoes. The authors believed that this combination allowed the athletes to retighten the brace periodically during activity, thus providing more constant support. Athletes with high-topped shoes tended to wear two pairs of socks, which also may have produced an adverse effect.

Lace-up braces are a cost-effective alternative to taping. They are safe, easy to apply, and reusable. They are not of much value in the acute stage of injury because they do not provide good uniform compression, although they can be applied over tape or elastic wrap. They are probably of some value in preventing ankle sprain, in preventing reinjury, and in treating chronic instability. Because athletes can become psychologically dependent on them, lace-up braces usually are not used for more than a few weeks after full function has been regained. Like tape, lace-up braces reduce athletic performance in some tasks, such as vertical leap, broad jump, and sprint, but this effect is small (< 5%) and may not affect functional ability in sports.[8]

Lace-up braces have been compared with ankle taping to determine which provides the better support. In one study tape was shown to offer the higher resistance to inversion when freshly applied. After activity, however, tape lost its advantage and was equivalent to the better ankle stabilizers.[7] A number of brands of lace-up braces are available. The Swede-O (Swede-O Universal, North Branch, MN), McDavid (McDavid, Chicago, IL), and Cramer (Cramer Products, Gardner, KS), among others, may offer similar benefits, although no controlled comparisons have been performed (Fig. 7). The Cramer brace incorporates a lace-up design with outside straps to provide a heel lock. The McDavid and Swede-O can accommodate steel or plastic stays for extra support. Other variations use Velcro closures.

Air-Stirrup

The most studied semirigid orthosis is the air-stirrup (Table 5)[29,38,48,55,61,69] (Fig. 8). In 1979 Stover reported on the development of the Aircast air-stirrup (Aircast, Summit, NJ),[60]

which is composed of an outer plastic shell that fits up both sides of the leg and is connected under the heel. It is lined with inner air bags and attached to the leg with Velcro. Other similar products are lined with foam or filled with gel. Regular shoes can be worn over the stirrup, which is designed to protect the ankle from excessive inversion and eversion while allowing functional dorsiflexion and plantarflexion. It is an off-the-shelf device that does not require custom fitting. At rest, the pressure of the air liner is 25 mm Hg. Weight-bearing increases the pressure to 50 mm Hg, and forced dorsiflexion to around 75 mm Hg. This is believed to provide intermittent compression during movement that aids in the "milking" out of edemous fluid.[61]

The air-stirrup can be used for acute ankle sprains, in the early postoperative period after stabilization procedures, after rigid casting, for treatment of some fractures, and in early return to activity to prevent recurrent sprain.[48,49,55,63,64] It is not currently used for prophylaxis or in chronic instability, although some newer variations of the splint have been designed for this purpose. As yet, their efficacy is unproven.

The air-stirrup has been advocated for treatment of all grades of ankle sprains.[48,62] It has been shown to have a better outcome than rigid casting for the treatment of stable lateral malleolar fractures[63] and for ruptures of the lateral ligaments.[39,48] It has been shown experimentally to provide support against ankle inversion compared with no brace and with tape.[29, 38] The air-stirrup is a well-tolerated, effective treatment for acute and subacute ankle sprains. It is probably best used in conjunction with taping in the early stages of a sprain. It is not used for prophylaxis and has been shown to decrease some athletic performance.[28]

Other Bracing (Table 6)

Other semirigid orthoses have not been studied adequately to make accurate comparison with taping or with air-stirrups, but the DonJoy Ankle Ligament Protector (DonJoy, Carlsbad, CA) (Fig. 9) shows promise in restricting range of motion at least as well as the air-stirrup and probably better than tape.[27,28] The Active Ankle (Active Ankle Systems, Louisville, KY) incorporates a stirrup and air cell liner with a hinged ankle (Fig. 10).

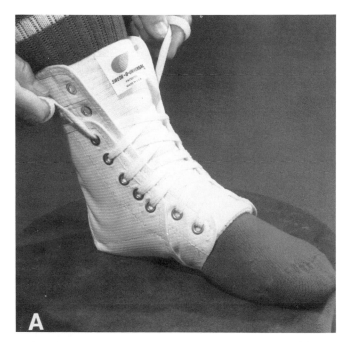

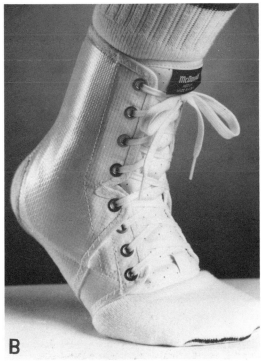

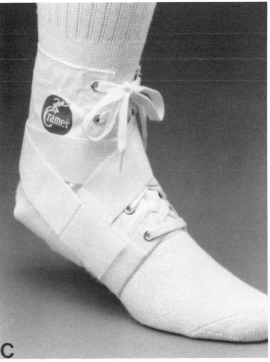

FIGURE 7. The Swede-O ankle lace-up brace *(panel A)* and similar designs by McDavid *(B)* and Cramer *(C).* (Photographs courtesy of Swede-O Universal, McDavid Knee Guard, and Cramer Products.)

The Malleoloc (Bauerfeind USA, Kennesaw, GA) (Fig. 11) is an interesting stabilizing ankle orthosis that uses a wrap-around ankle brace in conjunction with Velcro strap-wrapping. It offers excellent subjective ankle support with minimal bulk, but definitive proof of effectiveness is not yet available.

Other Ankle-Stabilizing Devices (Table 6)

Nonelastic Cloth Wrapping

Some athletic departments use a nonelastic cloth wrap applied over socks to prevent ankle injury. Commonly known as the Louisiana

TABLE 5. Overview of the Use of Air-Stirrups in Ankle Sprains

	Technique	Advantage	Disadvantage	Recommendation
Acute injury	Worn under shoes	Proven support Proven effective "Milking" effect on edema May be used with tape	Cost	Recommended
Prevent reinjury	Worn under shoes	Maintains support Possible proprioceptive feedback	May decrease performance	Recommended in early stages
Prophylaxis	Worn under shoes	Maintains support Possible proprioceptive feedback	Unproven Cumbersome	Not recommended
Chronic instability	Worn under shoes	Maintains support Possible proprioceptive feedback	Unproven Cumbersome	Not recommended

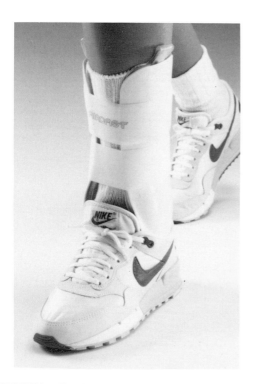

FIGURE 8. The Aircast air-stirrup ankle brace. (Photograph courtesy of Aircast.)

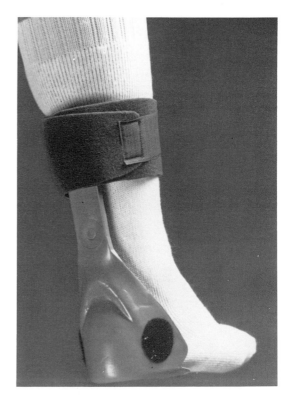

FIGURE 9. The DonJoy Ankle Ligament Protector. (Photograph courtesy of DonJoy.)

heel lock, this technique can be modified by using a roll-guaze wrap. The advantage of such a system is that the wrap can be washed and reused, thus reducing cost.

One study reported favorably on the use of a nonelastic cloth wrap applied over a limited tape wrap versus extensive tape wrapping alone.[13] The study was flawed in that subjects were not properly divided into control and study groups. In addition, all of the athletes performed special ankle exercises. It is impossible to determine whether or not the cloth wrap was solely responsible for the effects.

Cloth wrapping may improve proprioceptive feedback to the athlete, but it has not been adequately studied to make valid recommendations regarding its use for treatment or prophylaxis. It is unlikely to be more effective

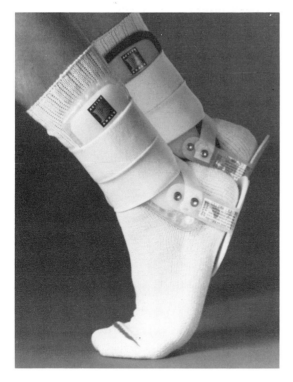

FIGURE 10. The Active Ankle. (Photograph courtesy of Active Ankle Systems.)

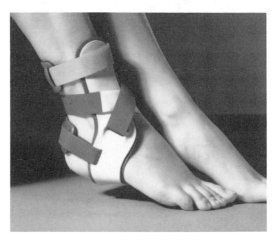

FIGURE 11. The Malleoloc. (Photograph courtesy of Bauerfeind USA.)

than tape or lace-up wrapping. The same can be said for numerous nylon or nylon/elastic wrap variations on the market (Fig. 12).

Orthoplast Stirrup

The orthoplast stirrup is a strip of thermoplastic material fitted to run under the heel and up both sides of the leg. The malleoli are padded, and stirrup is fitted with an elastic bandage. It has been successfully used to treat ankle sprains, but because it is relatively hard, it does not adapt to reduction in swelling. It has not been shown to decrease inversion range of motion more than tape[33] and is most appropriate in the acute or early rehabilitative stages.

Stabilizing Shoe

Several shoe designs have been advocated for prevention and treatment of lateral ankle sprains. One study showed that high-topped shoes increase effective ankle stiffness compared with low-tops.[68] Garrick's study[22] detected an advantage of high-topped over low-topped shoes. The effect was relatively small, and athletic shoes have certainly changed since he performed the study. No recent studies provide good information on the prophylactic benefits of various shoe types in sports.

Ankle fractures have also been treated with a special stabilizing shoe with apparently good results.[72] Whether or not the results are as good as or better than with other treatments is unknown.

The use of ankle-stabilizing shoes to treat ankle sprain or to prevent reinjury has not been studied adequately to date, although the Künzli line of shoes (Swiss Balance, Santa Monica, CA) (Fig. 13) shows promise.[32] These shoes incorporate an A-shaped pair of stays on each side of the ankle to provide support. Subjectively, they feel quite stable and allow adequate dorsiflexion and plantarflexion for most functional activities. Several models are

TABLE 6. Alternate Ankle-Stabilizing Devices*

Device	Recommendation
Active ankle	May be useful
Ankle ligament protection	Shows promise
Cloth or nylon wrap	Unlikely to be useful
Elastic ankle sleeves	Unlikely to be useful
Ice pack	Shows promise
Kunzli shoe	Shows promise
Malleoloc	Shows promise
Orthoplast stirrup	Limited use, not often necessary
Sarmiento cast brace	Unlikely to be useful

*These devices have not been studied adequately to make definite recommendations regarding their use. They are listed in alphabetical order.

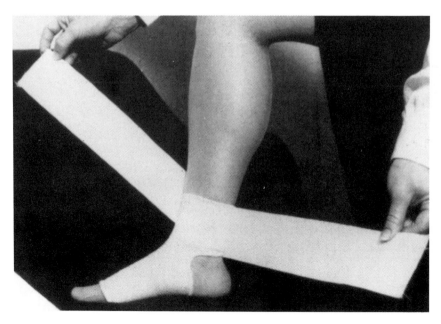

FIGURE 12. Elastic ankle sleeve with cloth or nylon/ elastic heel lock. (From Miller EA, Hergenroeder AC: Prophylactic ankle bracing. *Pediatr Clin* 37:1175–1185, 1990; with permission.)

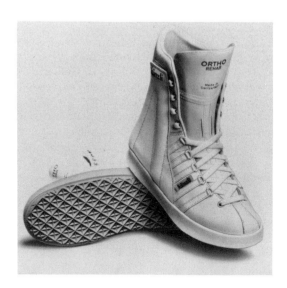

FIGURE 13. The Ortho Rehab Shoe from Kunzli. (Photograph courtesy of Swiss Balance Prosthetic and Orthotic Specialists.)

available for treating acute ankle injury and chronic ankle instability.

Cast-Brace

A number of hinged-casting techniques have been advocated for the treatment of ankle sprains. They allow weight-bearing as well as ankle motion in dorsiflexion and plantarflexion[11,35] and involve some sort of casting of the lower leg with ankle hinges and a heel stabilizer. The modified Sarmiento brace[11] is removable and fits in the patient's shoe. This technique has reportedly given good results in the treatment of sprains but has not been shown to offer any benefit over other forms of treatment. Because cast-braces require custom-fitting and are cumbersome and expensive, they are of questionable value.

Ice Pack with Air-Stirrup

This interesting device uses a U-pad (Cryo/ Strap, Aircast, Summit, NJ) for compression of the soft tissue around the malleolus. The pad contains a liquid that can be frozen and is held in place by an elastic strap. A modified air-stirrup is worn over the device. This system provides uniform compression and has been shown to decrease skin temperature for up to 90 minutes.[71] It is not known whether it improves long-term outcome.

IMPRESSIONS

Numerous difficulties arise in interpreting the studies of the various treatments for ankle sprains. First, most ankle sprains heal well regardless of the form of treatment; thus, almost all treatments produce good results. It is difficult to measure marginal differences among them. Secondly, difficulties arise in comparing different treatment protocols and brands of products. Research is needed to standardize forms of treatment and to compare the many products on the market. There is also much emphasis on which devices provide the best mechanical support of the ankle in laboratory stress testing, but it is not entirely clear that this emphasis is important. Perhaps the devices giving the most proprioceptive feedback are the best.

It is important to remember the potential for abuse of ankle supports. Certainly they are not to be recommended in all sports, regardless of risk of ankle injury. There are no well-studied guidelines for when not to use bracing or taping, but a few general rules seem to make sense:

1. Rigid casting or bracing should be avoided as long as swelling is fluctuating.
2. Circumferential taping in an area where swelling is likely to increase should be avoided.
3. Elastic wraps in areas where circulatory compromise is a potential problem should not be overtightened; they should be rechecked and rewrapped often to monitor the skin.
4. After pain has subsided and the athlete can walk without a limp, the brace or tape should be applied only during practice or high-risk activity. Leaving the brace or tape in place all the time only serves to restrict functional range of motion and to encourage psychological dependence.
5. There is generally no reason for prophylactic bracing or taping in low-risk activity, such as straight-ahead running on level surfaces.
6. Braces should not be used as a substitute for weak muscles; the athlete must have full strength and mobility to return to active participation.
7. Tape should be prescribed only if a person well-trained in its application is available to wrap it. Improperly applied tape may cause further injury.
8. Patients with single mild or moderate sprains should not be allowed to become addicted to external support.
9. It should be remembered that if used permanently, tape and braces become expensive.

RECOMMENDATIONS ON THE USES OF ANKLE SUPPORTS

There are as yet no commonly accepted parameters for how long braces or tape are to be applied after injury or for which form of treatment should be selected (see Tables 1–5). The length of time certainly depends on the serverity of the injury. Mild or moderate injuries should be treated with tape or semi-rigid support until the pain and swelling have subsided and the athlete can perform activity without pain. A few weeks of tape or lace-up bracing on initial return to activity may aid with proprioceptive feedback and psychological reassurance. Severe injuries are almost always treatable with functional support from day one.

Unstable fractures, large bone avulsions, osteochondral injuries, or gross deformities rarely occur. They should be evaluated by an orthopedic surgeon or other physician well-versed in the treatment of complicated sprains.

Severe simple ligamentous injury may be treated acutely with tape and air-stirrup alone. This treatment should continue for the next few weeks as rehabilitation proceeds and while pain and swelling are still present. When the patient enters the strengthening phase and returns to vigorous activity, a lace-up ankle brace is most beneficial. Its use may be continued until a few weeks after the athlete has regained preinjury status or possibly for the rest of the season. Unsuccessful outcomes with this approach may require secondary operative repair. This form of treatment is acceptable.

The issue of prophylactic bracing or taping is more difficult to address. Taping, lace-up bracing, and high-topped shoes have evidence supporting prophylactic use. Because of cost, inconvenience, and possible detraction from athletic performance, however, it is not clear that they should be advocated for routine use. Certainly, if the athlete tolerates them, high-topped shoes are to be recommended. Athletes in high-risk sports such as football, basketball, and racquetball may benefit from prophylactic lace-up bracing, especially to prevent reinjury after moderate-to-severe sprains. In other sports their use is basically up to the athletes, with advice from the physician and trainer. Lace-up braces may be more effective if used with low-topped shoes so that they can be retightened periodically.

Table 6 describes early impressions of some of the alternative devices available for use around the ankle. These devices have not been studied adequately to make definite recommendations regarding their use.

REFERENCES

1. Akeson WH, Frank CB, Amiel D, Woo SL: Ligament biology and biomechanics. In Finerman G (ed): *Symposium on Sports Medicine: The Knee.* St. Louis, CV Mosby, 1985, pp 11–51.
2. Balduini FC, Vegso JT, Torg E: Management and rehabilitation of ligamentous injuries to the ankle. *Sports Med* 4:364–380, 1987.
3. Bonci CM: Adhesive strapping techniques. *Clin Sports Med* 1(1):99–117, 1982.
4. Bostrom L: Sprained ankles I: Anatomic lesions in recent sprains. *Acta Chir Scand* 128:483–495, 1964.
5. Bostrom L: Sprained ankles V: Treatment and prognosis in recent ligament ruptures. *Acta Chir Scand* 132:537–550, 1966.
6. Bostrom L: Sprained ankles VI: Surgical treatment of "chronic" ligament rupture. *Acta Chir Scand* 132:551–565, 1966.
7. Bunch RP, Bednarski K, Holland D, et al: Ankle joint supports: A comparison of reusable lace on braces with taping and wrapping. *Physician Sports Med* 13(5):59–62, 1985.
8. Burks RT, Bean BG, Marcus R, et al: Analysis of athletic performance with prophylactic ankle devices. *Am J Sports Med* 19(2):104–106, 1991.
9. Capasso G, Maffulli N, Testa V: Ankle taping: Support given by different materials. *Br J Sports Med* 23: 1989, pp 239–240.
10. Carmines DV, Nunley JA, McElhaney JH: Effects of ankle taping on the motion and loading pattern of the foot for walking subjects. *J Orthop Res* 6:223–229, 1988.
11. Carne P: Nonsurgical treatment of ankle sprains using the modified Sarmeinto brace. *Am J Sports Med* 17(2):253–257, 1989.
12. Chapman MW: Sprains of the ankle. In *American Academy of Orthopedic Surgeons: Instructional Course Lecture,* vol 24. St. Louis, C.V. Mosby, 1975, pp 294–308.
13. Davis GJ: The ankle wrap: Variation from the traditional. *Athletic Training.* 12(4):294–297, 1977.
14. Diamond JE: Rehabilitation of ankle sprains. *Clin Sports Med* 8:877–891, 1989.
15. Evans GA, Hardcastle P, Frenyo AD: Acute rupture of the lateral ligament of the ankle. *J Bone Joint Surg* 66B:209–212, 1984.
16. Firer P: Taping the lateral ligaments of the ankle. *S Afr Sports Med* 4:7–8, 1980.
17. Firer P: Effectiveness of taping for the prevention of ankle ligament sprains. *Br J Sports Med* 24(1):47–50, 1990.
18. Freeman MAR: Treatment of ruptures of the lateral ligament of the ankle. *J Bone Joint Surg* 47B:661–668, 1965.
19. Freeman MAR: Instability of the foot after injuries to the lateral ligament of the ankle. *J Bone Joint Surg* 47B:669–677, 1965.
20. Freeman MAR, Dean MRE, Hanham IWF: The etiology and prevention of functional instability of the foot. *J Bone Joint Surg* 47B:678–685, 1965.
21. Fumich RM, Ellison AG, Geurin GJ, et al: The measured effect of taping on combined foot and ankle motion before and after exercise. *Am J Sports Med* 9:165–170, 1981.
22. Garrick JG, Requa RK: Role of external support in the prevention of ankle sprains. *Med Sci Sports* 5(3):200–203, 1973.
23. Garrick JG: The frequency of injury, mechanism of injury and epidemiology of ankle sprains. *Am J Sports Med* 5:241–242, 1977.
24. Gehlsen GM, Pearson D, Bahamonde R: Ankle joint strength, total work and ROM: Comparison between prophylactic devices. *Athletic Training* 26:62–65, 1991.
25. Glick JM, Gordon RB, Nishimoto D: The prevention and treatment of ankle injuries. *Am J Sports Med* 4:136–141, 1976.
26. Gray SD: Sports strapping and bandaging. *Aust Fam Physician* 20(3):276–282, 1991.
27. Green TA, Hillman SK: Comparison of support provided by a semirigid orthosis and adhesive ankle taping before, during, and after exercise. *Am J Sports Med* 18:498–506, 1990.
28. Green TA, Wight CR: A comparative support evaluation of three ankle orthoses before, during and after exercise. *J Orthop Phys Ther* 11:453–466, 1990.
29. Gross MT, Bradshaw MK, Ventry LC, et al: Comparison of support provided by ankle taping and semirigid orthosis. *J Orthop Sports Phys Ther* 9(1):33–39, 1987.
30. Halvorson G, Iserson KV: Comparison of four ankle splint designs. *Ann Emerg Med* 16:1249–1252, 1987.
31. Hergenroeder AC: Diagnosis and treatment of ankle sprains. *Am J Dis Child* 144:809–814, 1990.
32. Hintermann B, Holzach P, Matter P: Treatment of fibular ligament disruption with the ortho rehab shoe. *Swiss Med J* 38:1–7, 1990.
33. Hughes LY, Stetts DM: A comparison of ankle taping and semirigid support. *Physician Sportsmed* 11(4):99–103, 1983.
34. Jackson DW, Ashley RL, Powell JW: Ankle sprains in young athletes: Relation of severity and disability. *Clin Orthop* 102:201–215, 1974.
35. Jackson JP, Hutson MA: Cast brace treatment of ankle sprains. *Injury* 17:251–255, 1986.
36. Juvenal JP: The effects of ankle taping on vertical jumping ability. *Athletic Training* 7:146–149, 1972.
37. Kannus P, Renstrom P: Treatment for acute tears of the lateral ligaments of the ankle, operation, cast, or early controlled mobilization. *J Bone Joint Surg* 73A:305–312, 1991.
38. Kimura IF, Nawoczenski DA, Epler M, et al: Effect of the air stirrup in controlling ankle inversion stress. *J Orthop Sports Phys Ther* 9(5):190–193, 1987.
39. Klein J, Rixen D, Albring T, et al: Functional versus plaster cast treatment of acute rupture of the fibular ligament of the upper ankle joint. A randomized clinical study. *Unfallchirurg* 94(2):99–104, 1984.
40. Larsen E: Taping the ankle of chronic instability. *Acta Orthop Scand* 55:551–583, 1984.
41. Lassiter TE Jr, Malone TR, Garrett WE: Injury to the lateral ligaments of the ankle. *Orthop Clin North Am* 20:629–640, 1989.

42. Laughman RK, Carr TA, Chao EY, et al: Three dimensional kinetics of the taped ankle before and after exercise. *Am J Sports Med* 66:425–431, 1980.
43. Lindenfield TN: The differentiation and treatment of ankle sprain. *Orthopaedics* 2(1):203–206, 1988.
44. Mack RP: Ankle injuries in athletics. *Clin Sports Med* 1:75–85, 1982.
45. Malina RM, Plagenz LB, Rarick GL: Effect of exercise upon measurable supporting strength of cloth and tape ankle wraps. *Res Q* 34:158–165, 1962.
46. Mayhew JL: Effects of ankle taping on motor performance. *Athletic Training* 7:10–11, 1972.
47. McLean DA: Use of adhesive strapping in sports. *Br J Sports Med* 23(3):147–149, 1989.
48. Milford PI, Dunleavy PJ: A pilot trial of treatment of acute inversion sprains to the ankle by ankle supports. *J R Nav Med Serv* 76:97–100, 1990.
49. Miller EA, Hergenroeder AC: Prophylactic ankle bracing. *Pediatr Clin North Am* 37:1175–1183, 1990.
50. Moller-Larsen F, Wethlund JO, Jurik AG, et al: Comparison of three different treatments for ruptured lateral ankle ligaments. *Acta Orthop Scand* 59:564–566, 1988.
51. Myburgh KH, Vaughan CL, Isaacs SK: The effects of ankle guards and taping on joint motion before, during and after a squash match. *Am J Sports Med* 12:441–446, 1984.
52. Nicholas JA, Strizak AM, Veras G: A study of thigh muscle weakness in different pathological states of the lower extremity. *Am J Sports Med* 4:241–248, 1976.
53. Nitz AJ, Dobner JJ, Kersey D: Nerve injuries in grade II and III ankle sprains. *Am J Sports Med* 13(3):177–182, 1985.
54. Pope MH, Romstrom P, Donnermeyer D, et al: A comparison of ankle taping methods. *Med Sci Sports Exerc* 2:143–147, 1987.
55. Raemy H, Jakob RP: Functional treatment of fresh fibular ligament lesions using the aircast splint. *Schweiz Ztschr Sportmed* 31:53–57, 1983.
56. Rarick GL, Bigley G, Karst R, Malina RM: The measurable support of the ankle joint by conventional methods of taping. *J Bone Joint Surg* 44A:1183–1190, 1962.
57. Rovere GD, Clarke TJ, Yates CS, et al: Retrospective comparison of taping and ankle stabilizers in preventing ankle injuries. *Am J Sports Med* 16(3):228–233, 1988.
58. Rovere GD, Curl WW, Browning DG: Bracing and taping in an office sports medicine practice. *Clin Sports Med* 8:497–515, 1989.
59. Siegworth K, Draper D: A soft cast for compression following moderate ankle sprains. *Athletic Training* 23(1):37–38, 1988.
60. Stover CN, York JM: The aircast/airstirrup system for graduated management of lower extremity injuries. Presented at the American Association of Orthopaedic Surgeons, San Francisco, 1979,
61. Stover CN: Airstirrup management of ankle injuries in the athlete. *Am J Sports Med* 8(5):360–369, 1980.
62. Stover CN: Functional sprain management of the ankle. *Ambul Care* 6(11), 1986.
63. Stuart PR, Brumby C, Smith SR: Comparative study of functional bracing and plaster casting treatment of the stable lateral malleolar fractures. *Injury* 20:323–326, 1989.
64. Tillman BP, Stover CN, McCarroll JR, et al: Open fracture dislocation of the ankle with loss of medial malleolus in a college tennis player. *Physician Sportsmed* 14(4):81–88, 1986.
65. Tipton CM, Matthes RD, Maynard JA, et al: The influence of physical activity on ligaments and tendons. *Med Sci Sports* 7:165–175, 1975.
66. Tipton CM, Vailas AC, Matthes RD: Experimental studies on the influence of physical activity on ligaments, tendons, and joints: A brief review. *Acta Med Scand* 711(suppl):157–168, 1986.
67. Tropp H, Askling C, Gillquist J: Prevention of ankle sprains. *Am J Sports Med* 13:259–262, 1985.
68. Tsenter MJ, Shapiro MS, Mitchell P, et al: Effectiveness of ankle braces and tape in resisting ankle inversion [McDavid Product Information]. Chicago, McDavid.
69. Vaes P, DeBoeck H, Handelberg F, et al.: Comparative radiological study of the influence of ankle joint strapping and taping on ankle stability. *J Orthop Sports Phys Ther* 7(3):110–114, 1985.
70. Vailas AC, Tipton CM, Matthes RD, Gart M: Physical activity and its influence on the repair process of medial collateral ligaments. *Conect Tissue Res* 9:25–31, 1981.
71. Wilkerson GB: Treatment of the inversion ankle sprain through synchronous application of focal compression and cold. *Athletic Training* 26:221–234, 1991.
72. Zeegers AVCM, Van Raay JJAM, van der Werken C: Ankle fractures treated with a stabilizing shoe. *Acta Orthop Scand* 60:597–599, 1989.

Chapter 16

PEDIATRIC SPORTS ISSUES

Phillip R. Bryant, DO, and Barbara Koch, MD

Children participating in sports incur injuries that are often different from those that occur in adults. Children are more susceptible to certain types of injuries than adults because of the presence of growth cartilage and the process of growth itself. Because most of the disorders discussed here are also found in adults, the focus of this chapter is on features unique to the child. The reader is referred to other chapters for a more comprehensive discussion of disorders shared by adults and children.

The number of physically fit children has decreased in the last 20 years,[24] and in 1984 only 66% of children were participating in regular physical activities and exercise. In 1989 the Centers for Disease Control evaluated physical activities for the previous 10 years and in 1990 established objectives for physical fitness and the role of exercise in sports. The first of these objectives was to maintain a level of greater than 90% of adolescents participating in appropriate physical activities, particularly cardiorespiratory programs, which would be carried into adulthood. The second objective was to have 60% of children participate daily in school physical education, and the third objective was to have a standardized assessment of physical fitness for children 10–17 years of age. A report issued by the CDC stated that objective number two was not met.[24]

Certain questions were raised by the report. Are competitive sports for children the way to improve fitness? Do competitive youth sports contain too serious a risk of physical injury or emotional stress? Is there a risk in training? What are the best ways to train, condition, and protect young athletes from injury while fostering fun and play and obtaining the well-established benefits of exercise?

A number of health benefits of exercise have been documented in adults. Exercise is felt to reduce anxiety and tension as well as improve self-esteem.[24] Aerobic exercise has been shown to improve mood.[18,19] In general, improvement of muscle strength around a joint is protective of that joint.[3,4,13,21,25] Appropriate exercise also can contribute to joint stability and can increase bone density.[26,28,31] Exercise can minimize osteoporosis as well as improve cardiovascular fitness.[2,7,23]

The risk of injury in competitive sports remains a concern. Many physicians recommend that pre-adolescent children participate in physical activities that promote fun, fitness, and motor skills with minimal or no competition.[5] Others advocate diminishing an athlete's risk of injury by adhering to guidelines of *The Bill of Rights for Young Athletes* (Table 1). This document defines participation in athletics as both a privilege and a responsibility. The athlete has the responsibility to play fairly, to keep in training, to play his best, and to conduct himself proudly. In return, he has the right to good coaching, good officiating, good equipment and facilities, and good health supervision.

EPIDEMIOLOGY

The incidence of sports injuries per year in children has been reported to be 27–39%[15,27] in boys and 12–22% in girls.[27] However, one study reported that only 3 injuries per

1,000 children participating in sports occurred in children attending elementary school. In contrast, 7 of 100 injuries were reported in junior high school sports and 11 of 100 in high school sports. Higher injury rates were recorded in college and young professional athletes. Football, ice hockey, wrestling, baseball, tennis, track-running, and gymnastics have the highest incidence of injuries among children.

RISK OF DEATH AND RISK PREVENTION

Death on the playing field is rare. A community of 100,000 people will encounter 1 such unexpected death in children.[12] The majority of young people who have unexpected deaths have abnormalities of the heart muscle brought about by inflammation, fibrosis, dilatation, or hypertrophy of normal tissue.[6] Cardiac dysrrhythmias can also cause sudden death.[14] While many young athletes have no symptoms prior to their sudden death, some may benefit from preparticipation screenings to detect abnormalities (see Chapter 1).

Once a decision is made to participate in competitive pediatric sports, the young athlete needs competent medical care to deal with sport injuries. A concerted effort is required to minimize the risk of injuries. Prompt, complete treatment should be initiated so that the athlete can return to full health, and also return to play as early as possible. Since a stronger child generally runs and swims faster, jumps higher, and hits a ball

farther than a weaker one, safe strength training is potentially beneficial.[34] A common experience of coaches and clinicians is that strength improvements come about both through training and participation in sports. The child needs to be mature enough to follow safety rules in strength training,[34] and close supervision is mandatory. Any exercise-related back, shoulder, or joint pain needs to be evaluated fully before participation. Because there is an apparent developmental lag of shoulder, abdominal wall, and trunk musculature, routine strengthening of these muscle groups is considered beneficial.[36] Any previous injuries must be rehabilitated prior to the playing season.

PATHOPHYSIOLOGY OF PEDIATRIC INJURIES

Sports injuries are of two major types: (1) high impact, causing contusions or fractures, and (2) overuse, due to repetitive trauma. Overuse injuries are commonly seen in pitching, swimming, and gymnastics. They include Osgood-Schlatter disease, an apophysitis of the tibial tubercle; and Sever disease, an apophysitis of the calcaneus. The epiphyseal growth centers and the sites of tendon insertion (apophyses) are the most common sites of traumatic sports injury in children.[27,35]

Fortunately, the vascular supply to the growing epiphyseal cells is generally not compromised in most injuries. Crush injuries however, may be much more likely to compromise epiphyseal blood supply.[30] The epiphyseal plate is the weak link in growing bones and will succumb to stress before the ligaments or the joint capsule do.

Children's bones are softer and are more prone to deform than to fracture.[30] When they do fracture, the fracture is often as a "greenstick" fracture in which the cortex fails on one side but stays in continuity on the other side.

EMERGENCY MANAGEMENT OF SPECIFIC DISORDERS

In evaluating the patient for an acute injury, a brief but targeted history should be taken as to the site and nature of the injury. The position of the athlete at the time of the injury should be documented, as clearly as the patient and observers can relate. Was the injured arm or leg extended, flexed, or rotated, and what was the direction and force of the impact? Is the history more consistent with a repetitive injury instead? The patient's history is followed by a careful examination that includes a search for deformities, limitation in range of motion, and presence and degree of tenderness or ligamentous instability. In addition mental status, peripheral nerve function, and tendon function is noted.

Lacerations

Lacerations are common. Most are dirty because they occur on the playing field. If deep, a delayed closure may be indicated. Infiltration of the wound with xylocaine may be necessary, followed by thorough irrigation. If the wound is managed by primary closure, widely spaced sutures will allow for edema and purulent drainage that may develop at the surface.[29] "Steri-Strips" provide another option for approximating the edges of a laceration, particularly if the wound is clean and free of any foreign material. If the laceration is well covered with bandages, the child may return to most sports but not to wrestling, swimming, or judo until fully healed.

Strains and Sprains

Strains and sprains are graded as first, second, or third degree, depending on the severity of the injury. A strain is an injury to the musculotendinous unit. A sprain is an injury specifically involving ligaments. Both are graded as first degree if they are due to a mild stretching injury that does not result in hemorrhage. A second-degree injury involves a partial tear with localized swelling and pain as well as decreased function. Depending on the sport, the athlete with a first- or second-degree injury may be able to support the area with the use of an elastic cuff or proper taping, and return to play. A third-degree sprain involves disruption of the ligament, and a third-degree strain is a disruption or tear of the muscle-tendon unit. Swelling may be minimal, but, hemorrhage may extravasate into the surrounding soft tissues.[16] There may be excessive mobility due to opening of a growth center or disruption of a ligament.[17] The injured area should have stress radiographs and may subsequently require surgical repair.

Fractures

Fractures may occur in any situation involving significant blunt trauma. The injury site should be splinted and pulses checked. One should use half splints and padding rather than circumferential wrapping to accommodate the significant swelling that may occur and to avoid vascular compromise.[35] Ice, splinting, elevation, and confirmation of the fracture by x-rays are typically necessary.

Traumatic Brain Injury

Traumatic brain injuries should always be treated as serious or potentially serious injuries until proven otherwise by serial examination or diagnostic testing. The severity of head injury may range from a scalp laceration to a serious subdural or epidural hematoma. The history should include any changes in mental status, including loss of consciousness or memory loss. In severe traumatic brain injury, acute treatment will include 1.5–2.0 mg/kg of body weight of intravenous mannitol[16] if a long transport to a trauma center is required. This measure is designed to minimize the potential for serious complications of cerebral edema. Initial assessment should focus on maintaining a patent airway.

A patient in shock needs to be assessed for a hidden source of bleeding. This patient needs stabilization of the cardiovascular system and expeditious transfer to an appropriate medical facility.

While transferring the brain-injured child, regular assessments of pupil size, reactivity to light, and movement of extremities should be noted. The most important factor in the brain-injured patient is the level of consciousness. This needs to be recorded every few minutes until the child is in the emergency room. The Glasgow Coma scale measures eye opening, motor response, and verbal response.[37] Measurements are initially made in the emergency room and then at serial intervals. The 24-hour score is a reliable indicator of prognosis.

Nerve and Spine Injuries

Nerve injuries are another type of injury that need immediate attention. Common nerve injuries include brachial plexus stretch injuries (stingers) in football and traumatic injury to the ulnar nerve. Fracture or dislocation may injure nerves in the vicinity of the injury. Common examples include the axillary nerve in shoulder dislocations, the median nerve in elbow dislocations,[22] or the peroneal nerve in fibular fractures.

Although cervical spine injuries are rare, they are the most common cause of severe disability following sports trauma. Currently, no equipment exists that will guarantee adequate protection for the spinal cord. The risk of injury must be minimized by reducing the exposure to high-risk situations. The cervical spinal cord can be injured in all contact sports, and the best protection appears to be strong neck musculature. To avoid high-risk situations, children need to be counseled in pedestrian safety, bicycle safety, and the hazards of motorcycles and all-terrain vehicles. In addition, proper coaching in technique and in the appropriate use of equipment will minimize the incidence of spinal injuries.

Injury to the neck occurs relatively frequently, so knowledge and experience in the emergency management of this area are highly recommended. Signs of spinal injury include pain with movement, tenderness along the spine, deformity, impaired breathing, loss of active movement of the arms and or legs, sensory loss, loss of bladder or bowel control, and shock. Treatment should include avoidance of neck movement and adequate neck stabilization on a spine board. Administration of oxygen or ventilation may be indicated in some cases. Although a child may not complain of neck pain immediately, one who does must be removed from the game and examined. The headgear does not need to be removed unless it is interfering with the airway. The patient should then be carefully moved to a hospital for radiographic examination.

Cervical fractures and fracture dislocations may occur with or without neurological complications. These injuries all require acute medical management and many will benefit from rehabilitation. Patients with neurological damage will invariably require extensive rehabilitation.

Upper Extremity Injuries

The upper extremities are loosely connected at the shoulder to permit a wide plane of active motion. This looseness makes the shoulder a relatively unstable joint that is prone to injury. Careful examination of the shoulder is necessary in order to determine the site of injury. In general, pain on passive motion suggests an injury to the joint or capsule, while pain on resisted motion suggests a problem of the muscle or tendon responsible for that movement.[16]

Shoulder Instability

Shoulder dislocations are relatively common in young athletes. The most common direction of the dislocation is anterior-inferior. The humeral head is displaced forward, slips over the glenoid rim, and the arm drops toward the side. On physical examination the humeral head is palpable anteriorly below the acromion. The patient will resist adduction and internal rotation. Dislocation of the humeral head can be an emergency if there is an associated compromise of vascular function. Some physicians advocate reduction of the dislocation on the playing field, especially if this is a recurrent problem. However, because of the possible presence of a concomitant fracture, radiographic examination is always warranted after a reduction. Relocation on the field is dependent on the athlete's ability to relax the shoulder as well as the physician's experience and skill. A complete description of relocation techniques can be obtained elsewhere.[32] In general, excessive or overly abrupt traction force should be avoided to minimize the possibility of causing a brachial plexus injury. One should carefully check for any evidence of neurologic injury, both before and after reduction. Once a shoulder is dislocated, it is likely to have permanent damage and is at high risk of redislocation, especially in children. Aggressive rehabilitation with a strengthening program may reduce this risk of recurrence.

Acromioclavicular Sprain

Acromioclavicular (AC) sprain or joint injury may occur in sports in which an individual lands on the unprotected shoulder. This also may occur in football players who fall on an outstretched hand or flexed elbow. The humerus is driven against the glenoid and acromion. The clavicle remains in an anterior position with stress being applied to the acromioclavicular ligaments with tension and possible rupture. Depending on the degree of force, there will be a first-, second- or third-degree sprain.

Rotator Cuff Disorders

The rotator cuff comprises the infraspinatus, supraspinatus, teres minor, and subscapularis muscles. Injury may occur at the point where the supraspinatus portion of the rotator cuff passes under the acromial process. Bursitis occurs when there is friction between the two walls of the subdeltoid bursa. The high amplitude forces seen in wrestling, tackling, or throwing activities cause repetitive strain on the rotator cuff mechanism. In such cases, tenderness is typically along the greater tuberosity of the humerus. Pain will often occur at the shoulder or the deltoid insertion. Abduction against resistance will usually reproduce the pain.[16] Treatment includes relative rest and nonsteroidal antiinflammatory medication. This is followed by a rehabilitation program to return the shoulder strength and range of motion to normal.

Elbow Disorders

Fractures of the elbow can occur with relatively minor trauma. A quick throw may result in an avulsion of the medial epicondyle at the attachment of the origins of forearm flexor muscles. There will be tenderness and swelling at the medial humerus, and the diagnosis can be confirmed by x-ray. Open reduction is usually required. Fractures may also occur in the transcondylar or supracondylar area. The wide epiphyseal plate makes accurate interpretation of the x-ray difficult. Swelling and tenderness at the distal humerus should raise the level of suspicion for such an injury. It is of particular concern in pediatric injuries since the injury will probably be through the growth plate.[16]

Medial epicondylitis is an overuse injury that is common in young pitchers. The athlete begins throwing with a windup, cocks the arm back, accelerates the ball, releases it, and follows through. It is generally in the acceleration phase that the stress on the medial epicondyle occurs. This phase puts a stress on the medial elbow, and the flexor and pronator muscle are irritated. The repetitive motion of pitching strains the attachment of the aponeurosis to the bone. The microtraumatic

stresses on the ulnar collateral ligament will often manifest as pain before, during, and after the activity. To treat such overuse, the pitcher needs to rest the elbow and forearm in a foam splint that keeps the wrist in slight extension and the elbow in 90° of flexion.[42] A course of nonsteroidal antiinflammatory medication is also usually helpful. Preventing the injury or at least minimizing its occurrence has come about through changes in rules that limit the number of innings in which a young pitcher can participate per game.[16] Proper throwing technique is also important.

Wrist Disorders

A common wrist injury is a fracture of the scaphoid bone, which usually occurs when the athlete falls on an outstretched hand. The scaphoid lies next to the styloid tip of the radius, and with the fall it butts against the radius. The child will complain of pain on palpation of the anatomic snuff box or when attempting to make a fist. Treatment typically is with casting. Problems may arise because of the poor blood supply to the area, with secondary complications of nonunion or avascular necrosis. After the cast has been removed, the athlete should be given a protective splint for competition to protect him from re-injury for the remainder of the season. Mobilization and strengthening must also be carried out.

Lower Extremity Injuries

Pelvic, Hip, and Thigh Disorders

A common injury in young football players is a bruise of the pelvic crest (often referred to as a hip pointer). Since both abdominal muscles and hip flexors insert on the iliac crest, movement of these muscles aggravates the pain of this injury. Treatment consists of ice, possibly an injection of a local anaesthetic, and oral antiinflammatory medication. Pain will probably be severe for the first 24 hours. If a posttraumatic periostitis develops, the iliac crest will have prolonged tenderness.

If the iliac crest is avulsed, surgical intervention is indicated. These injuries may recur if the athlete returns to play prior to complete healing. The most severe injury occurs with blunt trauma sufficient to fracture the wing of the ilium. In this case, symptoms will be more severe, the patient will resist palpation of the injury, and diagnosis must be confirmed radiographically.

A slipped capital femoral epiphysis may occur with minimal trauma, causing the femoral head to slip in relation to the femoral shaft across the epiphyseal growth plate. This injury occurs primarily in people who are large, obese, sexually immature, and most commonly, in boys between the ages of 13 and 16 and in girls between the ages of 11 and 14. Children will often complain of anteromedial (referred) knee pain and will have a limp. The examination is characterized by limitation of internal rotation, abduction, and flexion of the hip with the child letting the leg fall passively into a position of external rotation. X-rays of the hip are the diagnostic tool of choice, and treatment is almost always surgical to keep the slip from progressing.

Intense trauma to the thigh may be followed by significant bleeding into the muscle. The player may sustain a large hematoma in the quadriceps muscle. These injuries usually resolve without incident, but occasionally the hematoma develops into a case of heterotopic ossification. Sometimes this mass must be differentiated from the early bone formation of osteogenic sarcoma.[16]

Fracture of the femur is one result of violent trauma. The condition may be serious because of the size of the injury, and the athlete may go into hypovolemic shock. In adolescents, the fracture may be through the epiphyseal plate of the femoral head. Symptoms include apparent shortening of the leg, pain in the hip, and abduction and external rotation of the hip. Meticulous care of this injury is important because this is a site of major linear growth in adolescents.

Knee Disorders

Although tears of the meniscus and injuries of the knee ligaments are rare in children, knee injuries can occur that involve ligaments, tendons, capsule menisci, cartilage, bone, or bursa. Careful examination and mild manipulation are necessary to determine if instability is present. Plain radiographs, arthrography, and arthroscopy may all be necessary to assess the integrity of these structures of the knee. Treatment will depend on which structures are involved.

Prepatellar bursitis is one of the more common disorders in young athletes, especially in wrestlers. It can be due to acute trauma or to repetitive irritation. Treatment is with a posterior splint and a warm wet dressing. Usually the bursitis will resolve in a few days unless the fluid has become infected, in which case the purulent material must be drained. Following acute bursitis, the knee must be protected with padding during future sporting events. Chronic bursitis develops with repeated attacks of acute bursitis and thickening of the bursal wall, oversecretion of inflammatory fluid, and filling of the bursal sac. Treatment includes aspiration of the fluid, injection of a corticosteroid, and the application of a firm pressure dressing.

Back

Low Back Pain

Low back pain is common in both athletes and nonathletes. In the sports setting it is usually due to chronic ligamentous or musculotendinous injury. Low back pain is often related to hyperlordosis of the spine. Many athletes have tightness involving muscles in the low back, hip girdle, and hamstrings. There may also be weakness of the abdominal muscles and hip flexors. Stretching of the tight musculature along with abdominal exercises, including pelvic tilts and stretching of the hip flexors, should be helpful in treating low back problems.

Anterior Disc Protrusion

Anterior disc protrusion may occur following trauma and may produce vertebral wedging. Although there may be pain, the condition usually responds to ice, rest, and antiinflammatory medications. The condition is self-limited. An elastic lumbar corset may relieve the symptoms but is not a substitute for rest. Recovery usually occurs in 2–3 weeks in uncomplicated cases.[16]

Spondylolysis and Spondylolisthesis

Stress reactions involving the spine are generally manifested as stress fractures of the pars interarticularis of the lumbar vertebrae. Many individuals have failure of fusion between the arch of the vertebra and between the articular processes. This is known as spondylolysis, and may be aggravated by repetitive exercise, particularly involving hyperextension of the lumbar spine. This structure is usually injured in repetitive stress activities such as gymnastics, diving, wrestling, football, weight lifting, pole vaulting, or hurdling. Plain radiographs may be negative early-on, whereas a bone scan will typically demonstrate the stress fracture. The main objective in the treatment of this condition is to rest the area for approximately 6 weeks, although full recovery may take up to 2 years.[16] The role of bracing is controversial, but the most effective brace is the Boston brace, which is designed to prevent lumbar hyperextension.[2] Ideally, the athlete can substitute an activity that will not stress the back during the time of healing. Gymnasts, football players, and others who are likely to continually stress the posterior elements of the spine may need to be counseled about seeking an alternative sport.

Spondylolisthesis occurs when, in the presence of spondylolysis, there is forward displacement of the superior vertebra on an inferior one. This condition may be treated by substituting nonaggravating activities. If pain persists despite conservative care, the athlete may need to be restricted from the sport that caused the injury. Occasionally, surgical correction of the defect is required.

Overuse Syndromes

One difference between skeletally mature adults and skeletally immature children is the nature of the overuse syndromes they develop. In children, overuse syndromes are characterized by inflammation at the sites of tendon insertion (apophyses) or at the cartilaginous physes.[1] A common form of overuse apophysitis in young athletes is Osgood-Schlatter disease, a disorder of the patellar tendon attachment to the tibial tubercle. This inflammation may lead to overgrowth of the tibial tubercle with enlargement and tenderness. Patients complain of pain that occurs during activity and goes away with rest. It generally responds to rest, ice, and nonsteroidal antiinflammatory agents. As the athlete matures, the condition typically resolves.

''Jumper's knee'' is an overuse syndrome of the patellar tendon attachment to the inferior pole of the patella. It is also known as Sinding Larsen syndrome. There is extreme pain on palpation of the inferior pole of the patella. The syndrome is characteristically found in basketball players with tight hamstrings. Heel pain, also known as Sever disease, is an overuse syndrome of the calcaneal apophysis.[1]

Medications

Aspirin is generally contraindicated in children because of its association with Reye syndrome. Children should be given acetaminophen for pain and other nonsteroidal medications for antiinflammatory effects. Not all of the nonsteroidal medications are approved for use in children. Tolmetin, naproxen, and ibuprofen are approved. Naproxen is probably not as effective as the other choices; however, it has the benefit of a long half-life so that it can be taken only twice a day. Ibuprofen is probably the most commonly prescribed nonsteroidal agent. It can be given in liquid form to younger children.

Training for Children Athletes

A common experience of coaches and clinicians is that children improve in strength with training and participation in sports; however, the amount of research is limited. In one study, children increased their strength 22–43% after strength training over 8–14 weeks as compared to a nontrained group. Heavy weight training is not generally recommended in skeletally immature athletes. However, this recommendation is based more on common sense and experience than on actual research.

Whether strength training is effective in preventing serious injuries is another unknown. Although this idea seems rational, the literature contains no evidence that strength training has any direct effect on the risk of sustaining a severe injury. Guidelines that help minimize risks of serious injuries are listed in Table 2.

Equipment

Each sport has different areas in which the body needs protection, and the reader is referred to other sources for this specific information.[29] One critical factor is that the equipment should fit properly. Since equipment is expensive, teams tend to pass on equipment

TABLE 2. Guidelines for minimizing the risk of serious injury

1	Begin strength training when the child is ready for competitive sports.
2	Children should be able to follow safety rules.
3	A preparticipation physical examination should be mandatory.
4	Pain after exercise precludes participation the next day. Pain for 2 days signifies a problem that warrants medical attention.
5	Resistance should be submaximal.
6	Resistance should be through the full range of motion.
7	It is important to maintain a normal lordotic curve to the spine.
8	Training sessions should be 3 times per week.
9	Strengthening should emphasize sports related use, upper body strength, and balance of opposing muscles. Strength training should minimize overuse injuries; however, it cannot protect against all serious injuries in sports.[11]

from year to year. The athlete typically receives equipment that comes as close to his size as the team has available, but it may not provide as much protection as equipment specifically fitted to the athlete. Ill-fitting equipment may provide little protection and may place the child at increased risk of injury. Ideally, properly fitted equipment should be available for all participants at all times, and it must be rechecked periodically as the child grows.

Steroid Use

Anabolic steroids are commonly abused by adolescent athletes. They are discussed in more detail in the chapter on weight lifting.

THE DISABLED ATHLETE

(See also the chapter on wheelchair athletics.) In discussing childhood sports, disabled individuals are often excluded. More recently, amputees, blind or hearing-impaired individuals, children with cerebral palsy, paraplegic or quadriplegic children in a wheelchair, mentally retarded children, and other groups with disabilities are beginning to participate in organized sports. The International Stoke Mandeville Games Foundation and the Special Olympics Foundation have international competitions so that individuals with disabilities can participate. Disabled athletes benefit from improved self esteem as well as improvements in physical fitness and function. Perhaps the main obstacles to training the disabled include exercise intolerance or anxiety, poor balance, and medical problems associated with the disability. Several authors have documented the effects of training

and improvements in strength and endurance. The disabled are becoming more active in competitive sports, and musculoskeletal injuries will occur more commonly. These injuries will need treatment, and standard treatment may require modification based on the nature of the athlete's disability. There seems to be no increased risk of serious musculoskeletal injuries in the disabled, and the injuries can usually be minimized by proper grouping of the athletes and by the use of the same safety guidelines put forth for other child athletes.[10,29]

REFERENCES

1. Andrish JT: Overuse syndromes of the back and legs in adolescents. Adolesc Med State Art Rev 2:213–244, 1991.
2. Blair SN, Kohl HW, Paffenbarger RS, et al: Physical fitness and all-cause mortality: A prospective study of healthy men and women. JAMA 262:2395–2401, 1989.
3. Brooks WH, Young AB: High school football injuries: Prevention of injury to the central nervous system. South Med J 69:1258–1260, 1976.
4. Burkett LN: Causative factors in hamstring strain. Med Sci Sports Exerc 2:39, 1970.
5. Committee on Sports Medicine and Committee on School Health: Organized athletics for preadolescent children. Pediatrics 84:583–584, 1980.
6. Denfield SW, Garson A Jr: Sudden death in children and young adults. Pediatr Clin North Am 37:215, 1990.
7. Ekelund LB, Haskell WL, Johnson JL, et al: Physical fitness as a predictor of cardiovascular mortality in asymptomatic North American men: The Lipid Research Clinic's mortality follow-up study. N Engl J Med 319:1379–1384, 1988.
8. Goldberg B, Rosenthal PP, Robertson LS, et al: Injuries in youth football. Pediatrics 81:255–261, 1988.
9. Gray J, Taunton JE, McKensie DC: A survey of injuries to the anterior cruciate ligament of the knee in female basketball players. Int J Sports Med 6:314–316, 1985.

10. Jackson RW, Davis GM: Sports and recreation for the physically disabled. In Sanders B (ed): Sports Physical Therapy. Norwalk, CT, Appleton and Lange, 1990.
11. Johnson MD: Steroids. Adolesc Med State Art Rev 2:79–92, 1991.
12. Kennedy HL, Whitlock JA: Sudden death in young persons—an urban study [abstract]. J Am Coll Cardiol 3:486, 1984.
13. Marroon JC, Steele PB, Berlin R: Football head and neck injuries: An update. Clin Neurosurg 27:414–429, 1980.
14. McFaul RC: Death on the playing field. Adolesc Med State Art Rev 2:93–107, 1991.
15. McLain LG, Reynolds S: Sports injuries in a high school. Pediatrics 84:446–450, 1989.
16. Micheli LJ: Pediatric and Adolescent Sports Medicine. Boston, Little, Brown & Co., 1984.
17. Molacrea RF: Injuries on the field. The pediatrician as team physician. Pediatr Ann 7:10, 1978.
18. Morgan WP: Affective beneficence of vigorous physical activity. Med Sci Sports Exerc 17:94–100, 1985.
19. Morgan WP, Roberts JA, Brand FR, et al: Psychological effects of chronic physical activity. Med Sci Sport Exerc 2:213–217, 1980.
20. Moseley CF: Growth. In Lovell WW, Winger RB (eds): Pediatric Orthopedics. Philadelphia, JB Lippincott, 1990.
21. Moskwa CA, Nicholas JA: Musculoskeletal risk factors in the young athlete. Phys Sportsmed 17(11):49–59, 1989.
22. O'Donoghue DH: Treatment of Injuries to Athletes. Philadelphia, WB Saunders, 1984.
23. Paffenbarger, RS, Hyde RT, Wing AL, et al: A natural history of athleticism and cardiovascular health. JAMA 252:491–495, 1984.
24. Raunikar RA, Strong WB: The status of adolescent physical fitness. Adolesc Med State Art Rev 2:65–75, 1991.
25. Reider B, Marshall JL, Warren RF: Clinical characteristics of patellar disorders in young athletes. Am J Sports Med 9:270–274, 1981.
26. Rippe JM: The health benefits of exercise. Part 1 of 2: Phys Sportsmed 15(10):115–132, 1987. Part 2 of 2: Phys Sportsmed 15(11):121–131, 1987.
27. Risser WL: Epidemiology of sport injuries in adolescents. Adolesc Med State Art Rev 2:109–124, 1991.
28. Safrit MF: Health-related physical fitness levels of American youth. In Effects of Physical Activity on Children. Champaign, IL, Human Kinetics, 1986, pp 153–166.
29. Sanders B: Sports Physical Therapy. Norwalk, CT. Appleton & Lange, 1990.
30. Sharrad WJW: Pediatric Orthopedics and Fractures. Oxford, Blackwell Scientific Publications, 1979.
31. Smith EL, Reddan W, Smith PE: Physical activity and calcium modalities for bone mineral increase in aged women. Med Sci Sports Exerc 13:60–64, 1981.
32. Tachdjian MO: Pediatric Orthopedics. Philadelphia, WB Saunders, 1990.
33. Teasdale G, Jennett B: Assessment of coma and impaired consciousness. A practical scale. Lancet 2:81–84, 1974.
34. Webb: Strength training in children and adolescents. Pediatr Clin North Am 37:1187, 1990.
35. Williams PE, Goldspink G: Longitudinal growth of striated muscle fibers. J Cell Sci 9:751–767, 1971.
36. Yessis MP: Pre- and post-pubescent weight training. Presented at California Strength and Conditioning Clinic, Los Angeles, March 20, 1987.

Chapter 17

THE ACTIVE WOMAN:
Part I. Anatomy and Physiology

Ralph M. Buschbacher, MD, and Lois P. Buschbacher, MD

The advent of women's widespread participation in recreational and competitive athletics is relatively recent. Most of the physiologic and athletic research in the past has focused on men, and only in the past 10 to 15 years have significant studies of women athletes emerged.

A number of questions have been generated: What issues are unique to women in sports? Is the physiology of women the same as for men, and should women train in the same manner as men? How does menstruation affect performance? How does exercise affect fertility, puberty, pregnancy, menopause, and bone density?

This chapter reviews women's historical role in sports and addresses anatomic, physiologic, and endocrinologic differences between men and women. Part II follows and addresses the reproductive and medical issues in women athletes.

HISTORY

In earlier ages, women rarely competed in athletic events. In ancient Greece, women were forbidden even to enter the arena where the Olympics took place. In the Middle Ages, athletics consisted mainly of martial practices such as jousting and fencing, mainly male preserves. Certainly, the average male peasant had little chance of participating in serious athletic competition; his female counterpart had even less opportunity.

In the early 19th century, the Turnverein movement in Germany and gymnastics in Sweden began to open the door for women to participate in athletics. Ballet, an art form, was also acceptable. Despite these advances, the first modern Olympic games, held in 1896, were exclusively male. In the 1912 Olympics, women were permitted to compete in tennis and swimming. By 1928, women could participate in short- and middle-distance track events, but only 5 of 11 participants finished the race that year.[19]

Until 1958, the longest running event for women in the Amateur Athletic Union was the 440-yard run. In 1965, women were threatened with banishment from international competition if they ran races longer than 1.5 miles, and it was 1984 before the first women's Olympic marathon took place.[10] Still, through it all, committed women persevered and slowly gained access and the right to compete in more and more sports. Despite these advances, the lay literature voiced concerns about women participating in athletics as late as the 1970s. Some articles discouraged women's participation in athletics with few or no supportive data. We now know that with appropriate training, women can compete safely and that they have improved their performances to the point of rivaling men in some events.

DIFFERENCES BETWEEN MEN AND WOMEN

A quick look at average people reveals certain major differences between the sexes. Other differences lie hidden beneath the skin, but overall men and women are more alike than different. The differences are important, however, and need to be understood for proper treatment and training of women.

Anatomy

On average, the adult female is 6 inches shorter than her male counterpart. Men typically weigh more, have more bone mass, and have proportionately less body fat than women; the body fat of the average sedentary male is around 10% to 15% of total weight, whereas it is typically around 20% to 25% in the average woman. Women's arms and legs are proportionately shorter than men's, and their center of gravity is a bit lower. Women also have narrower shoulders and a proportionately smaller thoracic cage.

A common misperception is that women have a wider absolute pelvic width than men. In fact, absolute pelvic widths in men and women are approximately equal. When measured relative to height, however, the pelvis is proportionately wider in women, who are on average shorter. When measured relative to shoulder width, the pelvis in women seems even wider.[23,24] The pelvis of most women differs in shape from that of men, with a wider pelvic inlet to accommodate childbearing.

Given an equally wide pelvis and shorter legs, women have a greater degree of normal valgus at the knee. They also have a greater Q-angle, i.e., the angle that the patellar ligament makes with the midline of the femur. Although it is commonly held that the greater valgus and Q-angle predispose women to a higher incidence of patellofemoral tracking disorders, few data support this assumption. Women who are well conditioned athletes, with a well-developed vastus medialis muscle, may have no more such problems than men.

Women are commonly reported to have a smaller heart, smaller thoracic cage, and lower blood volume than men.[10,22] This is said to reduce their maximal oxygen-carrying capacity. It is unclear from the literature, however, whether these differences are absolute or simply related to women's smaller physical size (especially fat-free size). There appears to be a difference in heart size even in childhood, before males become the larger sex (even in this population, boys appear to have greater lean body mass than girls).[12] One recent study concluded that the gender difference in heart size primarily reflects the smaller overall dimensions of women.[13] Women have a lower blood hemoglobin range than men (12–16 mg/dL vs 14–18 mg/dL), and this may affect performance.

Endocrine Differences

There are marked endocrine differences between men and women. Men have more testosterone and related androgens, which generate their typical secondary sexual characteristics, including muscle hypertrophy, increased skeletal mass, laryngeal changes, wider shoulders, and greater stimulation of hematopoiesis. In women the estrogens predominate. They regulate ovarian function and the menstrual cycle as well as stimulate breast development, cause widening of the pelvic inlet, and increase adiposity.

Strength

Women are approximately 56% as strong as men in the upper extremity, 72% as strong in the lower extremity, 64% as strong in the trunk, and 69% as strong in measures of dynamic (functional) strength.[14] Even when comparing athletically trained women with untrained men, the men are on average stronger, both in absolute strength and in strength relative to size.[15] Men's strength advantage is usually attributed to a greater lean body mass.

When strength is measured as maximal muscular tension relative to cross-sectional area of the muscle, there is no difference between men and women.[20] Because men on average are taller, however, they have a greater lever arm across their joints and can generate more torque, even when their muscular cross-sectional area is the same as in women.

Some data suggest that sex differences in the cross-sectional area of upper-extremity muscle relative to fat-free weight may be due to long-term differences in activity.[1,2] However, this activity differential appears to account for only a part of the difference in muscle mass. Most of the difference in muscle mass is probably due to major innate differences between the sexes. Men have a higher level of testosterone, which helps to increase muscle mass to a level not attainable by women. Weight-lifting exercise by women narrows the gap in strength but does not completely overcome it. There appears to be no difference in muscle fiber number or distribution between the sexes,[18,20] but muscle fibers in women are smaller.

In conclusion, it is clear that men, on average, are stronger than women. They have greater fat-free weight, better leverage, and, through the action of testosterone, more muscle cross-sectional area. The strength advantage of men is most pronounced in the upper extremities and in absolute muscle strength (not adjusted for lean body mass or height). Ultimately, strength is most closely related to muscle cross-sectional area. Functional strength is influenced by skill and training and thus may be higher in trained women than in untrained men. The great variation within both sexes should also be remembered. There is a tremendous overlap in size and strength, and the man should not always be assumed to be the stronger.

Performance ($\dot{V}O_{2max}$)

$\dot{V}O_{2max}$, the maximal rate of oxygen uptake, is a general measure of cardiovascular endurance and on average is lower in women than in men. Thus, women have a relative physiologic disadvantage in performing aerobic activity. Part of this disadvantage is due to the proportionately greater amount of body fat that women carry and possibly also to their generally lower level of conditioning.[21] However, even when measuring $\dot{V}O_{2max}$ relative to lean body mass in subjects with similar training, men have more aerobic capacity than women.[21] This appears to be due at least partially to absolute heart size[13] (in men, heart size has been shown to correlate with maximal aerobic power).[16]

Because women have smaller hearts, they have a smaller stroke volume. They compensate by increasing heart rate during exercise. But because maximal heart rate is unchanged between men and women, it means that women have a lower maximal cardiac output and thus also a lower $\dot{V}O_{2max}$.[22]

Other possible reasons for the sex difference in endurance performance include women's lower hemoglobin concentration[5] (and thus lower oxygen-carrying capacity) and lower muscle mass compared with men. Other as yet unknown sex-related differences, such as possible differences in mitochondrial density, may also be responsible, although their effects must be fairly small.

Energy Metabolism and Thermoregulation

In general, women are able to come closer to the levels achieved by men in endurance events than in strength events. In the past this was postulated to be due to a more efficient energy metabolism in women. However, there does not appear to be any such difference between the sexes in trained subjects. There may be a small difference between untrained men and women.[4,11]

When performing endurance exercise, men and women have similar responses in adaptability to a hot climate. Both sexes are equally susceptible to heat stress, and both respond by acclimatization.[7] Heat adaptation appears to be more efficient in athletes with better preexisting aerobic capacity.[3,8] Women seem to need a lower rate of sweating than men to maintain body temperature. This may indicate that women have a more efficient means of thermoregulation, but with endurance training, women's threshold for sweating becomes lower, closer to that of men.[3] The significance of this observation is unclear.

RESPONSE TO TRAINING

Strength

Almost all of the research in the physiology of women's exercise focuses on endurance training rather than strength training. The object of strength training is to increase strength through an increase in muscle mass. Because the absolute strength of a muscle is a function of its cross-sectional area, increasing muscle mass is the only way to increase absolute muscle strength. Women do not respond as well as men to a strength-training program. Androgens are needed to stimulate muscle hypertrophy, and thus women do not attain the sometimes phenomenal increase in muscle mass and strength seen in men.

Despite this lower level of response, strength training is valuable for women. Their muscles increase in size to some extent, and women may increase their relative strength to a similar proportion as men (in a moderately long period of regular weight-training).[6] Moreover, although they gain strength and muscle mass more slowly than men, women also develop an increase in the synchronization of muscle fiber activity and thus a greater functional strength. In addition, strength training may exert beneficial effects on bone mass and overall psychological well-being.

Endurance

Women's response to endurance training is similar to that of men. When men and women train at similar levels of effort for similar tasks, they have nearly identical rates of increase in $\dot{V}O_{2max}$, at least for up to 7 weeks of training.[9] Their heart rates at submaximal exercise loads also decrease similarly. Absolute $\dot{V}O_2$ is still higher among the men, and the maximal $\dot{V}O_2$ attainable by elite athletes also appears to be higher among men.

Endurance training increases the cross-sectional proportion of slow twitch (fatigue-resistant) fibers to a similar extent in both men and women, although the fibers in men are larger.[17,18] It also creates a proportionately similar change in body composition in men and women. Both sexes have a decrease in fat and an increase in lean body mass. However, unless they undergo rigorous strength and endurance training and an extremely strict diet, women's body fat percentages do not reach as low a level as men's.

How should women train?

It should be clear from the preceding discussion that the training differences between men and women are more quantitative than qualitative. Women respond to training like men, but perhaps a little slower and to a lesser extent. Thus, training principles should be approximately the same in both sexes. An individualized, sports-specific approach is recommended, regardless of gender.

REFERENCES

1. Bishop P, Cureton K, Collins M: Sex difference in muscular strength in equally-trained men and women. *Ergonomics* 30:675–687, 1987.
2. Bishop P, Cureton K, Conerly M, et al: Sex difference in muscle cross-sectional area of athletes and non-athletes. *J Sports Med* 7:31–39, 1989.
3. Cohen JS, Gisolfi CV: Effects of interval training in work-heat tolerance of young women. *Med Sci Sports Exerc* 14:46–52, 1982.
4. Costill DL, Fink WJ, Getchell LH, et al: Lipid metabolism in skeletal muscle of endurance-trained males and females. *J Appl Physiol* 47:787–791, 1979.
5. Cureton K, Bishop P, Hutchinson P, et al: Sex difference in maximal oxygen uptake. *Eur J Appl Physiol* 54:656–660, 1986.
6. Cureton KJ, Collins MA, Hill DW, et al: Muscle hypertrophy in men and women. *Med Sci Sports Exerc* 20:338–344, 1988.
7. Drinkwater BL: Women and exercise: Physiological aspects. *Exerc Sports Sci Rev* 12:21–51, 1984.
8. Drinkwater BL, Kupprat IC, Denton JE, et al: Heat tolerance of female distance runners. *Ann NY Acad Sci* 302:777–792, 1977.
9. Eddy DO, Sparks KL, Adelizi DA: The effects of continuous and interval training in women and men. *Eur J Appl Physiol* 37:83–92, 1977.
10. Fahey TD: Endurance training. In Shangold MM, Mirkin GM (eds): *Women and Exercise: Physiology and Sports Medicine.* Philadelphia, F.A. Davis, 1988, p 65.
11. Friedmann B, Kindermann W: Energy metabolism and regulatory hormones in women and men during endurance exercise. *Eur J Appl Physiol* 59:1–9, 1989.
12. Goble MM, Mosteller M, Moskowitz WB, et al: Sex difference in the determinants of left ventricular mass in childhood. *Circulation* 85:1661–1665, 1992.
13. Hutchinson PL, Cureton K, Outz H, et al: Relationship of cardiac size to maximal oxygen uptake and body size in men and women. *Int J Sports Med* 12:369–373, 1991.
14. Laubach LL: Comparative muscular strength of men and women: A review of the literature. *Aviat Space Environ Med* 47:534–542, 1976.
15. Morrow JR, Hosler WW: Strength comparisons in untrained men and trained women athletes. *Med Sci Sports Exerc* 13:194–198, 1981.
16. Osborne G, Wolfe LA, Burggraf GW, et al: Relationships beween cardiac dimensions, anthropometric characteristics and maximal aerobic power ($\dot{V}O_{2max}$) in young men. *Int J Sports Med* 13:219–224, 1992.
17. Prince FP, Hikida RS, Hagerman FC: Muscle fiber types in women athletes and non-athletes. *Pfluegers Arch* 371:161–165, 1977.
18. Saltin B, Henriksson J, Nygaard E, et al: Fiber types and metabolic potentials of skeletal muscles in sedentary man and endurance runners. *Ann NY Acad Sci* 301:3–29, 1977.
19. Sanders B: *Sports Physical Therapy.* Norwalk, CT, Appleton & Lange, 1990.
20. Schantz P, Randall-Fox E, Hutchison W, et al: Muscle fiber type distribution, muscle cross-sectional area and maximal voluntary strength in humans. *Acta Physiol Scand* 117:219–226, 1983.
21. Sparling PB: A metanalysis of studies comparing maximal oxygen uptake in men and women. *Res Q Exerc Sport* 51:542–552, 1980.
22. Wells CL, Plowman SA: Sexual differences in athletic performance: Biological or behavioral? *Physician Sportsmed* 11(8):52–63, 1983.
23. Wilmore JH, Behnke AR: An anthropometric estimation of body density and lean weight in young men. *J Appl Physiol* 27:25–31, 1969.
24. Wilmore JH, Behnke AR: An anthropometric estimation of body density and lean weight in young women. *Am J Clin Nutr* 20(3):267–274, 1970.

Chapter 18

THE ACTIVE WOMAN:
Part II. Medical, Gynecologic, and Reproductive Concerns

Lois P. Buschbacher, MD, and Ralph M. Buschbacher, MD

This chapter addresses reproductive and medical concerns in women athletes, including the relationships between exercise and menstruation as well as exercise and pregnancy, menopause, osteoporosis, nutrition, adolescent concerns, and gynecologic issues.

REPRODUCTIVE ISSUES

Menstruation

Effects of Exercise on Menstruation

The prevalence of menstrual abnormalities is about 3% to 5% in the general population of women.[55] In athletes, the prevalence is higher. Oligomenorrhea (infrequent or irregular menses) and amenorrhea (absent menses) occur in up to 10% to 25% of women athletes.[64,69,78] The prevalence appears to be higher in sports that require greater intensity, frequency, and duration of training. In high-level training, the prevalence may approach 50%.[18,20,63,78] When exercise intensity is reduced, a normal menstrual cycle often resumes.[2] However, the long-term effects of the interruption are unknown.

In 1982 Feicht-Sanborn et al.[63] found that the prevalence of amenorrhea in runners was greater than in swimmers or cyclists and that the rate was related to body weight. As body fat decreased, the rate of amenorrhea increased. The incidence of amenorrhea is higher in thin women and in women who lose weight.[79]

Shangold and Levine[69] studied the rate of infertility and amenorrhea among runners; 5% to 10% had problems of infertility. They found that amenorrheic runners were lighter and had a lower weight-to-height ratio than runners with normal menses. They also found that the best predictor of abnormal menses was a history of pre-running menstrual abnormality. Only 7% of women with normal menses developed an abnormality while running. Of women with irregular menses, 25% became regular after exercise was started. Women runners with menstrual irregularity tend to have a history of irregularity even before running.[12,15,64,69,78]

An insult to the female reproductive system disturbs menstruation. This disturbance probably follows an orderly sequence (Table 1).[3,70] Mild disturbances result in luteal-phase deficiency. A greater insult causes euestrogenic anovulation, and an even greater insult leads to hypoestrogenic amenorrhea.

The normal menstrual cycle of 28 days is split into a 14-day follicular (estrogen-secreting) phase followed by a 14-day luteal (progesterone-secreting) phase (Fig. 1). Ovulation occurs on day 14, between the two phases. The phases can be measured by monitoring daily basal body temperature or by measuring blood and urine hormones. When luteal-phase shortening or deficiency develops, infertility may result. Because menstruation and ovulation may still occur and appear normal, this condition is probably underdiagnosed.

TABLE 1. Progression of Menstrual Dysfunction

1. Luteal phase deficiency
2. Euestrogenic anovulation
3. Hypoestrogenic amenorrhea

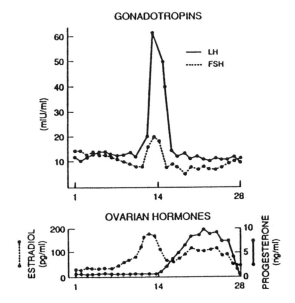

FIGURE 1. Hormone levels during the menstrual cycle. (From Gidwani GP: The athlete and menstruation. *Adolesc Med State Art Rev* 2:27–45, 1991; with permission.)

Euestrogenic anovulation is more severe than luteal-phase shortening. Menstrual bleeding may be irregular, but because it still occurs, this condition is also probably underdiagnosed. Because there is no ovulation, infertility is obviously a problem. Unopposed estrogen production may increase the risk for endometrial hyperplasia and adenocarcinoma, although this effect has not been proved.[71]

Hypoestrogenic amenorrhea, aside from leading to infertility, may also predispose the athlete to lower calcium absorption, osteoporosis, and musculoskeletal injury.[19,36] Osteoporosis is of special concern because regular weight-bearing exercise is usually said to reduce its severity. Exercise does not appear to prevent the bone loss associated with decreased estrogen production.[19] Therefore, women with menstrual irregularity should be counseled about this potential hazard.

The abnormalities of menstruation in women athletes have not been studied in great detail to date. Most of the research has relied on self-reports from volunteers. Shangold et al.[68] followed one runner through a series of 18 menstrual cycles, with varying running mileage among the cycles. Higher mileage correlated with a shorter luteal phase.

In 1982 Prior et al.[57] studied 14 women who recorded their daily temperatures and menstrual cycles over a total of 48 cycles. All the women were training for marathons and had normal menstrual cycle histories. Only one-third of the 48 cycles of these women were normal biphasic cycles. One-third had evidence of anovulation, and one-third had shortened luteal phases. The study was limited by its small sample size and reporting technique, but nevertheless it suggests a dramatically high rate of menstrual irregularity among avid women runners.

Numerous factors, both physiologic and psychologic, may affect menstruation, including weight loss, rate of weight loss, change in diet or inadequate diet, and physical and emotional stress. In addition, delayed menarche, excessive exercise, eating disorders, young age, prior menstrual dysfunction, and nulliparity may predispose to menstrual abnormality. A reduced-calorie vegetarian diet coupled with weight loss also appears more likely to cause luteal-phase irregularity than a nonvegetarian diet with a similar calorie count.[56,65] It is unclear whether or how any of these factors affect the hormonal stimuli to normal menstruation. Usually more than one factor is evident at any given time in an exercising person—or in a sedentary person, for that matter. It is probably safe to say that stress, generically speaking, increases the risk of menstrual abnormality. Exercise is probably a stressor that can be superimposed on other stressors already in place.

Many hormonal changes occur in the exercising woman, including changes in prolactin level, cortisol, estradiol, luteinizing hormone, gonadotropin-releasing hormone, progesterone, and testosterone.[51,58,81] Exactly how these changes affect menstruation is unknown.

Much has been written about the role of a critical fat percentage below which menstruation ceases. In 1974 Frisch et al.[24] postulated that 17% body fat is necessary for menarche to occur and 22% body fat is necessary for the restoration and maintenance of menstruation once it has been interrupted. Because fat cells convert an estrogen precursor to estrogen, the authors believed that an insufficient amount of body fat would result in amenorrhea. Their method of measuring body fat was relatively crude and inaccurate by modern standards. Other authors have suggested that the critical body fat level may be as low as 13%,[32] and there may be no such critical level at all. Because the amount of estrogen precursor converted to estrogen in fat is very small compared with total body estrogen, it is unclear why there should be a critical fat percentage. If such a percentage indeed exists, it probably varies widely from individual to individual.

When an athletic woman presents with complaints of oligomenorrhea, amenorrhea, or infertility, she deserves a full hormonal and physical evaluation, either by a gynecologist or other physician well versed in such problems. Assuming that all cases of amenorrhea in active persons are due to the exercise may result in missing other causes of menstrual dysfunction. When the diagnosis is made, treatment may involve fertility agents, oral contraceptives, and lifestyle or diet changes.

Effects of Menstruation on Exercise

Although many women feel that menstruation impairs athletic performance, no evidence suggests a consistent change in athletic performance at different points of the menstrual cycle.[11] Performance may increase in some women in some sports and may decrease in some women in some sports. Occasionally, women may perform better during the follicular phase of their cycle, and if they are elite athletes, manipulation of the cycle with birth control pills to coincide with major athletic competition is an option.[70] Performance benefits are small, however. Women may train as usual during menstrual bleeding; women swimmers can effectively use tampons during these times.

Pregnancy

During times of starvation, spontaneous abortion (miscarriage) occurs as a protective mechanism against potentially lethal stress on a woman's system. If the fetus were to develop further, it would sap more and more strength from the mother, who could not even support herself nutritionally, let alone a developing offspring. The miscarriage may sacrifice the life of the fetus to save the mother, who presumably would again become fertile in times of plenty. This rational has been used to argue that pregnant women should not exercise. Exercise, the argument goes, puts stress on the mother's system and if the stress becomes too great, her body may react like the starving woman's.

This argument lacks proof. Obviously in times past women had to continue their work and family roles despite being pregnant. There were seeds to sow, harvests to gather, and other children to care for. Somehow, women balanced the needs of livelihood with the needs of the fetus, although there may have been a higher rate of miscarriage. The basic questions, however, remain: Is exercise bad for pregnancy, and is it bad for the fetus? The answer to both is probably no, as long as exercise is done within reason.

Exercise Effects on the Fetus

The research to date on exercise and pregnancy is limited largely to animal experiments or human surveys. Exercise has been shown to decrease blood flow to the pregnant uterus.[47] However, the drop in blood flow is mainly restricted to the outer uterus (at least in goats).[30] Blood flow to the placenta is less reduced, and oxygen delivery to the fetus is probably unchanged.[38]

Other fetal factors that change during maternal exercise are temperature and blood glucose level. Temperature inside the uterus increases slightly with exercise and slowly returns to normal.[38] The significance of this change is unclear, but it is probably reasonable not to exercise heavily in conditions of environmental heat. It is important to avoid dehydration, which exacerbates heat stress. Blood glucose levels in the uterus rise slightly with exercise, though the increase is probably not clinically significant.

Data about the response of fetal heart rate to maternal exercise are conflicting and confusing. Fetal heart rate may decrease during strenuous exercise, but no frank evidence suggests any hypoxic stress on the developing fetus.[39]

In fact, no evidence suggests that mild-to-moderate exercise has any adverse effects on the developing fetus. Strenuous exercise at or above prepregnancy levels has not been shown to increase fetal mortality.[8,13,16] A study that reported decreased birth weight of infants and earlier delivery in women who exercised strenuously was not confirmed by other investigators,[8,16] and women who exercise may actually have less risk of preterm delivery than sedentary women.[8] It seems prudent for women with complications of pregnancy such as abnormal bleeding or hypertension and women with cardiopulmonary disease to avoid vigorous exercise (Table 2). Bouncing or jarring activities should probably also be avoided, especially near term. While pregnant, women should stay away from activities that predispose to abdominal trauma, and water skiing should be avoided. Women carrying twins may also be cautioned that the extra oxygen required by two fetuses may be compromised by overly vigorous exercise. For the great majority of healthy women, however, continued moderate activity such as biking, walking, and swimming are reasonable during pregnancy. Women who exercise typically have less excess weight gain, less deconditioning from a previously fit level, and improved psychological well-being. If they develop complications or symptoms that may be due to exercise, they should cease the activity and seek medical attention (Table 3).

There is no clear-cut limit for maximal heart rate or exercise intensity during pregnancy. The American College of Obstetri-

TABLE 3. Indications for Discontinuing Exercise*

Vaginal bleeding
Abdominal or pelvic pain
Chest pain
Severe shortness of breath
Palpitations
Headache
Tachycardia
Dizziness or lightheadedness
Nausea
Loss of muscle control

*Additional contraindications are left to the discretion of the physician. Data from the American College of Obstetricians and Gynecologists[4] and Revelli et al.[60]

cians and Gynecologists (ACOG)[4] recommends that the maximal heart rate during pregnancy should not exceed 140 beats/minute. They also recommend exercising 15 minutes or less, 3 times a week, with no bouncing or jarring motions. A meta analysis performed by Lokey et al.,[35] however, showed no change between the exercise and control groups in regard to maternal weight gain, gestation length, length of labor, birth weight, or Apgar scores, even in women who exceeded the ACOG guidelines. The authors found that even women who exercised on average up to 3 times a week for 43 minutes, achieving a heart rate of 144 beats/minute and performing bouncing activities, had no evidence of adverse effects. The heart rate of 140 beats/minute is probably quite conservative and could most likely be raised by 10 to 20 beats/minute, especially in women who were active prior to pregnancy. It is probably reasonable not to start new activities (except for a moderate walking program) during pregnancy.

Effects of Exercise on the Pregnant Mother

Pregnancy affects the body's response to exercise. Greater nonmuscular weight decreases exercise efficiency at any given load. Because a woman's metabolism increases with increasing gestational mass, greater cardiorespiratory effort is required for a given work load. Some training effect results from the pregnant state as the woman partially accommodates to the increased stress.

Blood volume increases during pregnancy, and cardiac output would be expected to rise. But the mechanical effect of the uterus pushing on the vena cava decreases venous blood return and may decrease stroke volume, espe-

TABLE 2. Contraindications to Exercise Training during Pregnancy*

Absolute contraindications
  Significant myocardial disease
  Pregnancy-induced hypertension
  Thromboembolic disease
  Active infection
  Ruptured membranes
  Multiple gestation
  Pelvic bleeding
  Fetal distress
  Placenta previa
  Incompetent cervix
  History of repeated miscarriage
  Intrauterine growth retardation
  Threatened premature delivery
Relative contraindications
  Hypertension
  Anemia or blood disorder
  Thyroid disease
  Diabetes
  Breech presentation in last trimester
  Excessive obesity
  Extreme underweight or malnutrition
  History of precipitous labor
  History of intrauterine growth retardation
  History of bleeding during pregnancy
  Extremely sedentary lifestyle

*Additional contraindications are left to the discretion of the physician. Data from the American College of Obstetricians and Gynecologists[4] and Revelli et al.[60]

cially during exercise.[48] The net effect is that exercise capacity is reduced. It is probably reasonable, especially during late pregnancy, not to exercise in the supine position, because the vena cava is most compressed while supine.

A nonpregnant woman responds to exercise by increasing cardiac output and systemic vascular resistance. Blood pressure rises. This response may be slightly greater in the pregnant woman.[48]

Pregnant women have mild changes in respiration compared with nonpregnant controls. Oxygen consumption at any active level, including rest, is greater. There is also a mild state of hyperventilation, but the pregnant woman's response to exercise is not significantly different from that in the nonpregnant state.[39] Pregnant women who are fit have a better capacity to carry out the workload of labor and delivery.[3]

Flexibility

A hormone called relaxin is produced in pregnant women. As its name suggests, it relaxes connective tissues and allows the pelvic bones to accommodate childbirth; it may also weaken some joints. During late pregnancy or the early postdelivery period, women should maintain their usual range of motion, but to avoid joint injury, they should not pursue a vigorous increase in flexibility.

Musculoskeletal and Back Pain

Pregnancy causes a number of mechanical changes in a woman's body. Larger breasts and abdomen change the center of gravity as well as the mechanical efficiency of the abdominal musculature and may predispose to back strain. About 50% of pregnant women develop backache,[7,42] which often is caused by dysfunction of the sacroiliac joint. The incidence of back pain increases with the age of the pregnant woman.[42] If back pain is severe during pregnancy, it often remains troublesome after delivery.[7] Back pain during pregnancy usually responds well to a period of relative rest.

Changes in posture and body habitus can lead to overuse syndromes and nerve compression. Water retention may predispose the woman to carpal tunnel syndrome or other compressive neuropathies.

No good evidence suggests that exercising women are more predisposed to developing pre- and postpartum musculoskeletal pain than sedentary women. It seems intuitively reasonable that a woman well-conditioned before pregnancy would tend to have a lower risk for such problems.

Heat

Excessive temperature rise in the pregnant uterus is believed to be harmful to the fetus and may have a teratogenic effect.[74] For this reason any deep heating agent such as ultrasound, microwave, or short-wave diathermy over the pregnant uterus is absolutely contraindicated. Therapies such as Hubbard tanks, which may raise core body temperature, are likewise contraindicated, along with steam rooms and saunas. Pregnant women also should be counseled not to undertake excessive physical activity in a hot climate to which they are not acclimated.

Medications

Before taking prescribed medication or over-the-counter drugs, a woman who is pregnant should be aware of the drugs' adverse effects. In general, most medications are best avoided, especially during early pregnancy.

Training After Delivery, Surgery, or Dilatation and Curettage

The following recommendations are made by Shangold.[70] They are to be viewed as the minimal waiting periods before resumption of activity, and only a few women are able to resume activity so quickly. Longer waits may improve healing but of course delay recovery of athletic ability. Exercise should not be pushed to the point of pain in the postpartum period or after dilatation and curettage. Shangold's[70] recommendations include:

1. After dilatation and curettage or first-trimester abortion, weight training and aerobic exercise, except water sports, may be resumed the same or the next day; water sports should be avoided until bleeding has ceased. Tampon use also should be avoided until bleeding has ceased.

2. After vaginal delivery or second-trimester abortion, weight training may be re-

sumed the same day; aerobic exercise, except water sports, may be resumed in 2 days; water sports may be resumed when bleeding has ceased. Tampon use should be avoided until bleeding has ceased.

3. After laparoscopy, aerobic exercise in and out of water and weight training may be resumed after 1 to 2 days.

4. After cesarean delivery or other abdominal surgery (requiring an incision), light aerobic exercise outside of water and light weight training may be resumed in 7 days; intense aerobic exercise (speed work), submaximal weight training, and water sports should be postponed at least 21 days.

GYNECOLOGIC ISSUES

Contraceptives

Contraceptive issues in women athletes are essentially the same as for nonathletes. Choices in contraception are individualized and based mainly on medical issues and lifestyle choices. Comfort during training may at times be affected by mechanical barriers such as diaphragms or sponges. Oral contraceptives have not been shown to have an adverse effect on athletic performance,[70] although they may reduce VO_{2max}.[53] A potential benefit of oral contraception in some women is that it may decrease anemia by reducing menstrual blood loss. It may also lower the risk of musculoskeletal injury by decreasing the effects of premenstrual syndrome.[46] In patients with ovulatory problems, oral contraceptives may help to prevent osteoporosis and subsequent fractures.[31]

Breasts

In the mid-1970s, Gillette[26] and Haycock[28] conducted surveys to investigate sports injuries in women. Both studies found that the overall injury profile was about the same for men and women and that breast injuries were the least common of all injuries. Because some women complain of breast pain during and after jogging and because of concern that jogging may accelerate breast sagging, research was undertaken to determine what type of breast support should be recom-

mended. Haycock found that women with a cup size of B or greater benefited from a supportive bra to reduce breast movement during running or bouncing activities. She recommends a firm, mostly nonelastic material that limits motion in all directions. Seams should be smooth and metal hooks covered. Lorentzon and Lawson[37] recommended a bra with nonelastic straps and a cup pad for contact sports. An underwire bra is also an option.

The influence of exercise on breast sagging is difficult to study because other factors contribute to sagging, including genetics, childbearing, and whether or not a woman has breast implants. Although no direct evidence suggests that exercise causes breast sagging, women in cultures that do not promote breast support seem to have more pendulous breasts.[70] It seems prudent to support the breasts during bouncing activities, especially if postexercise tenderness results.

Women with fibrocystic changes are predisposed to developing sore breasts during exercise. This condition is treated with a supportive bra and pain medication, as needed.

In contact sports or accidents the breast is sometimes traumatized. Minor bruising, which is the most common result, can be treated with compression, ice, and avoidance of further injury. If the skin is broken, it should be kept clean to avoid infection. Hematoma should be treated similarly, with ice and compression. If the hematoma increases in size, causes increased pain, or shows signs of infection, it may have to be surgically evacuated. Sometimes a hematoma may leave behind a hard lump or area of calcification. This condition is benign, but the lump may be removed for comfort and appearance. Serious breast trauma is rare, but in high-risk activities it may be prevented by adequate padding.

Recently the lay press has focused on the risks of breast implants. On rare occasions implants may be ruptured by trauma and are not recommended for women involved in contact sports. Because the implants increase nonmuscular body weight, they slightly reduce exercise efficiency. They also change breast movement during exercise and consequently are probably not to be recommended in elite athletes or in athletes who strive for their absolute best performance. Increased support may be necessary after implantation.

Nipple injury is seen in runners, both male and female, and is known simply as "runner's nipples." The nipples become irritated by the repetitive rubbing of clothing. Supportive care and prevention with a good bra are recommended. If the skin becomes abraded, a Band-Aid can be taped over the nipple. "Bicyclist's nipple" may be caused by exposure to cold. Supportive care with a warm covering is recommended.

Premenstrual Syndrome

Mood changes, headaches, and fluid retention occur in many women a few days before menstrual bleeding. Exercise does not appear to worsen the symptoms and in fact may lessen them.[52,59,77] Premenstrual syndrome (PMS) could impair athletic performance by affecting mood or by increasing body fluid.

Chronic Pelvic Pain

Women are more prone than men to developing chronic pelvic pain. Such pain is not necessarily more prevalent in athletes and may be less likely in active individuals. The causes are unknown but may include tension myalgia of the pelvic floor musculature, pelvic vein varicosities, and psychogenic expression.

Endometriosis

Endometriosis, a condition of abnormal abdominally located uterine tissue, is a relatively common cause of cyclic abdominal pain in women. The pain may first become manifest during exercise. Endometriosis is frequently well controlled by birth control pills, but it should always be evaluated by a gynecologist. Regular vigorous exercise, especially when started at a young age, may help to prevent the development of symptoms of endometriosis, possibly because of decreased estrogen production.[6,17]

MEDICAL ISSUES

Menopause and Osteoporosis

Menopause involves the cessation of the menstrual cycle with resultant loss of fertility. The medical effects are due to a decrease in circulating estrogen. Symptoms accompanying menopause include hot flashes and changes in mood and sleep habits. Atrophy of the vaginal mucosa may occur. In women, estrogen exerts a protective effect against atherosclerosis and coronary artery disease. When its production declines, women develop more cardiovascular disease. The decline also leads to osteoporosis, or loss of bone mass. Women at greatest risk for osteoporosis are white and thin and have had early menopause and few children. Smoking is a risk factor and possibly caffeine is also. Osteoporosis is a major health problem in elderly women. It leads to hip, wrist, and vertebral compression fractures.

Estrogen replacement therapy with a variant of the birth control pill is becoming increasingly popular as a method of preventing the effects of decreased estrogen production. Exercise is also useful.

The effects of aerobic exercise in maintaining cardiorespiratory fitness are well documented in men. There is no reason to believe that women will not also benefit from a lifetime of exercise. If started late in life, exercise should be initiated gradually and only after proper medical screening.

Bone mass begins to decline gradually after the age of 30 to 35 years. The decline is hastened by menopause. Thus, it is critical to have the maximal bone mass possible at approximately age 30 to 35 years. Weight-bearing exercise, such as running and walking, build up bone mass before this age and slow its decline afterward. Ideally women should exercise early in life to build bone and later in life to keep it strong. Exercise has been shown to increase the mineral content of vertebral[34] and arm[72] bone. The bone content is increased by both weight-bearing and other resistance exercise that stresses the bone.[54] It is best increased by a combination of aerobic and weight-training exercises rather than by weight-training alone.[9]

Once osteoporosis has developed, women should still be encouraged to exercise, except, of course, while an acute fracture is healing. Even in older women, light weight-bearing exercises such as walking are safe and effective.[75] Exercises that involve jarring motions and flexion of the spine should be avoided.

Nutrition

Nutritional requirements for women are essentially the same as for men with the exception of iron and calcium. Both men and women should eat a normal, varied diet, not too high in fat. No evidence suggests that female athletes need special diet supplements or vitamins.

Iron Status and Anemia

Because of iron loss during menstrual bleeding, menstruating women require 50% more dietary iron than men. Because iron is not as readily absorbed by the body as many other minerals and vitamins, women tend to become iron-deficient.

Women typically have lower blood levels of hemoglobin and are at greater risk for iron-deficiency anemia than men. One study of the bone marrow aspirates of college women revealed total body iron depletion in 25%.[66] Other studies have suggested that athletes, especially long distance runners, may have low iron stores.[14,76,82] Up to 40% to 50% of adolescent female athletes have iron depletion.[62] Athletes lose iron in sweat, through gastrointestinal blood loss,[44,76] and through hematuria and rhabdomyolysis. They may also have decreased iron absorption[29] and may ingest less iron[43] than nonathletes.

Iron deficiency has been shown in animal studies to impair muscular performance in endurance exercise. Iron deficiency, even without anemia, may cause animals to tire earlier.[21,22,50] The reduction in exercise tolerance is due to the depletion of iron-containing mitochondrial enzymes, which leads to increased lactic acid production.[21] When the deficiency becomes severe, anemia is the result. Anemia decreases the oxygen-carrying capacity of blood and impairs performance even further. In humans, iron repletion in a deficient athlete has been shown to decrease lactate production.[50] No change in $\dot{V}O_{2max}$ has been noted.

Iron-deficiency anemia must be differentiated from so-called "sports anemia," in which iron stores are normal. Exercise increases blood volume. If the mass of red blood cells remains constant, an increase in blood volume results in hemodilution, creating a false impression of anemia. This transient phenomenon is easily differentiated from the long-term anemia of iron deficiency by measuring body stores of iron.

All women need to ingest adequate amounts of iron. In athletes this is especially important to maximize performance. If iron deficiency is detected, a medical evaluation is indicated to rule out any worrisome sources of blood loss.

Calcium

To develop optimal bone strength and mass and to ward off osteoporosis, women need adequate amounts of calcium in the diet, estrogen in the blood stream, and weight-bearing exercise in their lifestyle. Estrogen is by far the most important of the three factors, but adequate intake of calcium is also essential. Exercise, though of lesser benefit by itself, acts synergistically with estrogen to develop bone strength.

Many women have inadequate dietary intake of calcium. This is especially so in women who shy away from dairy products for health reasons or because they do not tolerate them and in women with low levels of circulating estrogen. Estrogen aids in the absorption of calcium from the gastrointestinal tract. Thus, postmenopausal women or women with hypo-estrogenic amenorrhea should ingest even more calcium than euestrogenic women to compensate for poorer absorption. Adequate calcium intake, with supplements if necessary, is recommended for all women.

Gastrointestinal Issues

A number of gastrointestinal symptoms occur in athletes, especially in long-distance runners. Women typically report more such symptoms than men.[33] Lower gastrointestinal tract complaints are most common and occur in up to one-half of the high-level long-distance athletes who have been surveyed. The urge to have a bowel movement is most common.[49] Others have diarrhea, either during or after an event; bloody bowel movements may also occur. Occult blood loss detected by stool guaiac or Hemoccult testing has also been described.[44,76] It usually occurs within 36 hours of extreme exertion and resolves within 72 hours. If anemia is present, further medical evaluation is warranted.

Upper gastrointestinal tract symptoms can include nausea, vomiting, heartburn, bloating, and loss of appetite. These symptoms may occur in up to 35% or more of high-level athletes.[33,49,61] The symptoms are usually mild and self-limited; they often resolve with time or with a slight reduction in activity.

Hematuria

Hematuria induced by strenuous activity was first described in 1878 in soldiers. It can follow any vigorous sports activity, either traumatic or nontraumatic, and occurs with equal frequency in men and women.[10] After 1 marathon, 17% of the participants had hematuria and 30% had proteinuria.[10] In other reports, an incidence of hematuria from 50% to 80% has been noted following vigorous athletic activity.[1] The hematuria induced by exercise is most often microscopic, but sometimes it is gross. Etiology is unknown, but it may be due to such factors as hypoxic damage to the kidneys, kidney trauma, or bladder trauma. Such hematuria is almost always benign and self-limiting and usually resolves within 72 hours. Myoglobinuria, due to rhabdomyolyis, is also common after hard exercise. It may also occur as a result of red blood cell damage from foot-impact trauma in runners.[45] It too can cause urine to turn red. The condition is usually benign but occasionally may be life-threatening if it leads to renal failure. The kidneys of patients with compromised renal function may not tolerate vigorous exercise because of increased hemoglobin and myoglobin loads.

Drug Abuse

Men have received most of the attention of using illegal drugs to enhance performance, but the problem also exists among women. Anabolic steroids, like male sex hormones, help to increase muscle mass, but the price is quite high. They can have serious side effects such as heart and liver disease, personality change, increased hair growth, and clitoral enlargement. Steroids have no place in legitimate athletics, and their use should be highly discouraged. Stimulants such as amphetamines may increase subjective energy and heighten attention. They lead to dependence, produce lifestyle and personality changes, and may destroy an athlete's career.

CONCERNS IN PREBUESCENT AND ADOLESCENT FEMALE ATHLETES

Eating Disorders

Women are more likely to develop eating disorders than men. Adolescent girls are especially at risk. The prevalence of anorexia nervosa in adolescent girls is about 0.5% to 1%, and bulimia is present in approximately 10% of college women.[27] Both of these conditions are signs of significant psychologic dysfunction and can result in severe physiologic disturbance—even in death. Women in sports such as gymnastics and ballet may have an alarmingly high incidence of eating disorders. They should receive prompt treatment and counseling by a professional when they exhibit signs such as an abnormal preoccupation with food, weight, and body image.

No evidence suggests that exercise by itself is a cause of eating disorders, but women with such disorders may increase their exercise level in an attempt to lose weight.

Delayed Menarche

Delayed menarche has been associated with athletic participation.[18,23,25,40,41] Menarche occurs later in athletes and later in girls who start training before menarche[23,40] (Figs. 2 and 3). For each year of vigorous premenar-

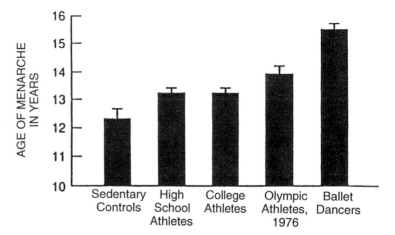

FIGURE 2. Menarcheal delay in athletes compared with controls. (From Gidwani GP: The athlete and menstruation. *Adolesc Med State Art Rev* 2:27–45, 1991; with permission.)

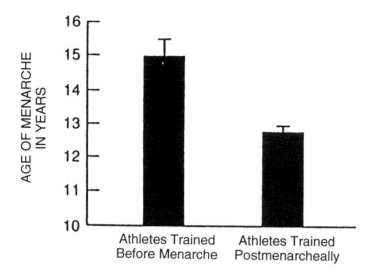

FIGURE 3. Age at menarche in girls who trained before menarche versus those that started exercise after menarche. (From Gidwani GP: The athlete and menstruation. *Adoles Med State Art Rev* 2:27–45, 1991; with permission.)

cheal training, menarche may be delayed by up to 5 months.[23] Whether the delay is due to exercise or whether girls with delayed menstruation are more drawn to athletics is unknown. It has also been postulated that exercise may delay the attainment of the critical fat percentage required to begin menstruation.[24] By delaying menarche, exercise may also cause girls to grow more and thus to attain a greater height, which may make them better athletes. In any case, the delay is not usually more than a few months to a year and almost always well within the normal age range for menarche. Delayed menarche is not generally considered harmful,[3] but it may increase the risk of developing stress fractures or scoliosis.[79,80] The ACOG recommends that if thelarche or pubarche has not begun by age 14 years or if menarche has not begun by age 16 years, a medical evaluation is in order.[3]

REFERENCES

1. Abarbanel J, Benet AE, Lask D, et al: Sports hematuria. *J Urol* 143:887–890, 1990.
2. Abraham SF, Beumont PJV, Fraser IS, et al: Body weight, exercise and menstrual status among ballet dancers in training. *Br J Obstet Gynaecol* 89:507–510, 1982.
3. American College of Obstetricians and Gynecologists: *Technical Bulletin: Women and Exercise.* Washington, DC, ACOG, 1985.
4. American College of Obstetricians and Gynecologists: *Exercise during Pregnancy and the Postnatal Period.* Washington, DC, ACOG, 1985.
5. Artal R: Exercise and pregnancy. *Clin Sports Med* 11:363–377, 1992.
6. Barbieri RL: Etiology and epidemiology of endometriosis. *Am J Obstet Gynecol* 162:565–567, 1990.
7. Berg G, Hammar M, Moller-Nielsen J, et al: Low back pain during pregnancy. *Obstet Gynecol* 71:71–75, 1988.
8. Berkowitz GS, Kelsey JL, Holford TR, et al: Physical activity and the risk of spontaneous preterm delivery. *J Reprod Med* 28:581–588, 1983.
9. Block JE, Genant HK, Black D: Greater vertebral bone mineral mass in exercising young men. *West J Med* 145:39–42, 1986.
10. Boileau M, Fuchs E, Barry JM, et al: Stress hematuria: athletic pseudonephritis in marathoners. *Urology* 15:471–474, 1980.
11. Brooks-Gunn J, Gargiulo J, Warren MP. The menstrual cycle and athletic performance. In Puhl JL, Brown CH (eds): *The Menstrual Cycle and Physical Activity.* Champaign, IL, Human Kinetics Publishers, 1986.
12. Cavanaugh DJ, Kanonchoff AD, Bartels RL: Menstrual irregularities in athletic women may be predictable based on pre-training menses. *J Sports Med Phys Fitness* 29(2):163–169, 1989.
13. Clapp JF III, Dickerson S: Endurance exercise and pregnancy outcome. *Med Sci Sports Exerc* 16:556–562, 1984.
14. Clement DB, Asmundson RC: Nutritional intake and hematological parameters in endurance runners. *Phys Sportsmed* 10(3):37–43, 1982.
15. Cokkinades VE, Macera CA, Pate RR: Menstrual dysfunction among habitual runners. *Women Health* 16(2):59–69, 1990.
16. Collings CA, Curet LB, Mullin JP: Maternal and fetal responses to a maternal aerobic exercise program. *Am J Obstet Gynecol* 145:702–707, 1983.
17. Cramer DW, Wilson E, Stillman RJ, et al: The relation of endometriosis to menstrual characteristics, smoking, and exercise. *JAMA* 255:1904–1908, 1986.
18. Dale E, Gerlach DH, Wilhite AL: Menstrual dysfunction in distance runners. *Obstet Gynecol* 54:47–53, 1979.
19. Drinkwater BL, Nilson K, Chestnut CH, et al: Bone mineral content of amenorrheic and eumenorrheic athletes. *N Engl J Med* 311:277–281, 1984.
20. Feicht CB, Johnson TS, Martin BJ, et al: Secondary amenorrhea in athletes [letter]. *Lancet* ii:1145–1146, 1978.

21. Finch CA, Gollnick PD, Hlastala MP, et al: Lactic acidosis as a result of iron deficiency. *J Clin Invest* 64:129–137, 1979.
22. Finch CA, Miller LR, Inamder AR, et al: Iron deficiency in the rat. Physiological and biochemical studies on muscle dysfunction. *J Clin Invest* 58:447–453, 1976.
23. Frisch RE, Gotz-Welbergen AV, McArthur JW, et al: Delayed menarche and amenorrhea of college athletes in relation to age of onset of training. *JAMA* 246:1559–1563, 1981.
24. Frisch RE, McArthur JW: Menstrual cycles: Fatness as a determinant of minimum weight for height necessary for their maintenance or onset. *Science* 185:949–951, 1974.
25. Frisch R, Wyshak G, Vincent L: Delayed menarche and amenorrhea in ballet dancers. *N Engl J Med* 303:17–19, 1980.
26. Gillette JV: When and where women are injured in sports. *Phys Sportsmed* 3(5):61–63, 1975.
27. Gordon RA: Anorexia and bulimia. *Anatomy of a Social Epidemic*. Oxford, Basil Blackwell, Oxford Press, 1990.
28. Haycock CE, Gillette JV: Susceptibility of women athletes to injury: Myths vs. reality. *JAMA* 236:163–165, 1976.
29. Haymes EM, Spillman DM: Iron status of women distance runners, sprinters, and control women. *Int J Sports Med* 10:430–433, 1989.
30. Hohimer AR, Bissonnette JM, Metcalf J, et al: Effect of exercise on uterine blood flow in the pregnant Pygmy goat. *Am J Physiol* 246:H206–H212, 1984.
31. Kanders B, Lindsey R, Dempster D, et al: Determinants of bone mass in young healthy women. In Christiansen et al (eds): *Osteoporosis: Proceedings of the Copenhagen International Symposia on Osteoporosis*. 1984, pp 337–339.
32. Katch FI, Spiak DL: Validity of the Mellits and Cheek method for body-fat estimation in relation to menstrual cycle status in athletes and non-athletes below 22 percent fat. *Ann Human Biol* 11:389–396, 1984.
33. Keeffe EB, Lowe DK, Goss JR, et al: Gastrointestinal symptoms of marathon runners. *West J Med* 141:481–484, 1984.
34. Krolner B, Toft B, Pors Nielsen S, et al: Physical exercise as prophylaxis against involutional vertebral bone loss: A controlled trial. *Clin Sci* 64:541–546, 1983.
35. Lokey EA, Tran ZV, Wells CL, et al: Effects of physical exercise on pregnancy outcomes: A meta-analytic review. *Med Sci Sports Exerc* 23:1234–1239, 1991.
36. Lloyd T, Triantafyllou SJ, Baker ER, et al: Women athletes with menstrual irregularity have increased musculoskeletal injuries. *Med Sci Sports Exerc* 18 374–379, 1986.
37. Lorentzen D, Lawson L: Selected sports bra: A biomechanical analysis of breast motion while jogging. *Phys Sportsmed* 15(5):128–139, 1987.
38. Lotgering FK, Gilbert RD, Longo LD: Exercise responses in pregnant sheep: Blood gases, temperatures and fetal cardiovascular system. *J Appl Physiol* 55(3):842–850, 1983.
39. Lotgering FK, Gilbert RD, Longo LD: Maternal and fetal responses to exercise during pregnancy. *Physiol Rev* 65:1–36, 1985.
40. Malina RM: Menarche in athletes: A synthesis and hypothesis. *Ann Hum Biol* 10:1–24, 1983.
41. Malina RM, Spirduso WW, Tate C, et al: Age at menarche and selected menstrual characteristics in athletes at different competitive levels and in different sports. *Med Sci Sports* 10:218–222, 1978.
42. Mantel MJ, Greenwood RM, Currey HLF: Backache in pregnancy. *Rheumatol Rehab* 16:95–101, 1977.
43. Martin DE, Vroon DH, May DF, et al: Physiological changes in elite male distance runners training for olympic competition. *Phys Sportsmed* 14(1):152–171, 1986.
44. McMahon LF, Jr., Ryan MJ, Larson D, et al: Occult gastrointestinal blood loss in marathon runners. *Ann Intern Med* 100:846–847, 1984.
45. Miller BJ, Pate RR, Burgess W: Foot impact force and intravascular hemolysis during distance running. *Int J Sports Med* 9:56–60, 1988.
46. Möller-Nielsen J, Hammer M: Women's soccer injuries in relation to the menstrual cycle and oral contraceptives. *Med Sci Sports Exerc* 21:126–129, 1989.
47. Morris N, Osborn SB, Wright HP, et al: Effective uterine blood flow during exercise in normal and preeclamptic pregnancies. *Lancet* 2:481–484, 1956.
48. Morton MJ, Paul MS, Campos GR, et al: Exercise dynamics in late gestation: Effects of physical training. *Am J Obstet Gynecol* 152:91–97, 1985.
49. Moses FM: The effect of exercise on the gastrointestinal tract. *Sports Med* 9(3):159–172, 1990.
50. Nilson K, Schoene RB, Robertson HT, et al: The effects of iron repletion on exercise-induced lactate production in minimally iron-deficient subjects [abstract]. *Med Sci Sports Exerc* 13(2):92, 1981.
51. Noel GL, Suh HK, Stone JG, et al: Human prolactin and growth hormone release during surgery and other conditions of stress. *J Clin Endocrinol Metab* 35:840–851, 1972.
52. Norris RV, Sullivan C: *PMS, Premenstrual Syndrome*. New York, Rawson Associates, 1983, p 225.
53. Notelovitz M, Zauner C, McKenzie L, et al: The effect of low-dose contraceptives on cardiorespiratory function, coagulation, and lipids in exercising young women: A preliminary report. *Am J Obstet Gynecol* 156:591–598, 1987.
54. Orwoll ES, Ferar J, Oviatt SK, et al: Swimming exercise and bone mass. In Christianson C, Johanson JS, Riis RJ (eds): *Osteoporosis*. Viborg, Sweden, Norhaven A/S, 1987, pp 494–498.
55. Pettersson F, Fries H, Nillius SJ: Epidemiology of secondary amenorrhea. Incidence and prevalence rates. *Am J Obstet Gynecol* 117:80–86, 1973.
56. Pirke KM, Schweiger U, Laessle R, et al: Dieting influences the menstrual cycle: Vegetarian versus nonvegetarian diet. *Fertil Steril* 46:1083–1088, 1986.
57. Prior JC, Caneron K, Ho Yuen B, et al: Menstrual cycle changes with marathon training: Anovulation and short luteal phase. *Can J Ap Sport Sci* 7(3):173–177, 1982.
58. Prior JC, Jensen L, Ho Yuen B, et al: Prolactin changes with exercise vary with breast motion: analysis of running vs. cycling [abstract]. *Fertil Steril* 36:268, 1981.
59. Prior JC, Vigna Y, Alojada N: Conditioning exercise decreases premenstrual symptoms: A prospective controlled three month trial. *Eur J Appl Physiol* 55:349–355, 1986.
60. Revelli A, Durando A, Massobrio M: Exercise and pregnancy: A review of maternal and fetal effects. *Obstet Gynecol Surv* 47 (6):355–367, 1992.

61. Riddich C, Trinick T: Gastrointestinal disturbances in marathon runners. *Br J Sports Med* 22:71–74, 1988.

62. Rowland TW: Iron deficiency in the young athlete. *Pediatr Clin North Am* 37:1153–1163, 1990.

63. Sanborn CF, Martin BJ, Wagner WW: Is athletic amenorrhea specific to runners? *Am J Obstet Gynecol* 143:859–861, 1982.

64. Schwartz B, Cumming DC, Riordan E, et al: Exercise associated amenorrhea: A distinct entity? *Am J Obstet Gynecol* 141:662–670, 1981.

65. Schweiger U, Laessle R, Pfister H, et al: Diet-induced menstrual irregularities: Effects of age and weight loss. *Fertil Steril* 48:746–751, 1987.

66. Scott DE, Pritchard JA: Iron deficiency in healthy young college women. *JAMA* 199:897–900, 1967.

67. Shangold MM: Sports and menstrual function. *Phys Sportsmed* 8:66–70, 1980.

68. Shangold M, Freeman R, Thysen B, et al: The relationship between long distance running, plasma progesterone and luteal phase length. *Fertil Steril* 31:130–133, 1979.

69. Shangold MM, Levine HS: The effect of marathon training upon menstrual function. *Am J Obstet Gynecol* 143:862–869, 1982.

70. Shangold MM, Mirkin G (eds): *Women and Exercise. Physiology and Sports Medicine.* Philadelphia, F.A. Davis, 1988.

71. Shangold M, Rebar RW, Wentz AC, et al: Evaluation and management of menstrual dysfunction in athetes. *JAMA* 263:1665–1669, 1990.

72. Simkin A, Ayalon J, Leichter I: Increased trabecular bone density due to bone-loading exercises in post-menopausal osteoporotic women. *Calcif Tissue Int* 40:59–63, 1987.

73. Sinaki M, Mikkelsen BA: Postmenopausal spinal osteoporosis: Flexion versus extension exercises. *Arch Phys Med Rehabil* 65:593–596, 1984.

74. Smith DW, Clarren SK, Harvey MA: Hyperthermia as a possible teratogenic agent. *J Pediatr* 92:878–883, 1978.

75. Smith EL Jr, Reddan W, Smith PE: Physical activity and calcium modalities for bone mineral increase in aged women. *Med Sci Sports Exerc* 13(1):60–64, 1981.

76. Stewart JG, Ahlquist DA, McGill DB, et al: Gastrointestinal blood loss and anemia in runners. *Ann Intern Med* 100:843–845, 1984.

77. Timonen S, Procope BJ: Premenstrual syndrome and physical exercise. *Acta Obstet Gynecol Scand* 50:331–337, 1971.

78. Wakat DK, Sweeney KA, Rogol AD: Reproductive system function in women cross country runners. *Med Sci Sports Exerc* 14(4):263–269, 1982.

79. Warren MP: The effects of exercise on pubertal progression and reproductive function in girls. *J Clin Endocrinol Metab* 51:1150–1157, 1980.

80. Warren MP, Brooks-Gunn J, Hamilton LH, et al: Scoliosis and fractures in young ballet dancers. Relation to delayed menarche and secondary amenorrhea. *N Engl J Med* 314:1348–1353, 1986.

81. White CM, Hergenroeder AC: Amenorrhea, osteopenia, and the female athlete. *Pediatr Clin* 37:1125–1141, 1990.

82. Wishnitzer R, Vorst E, Berrebi A: Bone marrow iron depression in competitive distance runners. *Int J Sports Med* 4(1):27–30, 1983.

Chapter 19

THE WHEELCHAIR ATHLETE

Leslie K. Schutz, MD

Members of the medical profession concerned with the treatment of deformities have always included physical exercise in the protocols. Galen (200 AD) was among the first advocates of medical "gymnastics." Maimonides, a famous medieval Jewish physician and a follower of Galen, wrote in his *Treatise of Hygiene* in 1199 AD, "Anyone who lives a sedentary life and does not exercise even if he eats good foods and takes care of himself according to proper medical principles—all his days will be painful ones and his strength shall wane."

With the increase in popularity of sports in the last 30 years and the development of sports medicine, it has become more widely recognized that even a major physical impairment may not necessarily preclude high-level performance in sports. This assumes that the disabled person has engaged in systematic training to mobilize and utilize his or her remaining abilities to compensate for the impairment.

The large number of disabled veterans after the Second World War provided the impetus for using team sports as an aid to rehabilitation. A pioneer in this effort was Sir Ludwig Guttman, a renowned neurosurgeon who trained in Germany and then left for Britain in 1938. In 1944 Guttman opened the National Spinal Injury Center at Stoke Mandeville Hospital in Aylesbury, England. There he introduced sports as medical treatment to paraplegics injured by war.[8] Shortly thereafter, other countries started their own sports clubs and competitions for people disabled by blindness, deafness, amputations, and paralysis. Ever since, sports have played an important role in the physical, psychological, and social rehabilitation of the physically disabled.

Sports not only increase physical fitness and skills, but also provide social interaction and motivation. In addition, sporting activities provide self-confidence and emotional stability both from pride in winning and from acceptance of losing as a part of life. Physicians and allied health personal are in a unique position to foster these attitudes. In addition, they must be aware of the medical problems and injuries associated with the wheelchair athlete. An understanding of the types, incidence, risks, prevention, and treatment of these injuries is vital for the enhancement of wheelchair sports at all levels.

The variety of athletic events available today for wheelchair athletes is remarkable. The choices include air-gun marksmanship and archery, basketball, bowling, football, racquetball, road-racing, rugby, track and field, winter sports such as skiing and slalom, softball, swimming, tennis, table tennis, weightlifting, and even mountaineering and scuba diving.[2,15,16] Many associations have been formed to organize both local and national competition in each of these sports and to further encourage their members to participate at a variety of skill levels (see Appendix A).

CLASSIFICATION

Classification systems for wheelchair athletes are used to promote fair competition. Emphasis on functional classification at international meets appears necessary to allow athletes with different diagnoses but similar dysfunction to compete in individual sports. Table 1 shows all current classification systems for adult and junior wheelchair sports.[11]

TABLE 1. International Wheelchair Sports Classification Systems

WHEELCHAIR COMPETITION

Spinal Cord Function	ISMGF	Adult Classification Functional[j] Track	Functional[j] Field	Junior Classification (USA only)	Cerebral Palsy	Les Autres	Amputee	Blind
C_4 C_5 C_6 C_7 C_8	IA 1B IC	T_1 T_2	F_1 F_2 F_3	J_1 Quadriplegic athlete with reduced function of arms/hands and zero sitting balance	CP_3 moderate involvement of 3 or 4 limbs, fair functional strength, and moderate control problems in upper extremities and trunk	L_1 wheelchair athlete with reduced functioning, mobility & balance	Ag combined upper and lower amputations	
T_1 T_2 T_3 T_4 T_5 T_6 T_7	II	T_3	F_4	J_2 high paraplegics with zero to poor sitting balance and normal upper extremities	CP_4 good upper extremity strength and minimal control problems of the trunk	L_2 wheelchair athlete with poor to moderate balance and a dominant arm or hand		
T_8 T_9 T_{10} T_{11} T_{12} L_1	III IV	T_4	F_5			L_3 wheelchair athlete with good balance	$A_{1,2,3,4}$ (competing without prosthesis)	
L_2 L_3 L_4 L_5 S_1 S_2	V VI		F_6 F_7	J_3 Lower paraplegics and all others with fair to normal sitting balance				

From Johnstone KS, et al: Sports for the handicapped child. *Phys. Med Rehabil State Art Rev* 5: 331–350, 1991, with permission.

BENEFITS AND COMPLICATIONS OF EXERCISE

Much has been studied and written about the benefits of exercise in sports. Investigators during the past 20 years also have looked at the positive effects of training in wheelchair athletes, which include an average improvement of 20% in maximal oxygen uptake ($\dot{V}O_{2max}$),[10] reduction of cardiovascular disease and respiratory infection,[1] improved self-image,[13] and fewer disturbances of psychological function compared with their less active counterparts.[7] It also has been shown that the mean number of hospitalizations per year was almost three times greater for paraplegic nonathletes compared with paraplegic athletes when all other demographics are similar.[24]

Additional studies have looked at the negative effects of sporting activities associated with wheelchair use, including medical illness and complications as well as sports-specific injuries.[2,5,17,18,23,24] Certainly, many variables contribute to each athlete's performance in sports, including genetics, age, sex, preserved motor and sensory function, nutrition, experience, practice, coaching, and training effects. Unfortunately, even in ideal situations, complications of exercise may arise. Even outstanding wheelchair athletes are at risk for both physical and emotional injury when they maximally stress their bodies and minds during training and competition.

INJURIES

Injuries and medical complications can be divided into three categories: mechanical, environmental, and impairment-related. Each can occur singularly or in combination with the others.

Mechanical Injuries

Sports requiring high speed and quick maneuvering of the wheelchair, or sports susceptible to contact with other objects or participating athletes, are most likely to cause mechanical injuries. Such sports include basketball, track and field, rugby, road-racing and skiing events. Sporting activities with less mechanical risk for injury include archery, bowling, pool, and table tennis.

Fortunately, major injuries such as bone fractures are rare. They may, however, disproportionately affect the already impaired athlete and cause a significant decline in function. Coaches, trainers, and physicians, as well as wheelchair athletes, should be familiar with the potential risks of such injuries.

The most prevalent mechanical injuries afflicting wheelchair athletes involve the soft tissues.[17,18] Muscle strains, ligamentous sprains, bursitis, and tendinitis are most common and primarily affect the upper extremities. The shoulder, elbow, and wrist are subject to overwork syndromes as a result of wheelchair propulsion. Kearney defines overwork as "an acute phase during which the training load, either volume or intensity, is significantly increased and produces a short-term deterioration of performance capabilities."[12] Regardless of the motion used for propulsion (shuttle-type in sprint athletes and circular pattern in distance competitors), many athletes still make unnecessary arm movements.[9,23] Hence, mechanical efficiency can be lost at the expense of soft-tissue anatomic structures.

Wheelchair athletes are particularly prone to develop pathologic conditions of the shoulder. Relying heavily on the upper extremities for mobility, they are unable to maintain nor-

mal dynamic patterns of motion. Increased energy is transmitted to the joint (shoulder) closest to the fixed structure (thorax). As a result, impingement syndromes and rotator cuff tendinitis may easily develop. Overhead sports such as basketball, shot put, discus, and swimming are especially aggravating to such conditions. Seldom does a frank tear of the rotator cuff occur without substantial force. Individuals who are older, with weak musculature of the rotator cuff, or who have not participated in a regular stretching program are at increased risk for a tear.

Magnified upper-extremity forces due to a fixed body can also be transmitted to the musculotendinous origins and insertions about the elbow and wrist. Consequently, medial and lateral epicondylitis as well as de Quervain's tenosynovitis can occur. These entities are more common in athletes with quadriplegia or poliomyelitis who have underlying muscular imbalance in the upper extremities.

Tearing and over-stretching of ligaments and musculotendinous structures can also occur as a result of falls or physical contact in the more aggressive sports. Skin abrasions, lacerations, and blisters frequently result from shear and frictional forces, due primarily to contact with the wheelchair seat back, brakes, push rims, or wheels. Figure 1 illustrates an abrasion of the biceps; Figure 2, thumb blisters. Both resulted from frictional contact with the wheelchair. Figure 3 depicts an elbow laceration in an athlete who collided with another wheelchair during competition. Figure 4 illustrates trochanteric

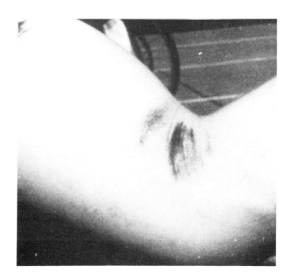

FIGURE 1. Biceps abrasion (photo courtesy of K. Johnstone).

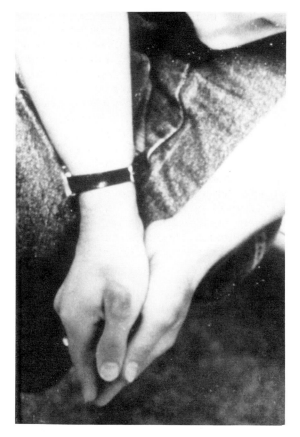

FIGURE 2. Thenar blisters (photo courtesy of K. Johnstone).

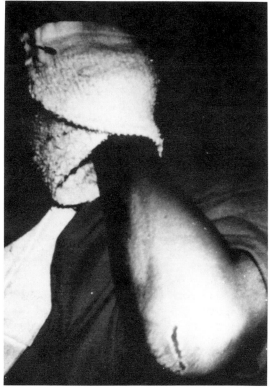

FIGURE 3. Elbow laceration (photo courtesy of K. Johnstone).

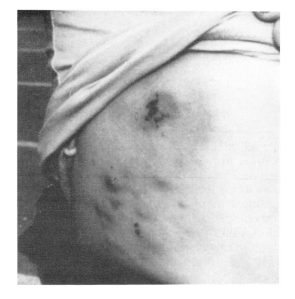

FIGURE 4. Trochanteric blisters (photo courtesy of K. Johnstone).

blisters due to body motion in a tight-fitting wheelchair. Although these injuries may seem relatively minor, they may have significant functional impact on an athlete. In addition, they may cause increased morbidity in athletes with insensate skin compared with athletes who have normal sensory function.

Nerve entrapment injuries of the upper extremities may occur in the wheelchair athlete and are believed to be exacerbated or caused by repetitive motions.[2] Athletes may complain of hand numbness and weakness as a result of median nerve compression at the wrist (carpal tunnel syndrome). This syndrome is typically caused by a repetitive pressure of the heel of the hand on the wheelchair push rim during each arm stroke. Median nerve entrapment may occur at various sites about the elbow, including the ligament of Struthers, lacertus fibrosus, and pronator teres.[4] Ulnar nerve entrapment at the elbow and wrist also may occur as a result of cumulative trauma. Radial tunnel syndrome occurs rarely, but it should be considered in recalci-

trant cases of lateral epicondylitis.[14] Electrodiagnostic testing should be ordered for confirmation of these injuries.

Treatment of mechanical injuries requires individualization. Each athlete should be given appropriate rest, anti-inflammatory medication, cold and heat modalities, stretching and strengthening exercises, and occasional steroid injections for inflamed joints or soft-tissue structures. Surgical release for entrapment neuropathies may be indicated in cases recalcitrant to splinting and conservative care.

Environmental Disorders

Environmental disorders seen in wheelchair athletics result primarily from abnormal thermoregulation in athletes with spinal cord injury, who have a reduced ability to tolerate extremes in temperature (hot and cold). This is due to loss of autonomic control over the vasomotor and sudomotor responses in the areas of insensate skin. In addition, persons with spinal cord injury have a reduced thermoregulatory effector response for a given core temperature and a loss of skeletal muscle pump activity from the paralyzed limbs. These factors contribute to an increased risk of hyperthermia and hypothermia.

Sawka[19] has described the differences in heat exchange for individuals performing upper-body exercise as opposed to the lower body. Upper-body exercise involves greater dry heat loss from the torso and no additional loss from the upper extremities.[19] If, for example, a paralyzed swimmer performs upper-body exercise in cold water, susceptibility to hypothermia is greater because of excessive heat loss. Similar situations apply to wheelchair athletes competing in cool air temperatures.

In athletes with spinal cord injury, vasomotor paralysis below the level of lesion and blood pooling in the lower extremities contribute to hypovolemia. The combination of hypovolemia and dehydration is a significant risk factor for hyperthermia, because there is a linear increase in core temperature with increasing dehydration.[20] Adequate hydration is thus vital for all wheelchair athletes in both warm and cold environments.

Impairment-Specific Injuries

The last category consists of injuries and medical complications related to wheelchair sports are impairment-specific. Most are reported in athletes with spinal cord injury. One such complication is autonomic dysreflexia, a syndrome manifested by headache, piloerection, sweating, paroxysmal hypertension, and bradycardia due to generalized sympathetic hyperactivity brought on by a noxious stimulus below the level of the lesion.[3] Provoking factors include a distended bowel or bladder, pressure ulcer, urinary tract infection, or tight-fitting clothing. Every effort should be made to remove the offending stimulus. The athlete should cease physical activity, be positioned with the head elevated, and be observed closely for progression of symptoms. Fortunately, most cases respond to immediate conservative management, but the potential is present for a medical emergency requiring hospitalization. Medications may be required to control the resulting hypertension, which can be life-threatening.

Pressure ulcers are a significant source of morbidity in athletes with spinal cord injury. Contributing factors include not only impaired sensation and motor function, but prolonged periods of unrelieved pressure during competition, skin moisture, and shearing forces created over the skin of the sacrum, ischial tuberosities, and greater trochanters. The design of racing wheelchairs—with the knees positioned higher than the buttocks—also creates increased pressure over the bony prominences, thus placing them at risk for breakdown (Fig. 5).

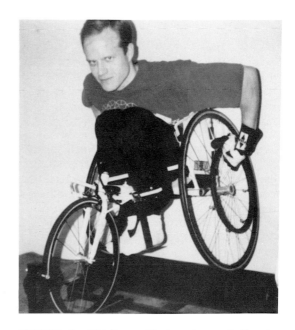

FIGURE 5. Athletic positioning demonstrating increased forces over ischial tuberosities in a racing wheelchair.

Urinary tract infections have been reported by wheelchair athletes with spinal cord injury.[18] Prolonged positioning in a wheelchair during competition, failure to empty the bladder in a timely fashion, or prolonged use of an indwelling catheter to compete without worry of incontinence may contribute to this problem.

Wheelchair athletes with amputated limbs or previously diagnosed poliomyelitis also have impairment-related injuries. Amputees are at risk for skin trauma to the residual limb unless it is properly protected with padding. Athletes with polio may be plagued by excessive fatigue and muscle imbalance between agonistic and antagonistic groups, which places them at risk for mechanical injuries. Fortunately, sensation is preserved in these athletes, enabling them to recognize skin problems in a timely fashion.

INJURY PREVENTION

Health care professionals, trainers, and coaches who work with wheelchair athletes should always stress the importance of injury prevention. Certainly, this begins with an appropriate training program that combines flexibility, strengthening, and endurance exercises to ensure adequate preparation for competition. Attention must be paid to the functioning of the upper-extremity musculoskeletal structures, which provide the majority of power and work in all sports. Trunk and back strengthening and flexibility programs are necessary for establishing stability in wheelchair positioning and propulsion, especially in track and field, road racing, rugby, basketball, and racquetball.

Wheelchair athletes themselves must be vigilant to obtain adequate rest, nutrition, and hydration at all levels of competition. All practices and competitions should be preceded by careful stretching and warm-up and followed by stretching and cool-down. These activities enhance extensibility of soft-tissue structures for prevention of sprains and strains. Appropriate personal hygiene, including bowel and bladder management, are mandatory for prevention of autonomic dysreflexia and urinary tract infections. Careful skin surveillance and frequent position changes in the wheelchair are necessary for the avoidance of pressure ulcers. Intentional callus formation over bony prominences may help to prevent skin breakdown.

Appropriate clothing should not be taken for granted. Moisture-absorbent fabrics should be worn by all competitors to decrease friction and to minimize skin breakdown. Insulated clothing is necessary in colder temperatures to avoid hypothermia. Even in warmer temperatures, a shirt should be worn to prevent skin abrasions from the wheelchair seat back.

Protective equipment may be necessary, depending on the sport. Padded gloves are often worn by road racers and by athletes competing in track. Arm and leg pads may be beneficial in contact sports such as football and rugby. Protective eye gear is recommended in racquetball. Additional protective measures and equipment are obviously indicated for the more exotic pursuits such as mountain climbing or scuba diving.

WHEELCHAIR DESIGNS

Wheelchair designs have changed markedly over the years, both to enhance competition and to prevent injuries. One of the most important developments with regard to performance is the lightweight wheelchair. Materials such as aluminum, chromoly, titanium, and carbon fiber are now used to make racing chairs that weight as little as 12 pounds. A low center of mass provides enhanced maneuverability. Typically, the frame is narrowed, the seat is lowered, and the arm rests and handles are eliminated (Fig. 6). Sprint athletes prefer small-diameter push rims for a high drive ratio, increased speed, and efficiency, despite some loss of maneuverability.[6] Drive wheels have an inward camber to improve the efficiency of pushing and to minimize arm and hand abrasions.[21,22] Reinforced padding of seat posts and adequate cushioning provide extra skin protection. Roll bars can be added to prevent collapse of the chair in a fall.

CONCLUSION

A positive relationship between involvement in wheelchair sports and health maintenance has been established.[24] This should encourage health care professionals to promote sports activities for the disabled. After acute rehabilitation, adaptive sports may further enhance the residual functional capacity of the participants as well as provide social, avoca-

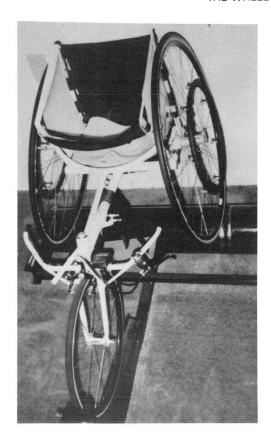

FIGURE 6. Racing chair design shows narrow frame, low seat, absent arm rests.

tional, and emotional enrichment. Athletes, trainers, coaches, therapists, and physicians should work together to provide optimal athletic performance and to prevent injury, thus enhancing the benefits.

APPENDIX A
ASSOCIATIONS AND RESOURCES FOR WHEELCHAIR ATHLETICS

American Wheelchair Bowling Association
   3620 Tamarack Drive
   Redding, CA 96003
   (916) 241-6297

International Wheelchair Aviators
   1117 Rising Hill Way
   Escondido, CA 92029
   (619) 746-5018

Handicapped Scuba Association
   7172 W Stanford Ave.
   Littleton, CO 80123
   (303) 933-4864

International Wheelchair Road Racers Club
   30 Myano Lane
   Stamford, CT 06902
   (203) 325-1429

National Foundation of Wheelchair Tennis
   940 Calle Amanecer, Suite B
   San Clemente, CA 92672
   (714) 361-6811

National Handicapped Sports and Recreation
   Association (multiple disabilities)
   451 Hungerford Drive, Suite 100
   Rockville, MD 20850
   (301) 217-0960

National Wheelchair Athletic Association (spinal
   cord disabilities)
   3595 E. Fountain Blvd., Suite L-1
   Colorado Springs, CO 80910
   (719) 574-1150

National Wheelchair Basketball Association
   110 Seaton Building
   University of Kentucky
   Lexington, KY 40506
   (606) 257-1623

National Wheelchair Softball Association
   1616 Todd Court
   Hastings, MN 55033
   (612) 437-1792

U.S. Cerebral Palsy Athletic Association
   500 S. Ervay, Suite 452B
   Dallas, TX 75201
   (214) 761-0033

U.S. Quad Rugby Association
   1605 Matthew St.
   Fort Collins, CO 80525
   (303) 484-7395

U.S. Les Autres Sports Association
   1101 Post Oak, Suite 9-486
   Houston, TX 77056
   (713) 521-3737

Wilderness Inquiry (canoeing, kayaking)
   1313 Fifth St. SE Box 84
   Minneapolis, MN 55414
   (800) 728-0719

REFERENCES

1. Cowell LL, Squires WG, Raven PB: Benefits of aerobic exercise for paraplegic: Brief review. *Med Sci Sports Exerc* 18:501–508, 1986.
2. Curtis KA, Dillon DA: Survey of wheelchair athletic injuries: common patterns and prevention. *Paraplegia* 23:170–175, 1985.

3. Erikson RP: Autonomic hyperreflexia: Pathophysiology and medical management. *Arch Phys Med Rehabil* 61:431–440, 1980.
4. Eversmann WW: Compression and entrapment neuropathies of the upper extremity. *J Hand Surg* 8:759–766, 1983.
5. Ferrara MS, Buckley WE, McCann BC: The injury experience of the competitive athlete with a disability: Prevention implications. *Med Sci Sports Exerc* 24:184–188, 1992.
6. Glaser RM, Sawka MN, Brune MF: Physiological responses to maximal effort wheelchair and arm crank ergometry. *J. Appl Physiol Resp Exerc Environ Physiol* 48:1060–1064, 1980.
7. Goldberg G, Shephard RJ: Personality profiles of disabled individuals in relation to physical activity patterns. *J Sports Med Phys Fitness* 22:477–484, 1981.
8. Guttman L: *Textbook of Sport for the Disabled*, Bucks, England, HM&M Publishers, 1973.
9. Higgs C: Propulsion of racing wheelchairs. In Sherill C (ed): *Sport and Disabled Athletes*. Champaign, IL, Human Kinetics Publishers, 1986, pp 165–172.
10. Hoffman MD: Cardorespiratory fitness and training in quadriplegics and paraplegics. *Sports Med* 3:312–330, 1986.
11. Johnstone KS, Perrin JCS: Sports for the handicapped child. *Phys Med Rehabil State Art Rev* 5:331–350, 1991.
12. Levin S: Overtraining causes olympic sized problems. *Physician Sports Med* 19:112–118, 1991.
13. Lewko JH: Social and psychological considerations in physical recreation for the disabled. In *Report of the Research Priority Development Conference,* March 1981, Fitness and Amateur Sport, Ottawa, 1981.
14. Lister GD, Belsole RB, Kleinert HE: The radial tunnel syndrome. *J Hand Surg* 4:52–59, 1979.
15. Madorsky JGB, Madorsky AG: Scuba diving: Taking the wheelchair out of wheelchair sports. *Arch Phys Med Rehabil* 69:215–218, 1988.
16. Madorsky JGB, Kiley DP: Wheelchair mountaineering. *Arch Phys Med Rehabil* 65:490–492, 1984.
17. Madorsky JGB, Curtis KA: Wheelchair sports medicine. *Am J Sports Med* 12:128–132, 1984.
18. Nilsen R: Complications that may occur in those with spinal cord injuries who participate in sport. *Paraplegia* 23:152–158, 1985.
19. Sawka MN: Temperature regulation during upper body exercise: Able-bodied and spinal cord injured. *Med Sci Sports Exerc* 21:S132–S140, 1989.
20. Schaefer RS: Sports medicine for wheelchair athletes. *Am Fam Physician* 39:239–245, 1989.
21. Schuman S: Wheelchair frame modifications. *Sports 'n' Spokes* 5:5–6, 1979.
22. Shephard RJ: *Physical Activity for the Disabled*. Champaign, IL, Human Kinetics Publishers, 1988.
23. Shephard RJ: Sports medicine and the wheelchair athlete. *Sports Med* 4:226–247, 1988.
24. Stotts KM: Health maintenance: Paraplegic athletes and nonathletes. *Arch Phys Med Rehabil* 67:109–114, 1986.

Chapter 20

EXERCISE AND SPORTS IN PERSONS WITH MEDICAL ILLNESS:
Guidelines and Precautions

Phillip R. Bryant, DO

Physical activity provides improved cardiovascular fitness and strength, as well as a sense of well-being, for adults and children who have no documented medical problems. More recently it has been recognized that it also provides substantial benefits for individuals with medical illnesses. Habitual physical activities, particularly sustained aerobic exercise, have been documented to produce a number of positive health effects (Table 1)[2,6,11,17,21,23]

Regular physical activity clearly has a significant role in helping to maintain good health. Persons who do not exercise miss the positive benefits. They also are at increased risk of developing medical illnesses, particularly coronary heart disease.[29] Berlin and Colditz[4] performed a meta analysis of data from 40 studies, which indicated that coronary heart disease is 1.9 times more likely to develop in physically inactive than in active persons. Other studies have demonstrated significant reductions in the morbidity and mortality of cardiovascular disease in the physically active versus sedentary controls.[18,24,26]

In a longitudinal study of 17,000+ Harvard alumni, Paffenbarger and Hale[26] revealed that men expending 2,000+ kcal/week in walking, stair climbing, or sports participation had a 39% lower risk of developing coronary heart disease than their classmates who expended less than 500 calories/week in physical activity. When other risk factors were statistically controlled in this study, the more active individuals lived longer. Exercise training appears to reduce the morbidity and mortality associated with atherosclerosis both by direct impact on the cardiovascular system and by the indirect effects of reducing or eliminating risk factors.[15]

This chapter discusses general principles of the exercise prescription and the various means of determining appropriate exercise intensity. Also included are guidelines for prescribing safe and effective exercise programs for individuals with selected medical problems.

PRINCIPLES OF EXERCISE PRESCRIPTION

An exercise prescription is defined as an individualized program of physical activity designed to restore, maintain, or enhance the level of physical fitness and health. Specifically it should include clear delineation of the type, intensity, duration, frequency, and progression of physical activity. A warm-up and cool-down period should be an integral part of the exercise program. Short-term and long-term goals should be established and periodically revised as necessary, depending on an individual's physical and emotional response to the exercise program.

In healthy, asymptomatic individuals, well-established guidelines for progressive conditioning and strengthening are available. Individuals with medical illnesses or chronic conditions, on the other hand, require more careful tailoring of the exercise prescription

TABLE 1.   Health Benefits Associated with Exercise

Increased maximal oxygen uptake
Increased cardiac efficiency by increasing stroke volume and reducing heart rate and blood pressure (reduced heart rate × blood pressure product)
Decreased myocardial oxygen demand
Improved myocardial vascularization
Decrease in cardiac-related morbidity and mortality
Increased capillary density in skeletal muscle
Increased mitochondrial density in skeletal muscle
Reduced peripheral vascular resistance
Enhanced vasodilatory capacity
Increased regional blood flow and oxygen delivery to tissues
Reduced lactate production at a given percentage of maximal oxygen uptake
Reduced perceived exertion at a given oxygen uptake
Enhanced ability to utilize free fatty acids as substrate during exercise
Increased triglyceride clearance
Increased high-density lipoprotein formation
Improved endurance during exercise
Increased metabolism
Reduction or resolution of obesity
Increased muscular strength and endurance
Increased production of endorphins
Increased sweat production during exercise with resulting improved tolerance to hot environments
Inhibition of osteoporosis if weight-bearing exercise activity performed
Increased glucose tolerance
Increased work tolerance and reduction in dyspnea in patients with chronic obstructive pulmonary disease

to ensure that goals are achieved without compromising their safety.

Physiologic and psychological responses to physical activity vary among individuals. Responses may be even more variable among those with medical illnesses. When prescribing exercise for such a population, it is important to have a clear appreciation of the disease process and the physiologic impact of exercise on the patient's condition. Moreover, individuals with the same medical condition may adapt differently or at different rates to comparable exercise programs. Awareness that exercise may cause differential effects offers the physician the opportunity to tailor the prescription appropriately to the tolerance and needs of each patient.

Clear delineation of the individual's past medical history, risk profile, lifestyle, motivation, interests, and current medications is a prerequisite for proper exercise prescription. A list of current medications and recognition of their influence on the response to exercise are also important.

A workable exercise prescription must be practical. Many factors are involved in whether a patient initiates or maintains an exercise program, including individual interests, short- and long-term goals, time constraints, and access to exercise facilities or equipment. Age, geographic location, and even cultural perspectives may play a role in the willingness to perform particular types of exercise. Insight into the influence of these factors may significantly enhance compliance with the prescription.

Typical reasons for initiating an exercise program include the following:

1. to prevent progressive deconditioning;
2. to improve overall physical fitness, appearance, and well-being;
3. to minimize risk for disease progression or recurrence; and
4. to improve one's functional capacity at work, home, and play.

Of particular importance is the realization that the amount and intensity of exercise necessary to reduce disease risk may be considerably less than that required to improve and maintain high levels of physical fitness.[5] This principle implies that individuals with selected medical conditions may receive significant health benefits with a regular exercise program of relatively low intensity. A low-intensity program minimizes the risks associated with more vigorous physical activity. Although optimal physical fitness may be desirable, public health surveys reflect that only a small percentage of adults actually achieve high levels of fitness.[1] The low-intensity program is a more realistically attainable goal for a much greater number of individuals, particularly those with medical conditions and illnesses.

The American College of Sports Medicine (ACSM) distinguishes between physical activity primarily designed to enhance health and an exercise program intended to achieve improved physical fitness. They have provided recommendations for programs with improved health as the primary goal (Table 2). The ACSM guidelines concerning the quantity and quality of exercise training for developing and maintaining cardiorespiratory fitness and proper body composition in a healthy adult differ from those designed only to enhance health primarily in terms of the intensity of the exercise.

The intensity of exercise prescribed is crucial, especially for patients with coronary artery disease. Most exercise programs include intensity prescriptions ranging from 40% to

TABLE 2. **American College of Sports Medicine Recommendations for Improving Health**

1. Rhythmic, aerobic activity that uses large muscle groups. Examples include walking, jogging, swimming, bicycling, rowing, machine-based stairclimbing, and cross-country skiing.
2. Physical activity corresponding to 40–85% VO_{2max} or 55–90% of maximal heart rate.
3. 15–60 minutes of continuous or discontinuous aerobic activity.
4. Exercise 3–5 days/week.
5. Rate of progression tailored to the individual's current medical condition and response to exercise. Modification of the exercise program may be achieved by altering the timing, intensity, duration, frequency or type of physical activity.

Data from American College of Sports Medicine: *Guidelines for Exercise Testing and Prescription,* 4th ed. Philadelphia, Lea & Febiger, 1991.

85% of functional capacity. The previously sedentary individual or patient with a medical illness obviously requires initiation of exercise intensity at a lower level and initially may require discontinuous rather than continuous physical activity. Healthy adults are typically started at an intensity of 60% to 70%, with progression up to 85%, of functional capacity. Those with lower functional capacities typically initiate their conditioning at 40% to 60%. Overweight individuals and those suffering from musculoskeletal injuries also generally require a lower level of intensity. This helps to prevent precipitation of a new injury or aggravation of an existing problem.

Any activity that utilizes large muscle groups in a rhythmic, aerobic fashion 3 to 5 days/week is recommended if a moderate or high level of cardiorespiratory fitness is to be achieved. The activity must be continuous for 20 to 60 minutes.

The lower the intensity of exercise, the longer the duration required for achieving comparable aerobic benefits. The total work performed is the critical factor and can be estimated from the total caloric expenditure for a given physical activity. In continuous exercise, the total work can be increased by increasing the intensity and/or the duration of physical activity. The rate of progression must be individualized. Most healthy adults obtain their most notable conditioning responses during the first 6 to 8 weeks of a regular exercise program. After this time the program can be modified to maintain the conditioning or to continue to improve the conditioning status.[30]

Some forms of physical activity provide relatively consistent levels of intensity, such as walking, jogging, and cross-country skiing. Other forms of exercise are more variable in intensity, such as basketball, tennis, and racquetball. A physician should prescribe cautiously any physical activity that is inherently variable in intensity, particularly for the sedentary or high-risk, symptomatic patient. Highly competitive or contact sports should be minimized or avoided by these patients.

The recommended exercise intensities for the healthy adult population are 50% to 85% of maximal oxygen uptake, 50% to 85% of maximal heart rate reserve, or 60% to 90% of maximal heart rate. Most individuals are prescribed a level between 60% and 80% of $\dot{V}O_{2max}$. The actual training effect of such exercise differs among individuals. For instance, sedentary individuals begin to receive a positive training effect at a lower level of intensity. An elite athlete, on the other hand, must exercise at a higher level of intensity if a significant training effect is to be achieved.

DETERMINATION OF EXERCISE INTENSITY

There are several methods of calculating and prescribing an appropriate level of intensity based on a percentage of the individual's functional capacity. The goal is to achieve a predetermined level of health and/or fitness while minimizing risk to the participant. The methods most commonly used include the following:

1. Exercise prescription based on a target heart rate range

These methods are based on the relatively linear relationship between heart rate and exercise intensity. The heart rate–exercise intensity relationship is determined for any given individual by performing a graded exercise test.

a. Heart rate response to exercise. This method involves determination of a target heart rate range by monitoring the heart rate at each stage of a maximal graded exercise test. A given heart rate can then be plotted against the $\dot{V}O_2$ (or MET, see below) equivalents at each stage of the test. The maximal heart rate is the heart rate measured at the highest exercise intensity attained during the test. One can then determine a range of heart rates associated with given percentages of functional capacity. A healthy adult would be prescribed an exercise intensity between 50–85% of $\dot{V}O_{2max}$. The heart rates that correspond to 50% and 85% of the $\dot{V}O_{2max}$ are then determined from the graph and serve as the training heart rate range (Fig. 1).

b. Exercise prescription using heart rate reserve. This method, developed by Karvonen, is considered one of the best means of determining a training heart range for aerobic activities. It does not have the same value for nonaerobic or only partially aerobic activity because heart rate does not always accurately reflect cardiovascular work in the latter activities. The target range for heart rate is determined by the following calculations:

HRR = maximal HR - resting HR
THR = (maximal HR - resting HR) x 0.60 (and x 0.80) + resting HR

where HR = heart rate, HRR = heart rate reserve, and THR = training heart rate.

This method has particular value in cardiac patients because calculated heart rates closely approximate heart rates determined by using the relationship to oxygen uptake. Also, if the resting heart rate is not included in the formula for calculating a training heart rate range for cardiac patients, then the training heart rate may actually be lower than the resting heart rate for some patients.[3]

c. Maximal heart rate prediction by age. This method is based on the finding that 70–85% of maximal heart rate is equal to 60–80% of functional capacity ($\dot{V}O_{2max}$).

Maximal HR = 220 - age (in yrs)
THR range = maximal HR x 0.70 (and x 0.85)

The aforementioned calculations to determine a training heart rate range assume that physical activity is performed in a continuous fashion without extremes of temperature or humidity. When exercise is done in a discontinuous fashion, the heart rate range is more variable. The duration of the exercise should be prescribed so that the average heart rate approximates the midpoint of the prescribed range

2. Exercise prescription based on rating of perceived exertion

This method, developed by the Swedish psychologist Gunnar Borg, involves use of a 15-point numerical scale from 6 to 20. A rating of perceived exertion (RPE) of 12 to 13 corresponds to about 60% of $\dot{V}O_{2max}$. A rating of 16 corresponds to 80–85% of $\dot{V}O_{2max}$. Healthy adults are typically prescribed an RPE from somewhat-hard to hard (12–16 on the 15-point scale). There is a comparable 10-point Borg RPE scale, on which 4–6 corresponds to 12–16 on the 15-point scale (Table 3).

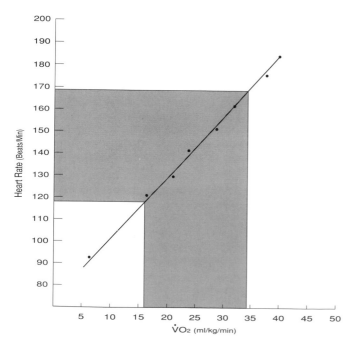

FIGURE 1. Calculation of Target Heart Rate Range.
1. Maximal exercise test performed with heart rate recorded at selected points during the test.
2. A line of best fit is drawn through heart rate data points.
3. $\dot{V}O_{2max}$ is 40mL/kg/min in this example. The goal in this case is to exercise between 40–85% of $\dot{V}O_{2max}$.
   40% of $\dot{V}O_{2max}$ = 16mL/kg/min
   85% of $\dot{V}O_{2max}$ = 34mL/kg/min
4. The target heart rate range for this patient is approximately 118–168 beats/min.
(From American College of Sports Medicine: *Guidelines for Exercise Testing and Prescription,* 9th ed. Philadelphia, Lea & Febiger, 1991.)

TABLE 3. **The 15-Point and 10-Point Borg RPE Scales**

Category	RPE Scale	Category/Ratio	RPE Scale
6		0	Nothing at all
7	Very, very light	0.5	Very, very weak
8		1	Very weak
9	Very light	2	Weak
10		3	Moderate
11	Fairly light	4	Somewhat strong
12		5	Strong
13	Somewhat hard	6	
14		7	Very strong
15	Hard	8	
16		9	
17	Very hard	10	Very, very strong
18		*	Maximal
19	Very, very hard		
20			

From Borg GA: *Med Sci Sports Exerc* 14:377–387, 1982.

The RPE method can be used to modify an exercise program because it offers a readily detectable measure of change in cardiorespiratory fitness.[30]

RPE response to graded exercise correlates highly with $\dot{V}O_{2max}$, heart rate and ventilation. RPE can be used in conjunction with heart rate prescriptions. Individuals can determine their RPE at a selected heart rate level during exercise activity. This enables them to establish a reliable heart rate-RPE relationship. Subsequently, they are able to rely less on the heart rate and more on the RPE to determine an appropriate level of exercise intensity.

RPE is a valid indicator of the level of physical exertion during continuous exercise. It is, therefore, a useful means of establishing an exercise intensity level for endurance training. This method is particularly useful for individuals who have been engaged in an exercise program for some time. It is less reliable in individuals just beginning an exercise program. It is also useful in individuals undergoing a change in dosage of beta-blocker or calcium channel blocker. Although modification of dosage may alter the heart rate response, the RPE is not affected.[3]

3. Exercise prescription by METs.

A MET (metabolic equivalent of the task) is defined as the rate of oxygen consumption at seated rest. One MET is equivalent to oxygen consumption of 3.5 mL/kg/min. There are established MET values for a variety of physical activities. For example, the MET value for running 10 minutes/mile is 10.2. Dancing has a MET value range of 6–9, whereas soccer ranges from 5–12 depending on the level of intensity exerted. One determines the range of percentages of functional capacity (percentage of the maximal MET level) desired for a given individual and then identifies activities that fall within the desired range. Typically, a range of 40–85% of functional capacity is prescribed.

If an individual is known to have a symptom-limited endpoint of 10 METs and 50–85% of this endpoint is a desirable range of exercise intensity for that individual, then the individual is instructed to perform a physical activity that requires between 5 and 8.5 METs.

The disadvantage of this method is the considerable variation in energy use among individuals performing a similar activity. Environmental conditions, such as excessive heat, cold, or humidity, can also significantly increase the workload of the cardiovascular system at the predetermined MET level.

Despite their limitations, all the aforementioned methods of determining the appropriate level of exercise intensity for a given individual are considered acceptable when applied to the proper group of patients. Whatever method is practiced, one should bear in mind that the average exercise intensity is the critical factor in determining whether or not a proper training effect is achieved. As a safety precaution, it is important that the upper limit of intensity not be exceeded for any significant length of time.

Many individuals with medical illnesses can achieve improved health, and sometimes significant physical fitness as well, through participation in an appropriate exercise program. When prescribing a formal exercise program for such patients, it is important to be aware that the integrity of the following physiologic processes affects the capacity for oxygen uptake and utilization during physical activity:

1. Pulmonary ventilation
2. Diffusion of oxygen from lung alveoli to pulmonary capillary blood
3. Cardiac performance
4. Redistribution of blood flow to skeletal muscle vascular beds
5. Utilization of oxygen and extraction from arterial blood by contracting skeletal muscle

CORONARY ARTERY DISEASE

Cardiac rehabilitation, including a formal exercise program, is prescribed for patients with coronary artery disease to enhance their overall health and level of physical fitness, to minimize progression of the disease process, and to restore as much function as possible. The primary intent of an exercise program is to improve a patient's functional capacity. Typically the patient's training should include a workload of 40% to 60% of maximal oxygen uptake, 50% to 70% of maximal heart response, or an expenditure of 300 kcal/exercise session. The deconditioned patient with cardiac disease, however, may need to initiate exercise at a lower workload to avoid excess or premature stress on the compromised cardiac system.

Safety should be the primary focus when prescribing exercise for a cardiac patient. To provide reasonable and safe exercise recommendations for a patient with coronary artery disease, intensity designation should be based on determination of the level of exercise activity at which the patient develops signs and/or symptoms of physiologic intolerance. This process involves a graded exercise stress test and allows one to establish a symptom-limited endpoint for a particular patient.[3]

The contraindications for beginning an exercise program in a patient with coronary artery disease are listed in Table 4. Table 5 lists the situations in which physical activity should be discontinued.[3] Additional criteria for when exercise should be stopped have been established by the American College of Sports Medicine (Table 6).[1]

Medications

When prescribing exercise for patients with coronary artery disease, it is imperative to determine exactly what medications are being

TABLE 4. Contraindications for Entry into Exercise Programs for Patients with Coronary Artery Disease

Unstable angina
Resting systolic blood pressure >200 mm Hg or resting diastolic blood pressure >100 mm Hg
Orthostatic blood pressure drop of ≥20 mm Hg
Moderate to severe aortic stenosis
Acute systemic illness or fever
Uncontrolled atrial or ventricular dysrhythmias
Uncontrolled sinus tachycardia (>120 beats/min)
Uncontrolled congestive heart failure
Third-degree heart block
Active pericarditis or myocarditis
Recent embolism
Thrombophlebitis
Resting ST displacement (>3 mm)
Uncontrolled diabetes
Exercise limiting orthopaedic problems

Data from American College of Sports Medicine: *Guidelines for Exercise Testing and Prescription,* 4th ed. Philadelphia, Lea & Febiger, 1991, p 126.

TABLE 5. Guidelines for Discontinuing Exercise in Patients with Coronary Artery Disease

1. When the patient experiences pain or discomfort in the chest, abdomen, back, neck, jaw, or arms during exercise. Even a trace of angina-like symptoms precipitated with exercise should receive serious consideration. Patients should be instructed to slow their activity gradually and then discontinue it. If symptoms persist despite stopping the exercise, then use of nitroglycerin may be indicated. Typically, an individual takes the first nitroglycerin tablet (or oral spray) if symptoms persist for 2 to 3 minutes after onset. The patient takes a second nitroglycerin dose if discomfort continues another 5 minutes. A third tablet is taken if symptoms persist, and a physician should be contacted.
2. When the patient experiences an unusual degree of dyspnea.
3. When a patient experiences notable nausea, dizziness, or a sense of feeling "faint."
4. When an unusual change occurs in the patient's pulse, especially an irregular pulse during the exercise session. This may manifest as extra heartbeats or missed beats and suggests that premature contractions (PVCs) may be present. The exercise session should be discontinued if the patient has 3 or more consecutive PVCs or multifocal PVCs (30% or more of the complexes).

TABLE 6.   Additional Conditions in Which Physical Activity Should be Discontinued in Patients with Coronary Artery Disease

Excessive fatigue

Failure of monitoring

Light-headedness, confusion, ataxia, pallor, cyanosis, dyspnea, nausea, or peripheral circulatory insufficiency

Syptomatic supraventricular tachycardia

ST displacement of 3 mm horizontal or downsloping from rest

Exercise-induced left bundle branch block

Onset of second degree and/or third-degree atrioventricular block

One or more R-on-T premature ventricular contractions

Exercise hypotension (>20 mmHg drop in systolic blood pressure during exercise)

Excessive blood pressure rise (systolic ≥220 mmHg or ≥110 mmHg)

Excessive bradycardia (drop in heart rate >10 beats/min) with increase or no change in work load

Data from American College of Sports Medicine: *Guidelines for Exercise Testing and Prescription,* 4th ed. Philadelphia, Lea & Febiger, 1991.

taken. In the interest of safety and a more accurate appraisal of the effects of medication on a patient's physiologic response, a formal graded exercise test should be performed before instituting an exercise program, with the patient taking medications as normally prescribed. Exercise performed several hours after taking selected medications may result in higher heart rate responses to physical activity than exercise performed shortly after taking the medication. Therefore, it is preferable to perform the test at about the same time the patient expects to perform exercise activity.

The American College of Sports Medicine notes that patients with coronary artery disease appear to improve cardiorespiratory fitness with exercise training, regardless of the type of beta-blocker used.[1] Therefore, training heart rates for patients receiving beta-blocker therapy should be based on the results of graded exercise testing while the patient is taking the medication.

Nitrates may improve exercise capacity by increasing the anginal threshold. Use of sublingual nitroglycerin immediately before prescribed physical activity may reduce or eliminate anginal symptoms during the exercise session. Transdermal or oral long-acting nitrates appear to reduce angina. A potential complication associated with nitrates, however, is significant hypotension when exercise is abruptly halted. This is due to venous dilatation and diminished arterial pressure. A cooldown period should always be included in the

exercise session to avoid this potential problem.

Calcium channel blockers also reduce angina by improving myocardial oxygen supply and by lowering myocardial oxygen demand. As in the case of patients taking beta-blockers, exercise prescriptions should be based on a graded exercise test with the patient taking the calcium channel blocker as prescribed.

Vasodilators are frequently prescribed in cardiac patients. Because all drugs in this category can cause significant hypotension after exercise, a cool-down period of an appropriate duration should consistently be included in the exercise program. Angiotensin-converting enzyme (ACE) inhibitors (captopril, enalapril, and lisinopril) also have the potential of causing postexercise hypotension. They do not, however, have a direct effect on the electrocardiogram, and there is no need to modify the exercise prescription when ACE inhibitors are used, except to ensure that the cool-down period is of adequate duration. Lipid-reducing medications are often used in patients with coronary artery disease, but none of these medications directly affects exercise testing or training.[1]

Cardiac Rehabilitation Program

A comprehensive cardiac rehabilitation program typically includes four phases. Phase I consists of the first few days of hospitalization. Phase II is the early outpatient period; Phase III, the later outpatient phase; and Phase IV, the maintenance phase. Full discussion of the various phases of cardiac rehabilitation is beyond the scope of this chapter. However, one should be aware that the phases are designed to take a patient with cardiac disease from the inpatient setting to an outpatient program in a gradually progressive fashion with careful attention to minimizing risk to the patient. For example, 1 to 3 days after a myocardial infarction, only low-intensity activities on the order of 2 to 3 METs are permitted. This level consists of self-care activities and gentle range-of-motion exercises. Despite the low intensity, this activity minimizes orthostatic hypotension, maintains joint mobility, and helps to reduce the risk of thrombus formation. The patient is progressed to walking 3 to 5 days after the infarction, assuming no complications have occurred. Initially the exercise sessions, including warm-up and cool-down periods, may be quite short, but they should be slowly lengthened over the course of the hospital stay to 20 to 30 min/session, if possible. The exercise intensity is typically begun as low as 40% to 60% of the patient's documented or suspected functional capacity. Use of the heart rate as a means of determining exercise intensity in patients taking beta-blockers or calcium channel blockers may be misleading. Standing resting heart rate plus 10 to 20 beats/min or an RPE of 11 to 13 on the Borg scale may be a more appropriate means of gauging the proper intensity for these patients. A graded exercise test should be performed before increasing the patient's exercise intensity to greater than 5 METs.

Patients who have experienced recent **myocardial infarctions** or have had recent **coronary artery bypass** surgery are at greater risk for developing angina pectoris, dysrhythmias, and dyspnea. Bypass patients appear to have a greater incidence of light-headedness and supraventricular dysrhythmias, whereas postinfarction patients more frequently develop ST-segment changes. This highlights the need to monitor closely these patients during exercise programs.[1]

Aerobic exercise rather than strength training is favored in patients with cardiac disease. However, patients with relatively good left ventricular (LV) function usually respond to resistive training, including isometric exercise, much like individuals without cardiac pathology. In hypertensive and cardiac patients with normal LV function at rest, mild-to-moderate intensity resistive training increases LV mass index without deleterious effects on LV systolic and diastolic function. In patients with poor LV function, on the other hand, isometric activity may cause LV decompensation. Consequently, resistive training at mild or moderate intensity can be prescribed as an adjunct to the aerobic exercise activities without adversely affecting LV function in cardiac patients without premorbid LV dysfunction. However, resistive exercises should be cautiously prescribed, if at all, in patients with abnormal LV function at rest.[1,14]

Specific exclusion criteria for resistive training are listed in Table 7.[1] If not contraindicated, a starting weight for resistive training can be determined by one of the following means.[1]:

1. 40% of the one-repetition maximum for each exercise
2. 40% of the three-repetition maximum for each exercise (more conservative)

TABLE 7.   Exclusion Criteria for Resistive Training in Patients with Cardiac Disease

Abnormal hemodynamic responses or ischemic changes on the ECG during a graded exercise test
Poor left ventricular function
Peak exercise capacity < 6 METs
Uncontrolled hypertension
Dysrhythmias

3. Start with lowest weight for a given exercise on a weight machine. Monitor target heart rate and rate-pressure product during the effort. If well tolerated, increase weight to next level.

The goal is to gradually work up to 3 sets of a given resistive exercise with up to 12 to 15 repetitions/set.

Patients with **stable angina pectoris** who are not candidates for coronary artery bypass or percutaneous transluminal coronary angioplasty and/or those with an angina threshold ≥ 4 METs are considered eligible for an exercise program. The goal is to maximize the amount of exercise before angina limits further exertion. Typically, exercise intensity is set at 10 to 15 bpm lower than the ischemic threshold. These patients may be best managed with intermittent exercise regimens that alternate work and rest periods. Breath-holding should be discouraged. If angina occurs with exercise, the activity should be discontinued. A warm-up and cool-down period are necessary. The cool-down should be gradual and prolonged (>10 min) to avoid blood pooling in the lower extremities. If a patient continues to experience angina despite cessation of exercise, up to three sublingual nitroglycerin tablets may be taken at 5 minute intervals. If the third tablet is required, the patient should be taken immediately to the nearest hospital emergency room.

Patients who have undergone **percutaneous transluminal coronary angioplasty** may be candidates for an exercise program. It is important to be aware of the significant rate of early restenosis (23% to 30%) within the first 5 to 6 months after the procedure. Patients experiencing this complication may develop abrupt onset of signs and symptoms of restenosis during an exercise session. Consequently, these patients require close observation and ECG monitoring in phases II and III of cardiac rehabilitation.

Patients with **pacemakers** pose a special challenge to those prescribing exercise. One must be aware of the type and operation of the patient's pacemaker and understand the underlying cardiac pathology to safely prescribe physical activity. A detailed presentation of the various types of pacemakers and their function during exercise is discussed in the American College of Sports Medicine *Guidelines for Exercise Testing and Prescription.*[1] As a general rule, patients with pacemakers should have a graded exercise test, and their exercise prescription should be based on the results, which should include pacemaker response, blood pressure changes, RPE, and onset of symptoms. Standard exercise heart-rate formulas are not appropriate for this patient population. Target MET levels or upper heart rate limits 12 beats below the upper tracking rate offer more reliable guidelines.

Patients who have undergone a **heart transplant** also obtain physiologic and psychological benefits from a comprehensive and individualized exercise program. Physiologic benefits include increases in lean body mass, peak oxygen uptake, and peak heart rates, along with reductions in resting blood pressure and submaximal exercise blood pressure. However, because of denervation of the ventricle, secondary to loss of innervation by the autonomic nervous system, these patients have an altered cardiac response to exercise. Early exercise results in increased venous return, increased stroke volume and an associated increase in cardiac output. However, patients with heart transplants do not experience the same submaximal or maximal heart rate responses as patients with normal cardiovascular function. Transplant patients have a resting heart rate approximating the intrinsic rate of the sinoatrial node (90 to 100 beats/min.) In addition, they have a reduced peak heart rate, delayed recovery of heart rate and stroke volume response, elevated blood pressure (as a complication of immunosuppressive drug therapy), diminished maximal capacity due to a reduced cardiac output, absence of anginal symptoms due to sensory denervation, and limited aerobic capacity.

Exercise prescriptions should be individualized and typically begin at 60% to 70% of the maximal METs. Borg's RPE scale and the dyspnea scales are applicable for these patients because the heart rate response does not adjust to exercise intensity. Longer warm-up and cool-down periods are necessary. Hypertension is often seen in patients on cyclosporine, an immunosuppressive drug commonly used in patients with transplants. Prednisone, also commonly prescribed,

TABLE 8. Factors Contributing to Limited Exercise Capacity in Congestive Heart Failure Patients

Ventricular dysfunction
Restricted cardiac function
Impairment of skeletal muscle vasodilator capacity due to neurohumoral mediators of vasoconstriction
Decreased skeletal muscle aerobic metabolic capacity secondary to chronic disuse
Increased pulmonary pressure

causes a multitude of well-established side effects. An awareness of the results of cardiac biopsies is important because rejection is associated with decreased exercise tolerance.[1]

Patients with **congestive heart failure** have a limited exercise capacity; contributing factors are listed in Table 8. Nevertheless, patients with congestive heart failure experience physiologic benefits from exercise (Table 9).[3] Peripheral adaptation appears to be the primary explanation for the changes since resting left ventricular performance has not been shown to be improved by training.

Before patients with congestive heart failure are started on an exercise program, they should be medically stable. They also should have a resting left ventricular ejection fraction greater than 20% and exercise capacity greater than 3 METs. Patients with signs and symptoms of exercise-induced ischemia or dysrhythmias are considered to have a poor prognosis for successful participation in an exercise program. The risks of exercise training in patients with congestive heart failure are listed in Table 10.

Patients with congestive heart failure are typically started on at an exercise intensity at 40% to 60% VO_{2max}. Duration is initially limited to intervals of 2 to 6 minutes with 1 to 2 minutes of rest between intervals. Heart rate as a measure of appropriate exercise intensity may be misleading in these patients because their heart rate response may be abnormal. Thus RPE ratings are favored and a rating of 12 to 14 is a reasonable starting point.

TABLE 9. Physiologic Improvements with Exercise in Congestive Heart Failure Patients

Improvement in peak VO_2
Decrease in heart rate response at standard exercise intensities
Increase in maximum arterial-venous O_2 difference
Reduction in arterial lactate level
Reduction in ventilatory threshold
Increase in maximal cardiac output

TABLE 10. Risks Associated with Exercise Training in Patients with Congestive Heart Failure

Dysrhythmias (including malignant ventricular dysrhythmias due to chronic use of digoxin, and dysrhythmias secondary to altered electrolytes associated with chronic diuretic therapy)
Hypertension
Aggravation of the congestive heart failure

TABLE 11. Dyspnea Scale

+1	Mild, noticeable to patient but not observer
+2	Mild, some difficulty, noticeable to observer
+3	Moderate difficulty, but can continue
+4	Severe difficulty, patient cannot continue

Data from American College of Sports Medicine: *Guidelines for Exercise Testing and Prescription*, 4th ed. Philadelphia, Lea & Febiger, 1991, p 73.

CHRONIC OBSTRUCTIVE PULMONARY DISEASE

Chronic obstructive pulmonary disease (COPD) includes emphysema and chronic bronchitis. It is the fifth leading cause of death and the second leading cause of morbidity in the United States. The primary complaints of these patients are dyspnea and exercise intolerance. Carter et al.[11] noted that most of their patients with chronic obstructive pulmonary disease responded favorably to exercise training, as manifested by a reduction in dyspnea and an increased tolerance of both exercise and activities of daily living. Of interest, all these changes occurred in the absence of any change in pulmonary function indices. Therefore, the exact mechanism by which the improvements occur remain obscure at this time.[11]

According to the American College of Sports Medicine guidelines, all patients with chronic obstructive pulmonary disease should receive complete pulmonary testing. In addition, it is recommended that they undergo formal exercise testing to calculate a target heart rate, to determine if oxygen may be required during exercise, to determine the level of impairment that may preclude the patient from a given type of employment, to detect any dysrhythmias during exercise, and to clarify whether other factors such as peripheral vascular disease contribute to exercise limitations and dyspnea.

Severely limited patients experience dyspnea with only mild exercise. The exercise intensity of these patients can be rated by the dyspnea scale (Table 11). Some may require supplemental oxygen. If so, the oxygen should be delivered at high flow rates at an FIO_2 of 24% to 28%. The exercise sessions may be of variable duration depending on the patient's tolerance. Although 20 to 30 minutes of continuous aerobic activity is favored, more frequent exercise sessions of shorter duration may be more realistic.

HYPERTENSION

Patients with mild-to-moderate hypertension respond to dynamic exercise differently from normotensive patients. They have greater increases in cardiac output and a greater rise in systolic and diastolic pressure. Severe hypertensives, on the other hand, show a decrease in cardiac output in response to exercise because of a drop in stroke volume. Isometric exercises cause more pronounced increases in both systolic and diastolic pressure in hypertensive compared with normotensive patients.[1]

Moderate daily exercise is recommended by the American College of Sports Medicine, although exercising at least 4 times/week is acceptable. Duration should be gradually increased to 30 to 60 minutes with an intensity of 40% to 65% of the target heart range. High-intensity and moderate-to-heavy isometric exercise is strongly discouraged. However, as previously noted, mild-to-moderate resistive exercises can generally be safely performed as an adjunct to an aerobic program. If resistive exercises are done, low resistance with high repetitions is recommended. A warm-up and especially an adequate cool-down period should always be included in the exercise session. The cool-down period is particularly important for these patients, who frequently take medications that can cause postexercise hypotension. If the patient is taking medications that limit cardiac output response to exercise, the RPE scale rather than heart rate measures should be used to determine the proper intensity.

PERIPHERAL VASCULAR DISEASE

Peripheral vascular disease is a common complication of arteriosclerosis. Arterial stenosis, Raynaud's syndrome, and Buerger's disease represent other forms of peripheral vascular insufficiency. Patients experience claudication with physical activity. This ischemic pain is typically relieved with cessation of physical activity, except in severe cases. Exercise is prescribed for the purpose of increasing the patient's symptom-limited functional capacity. A progressive walking program is commonly prescribed, because it allows easy measurement of exercise in terms of distance and time and has direct functional significance. Nevertheless, non-weight-bearing activities can supplement the walking program and typically allow the patient to exercise for a longer duration at a greater intensity. Daily exercise is advocated, beginning with sessions of short duration at least twice daily to the point of pain tolerance. Gradual progression to 40 to 60 minutes of total exercise in one daily session is the recommended goal.[1]

DIABETES MELLITUS

Regular aerobic exercise, performed in coordination with proper diet, rest, and attention to optimal glycemic control, has been established to have metabolic and cardiovascular benefits in patients with both type I and type II diabetes mellitus. Of interest, in societies in which consistent, relatively high levels of physical activity are the norm, primarily in the less industrialized countries of the world, the incidence of type II diabetes is low.[27]

The rest of this discussion focuses on the effects of exercise on type II diabetes. The primary effect of exercise in type I diabetics is to decrease insulin requirements because of greater utilization of glucose.

Potential exercise benefits in type II diabetes are listed in Table 12. Patients experience an improved insulin sensitivity that is lost when the exercise program is discontinued.[8] Although insulin resistance is decreased with

exercise, the specific mechanism for this phenomenon remains obscure. It is known that the number and activity of glucose transporter proteins are increased in adipocytes and myocytes with exercise activity.[16] This results in an increase in insulin-stimulated glucose transport into cells.[19]

Marked blunting of insulin secretion occurs, possibly because of reduced ability of the beta cells of the pancreas to synthesize insulin. This short-term effect is quickly lost after regular exercise ceases.[17]

Exercise prescription in diabetics is complicated by the fact that some patients may have an autonomic neuropathy that prevents them from achieving age-predicted maximal heart rates. Thus, intensity levels based on heart rate may be unreliable. Diabetics also suffer complications that directly or indirectly affect the efficacy of an exercise program. Three potentially critical complications merit discussion:

1. Diabetics have a high incidence of silent ischemic cardiac injury due to diabetic sensory neuropathy. Nesto et al.[25] found that 36 (72%) of 50 diabetic patients developed ischemia on an exercise thallium scintigraphy test but had no symptoms of chest pain during the test. This percentage is significantly higher than that noted with nondiabetic patients. Thus, it is imperative to perform a careful cardiac screen before initiating a formal exercise program for diabetic patients.

2. Many diabetics develop diabetic neuropathy with sensory and/or motor nerve impairment. This may result in a claw-foot deformity of the feet, which causes maldistribution of pressure with more focal and increased weight on the metatarsal head areas and thus increased potential for formation of pressure sores. Because many patients have insensate feet, they may develop severe ulceration and infection with weight-bearing exercise. This potential is increased if improperly fitting shoes and socks are worn during exercise. For this reason, non–weight- or low–weight-bearing exercise, such as swimming or bicycling, is preferred. Weight-bearing activities, such as jogging, or sports that require sudden, quick pivots and turns, such as basketball or tennis, place the diabetic at increased risk of skin breakdown. Inspection and meticulous hygiene of the feet are imperative after any exercise session.

3. The insulinlike effect of exercise explains why exercise-induced hypoglycemia is the most common problem encountered by

TABLE 12. Potential Benefits of Exercise in (Type II) Diabetes Mellitus

Improved insulin sensitivity.

Marked blunting of insulin secretion (short-term effect).

Normalization of glucose tolerance in elderly individuals and enhanced muscle sensitivity to insulin.

Improvement in lipid profile characteristic of patients with type II diabetes. Decrease in very low-density lipoprotein, increase in high-density lipoprotein, and small decrease in low-density lipoprotein cholesterol levels.

Decrease in the level of anxiety and increase in self-esteem.

TABLE 13. American College of Sports Medicine Guidelines for Avoiding Hypoglycemic Episodes in Diabetics

1. Closely monitor the serum glucose at the beginning of an exercise program.
2. Decrease the preexercise insulin dose by 1–2 units or increase the carbohydrate intake by 10–15 g/0.5 hour of exercise prior to the exercise session.
3. Use an area of the body, such as the abdomen, not directly exercised to inject the insulin.
4. Avoid exercise activity during periods of peak insulin activity.
5. Eat carbohydrate snacks pre- and postexercise.
6. Be aware of the typical signs and symptoms of hypoglycemia. One should be aware that diabetic patients taking beta-blocking medications may not manifest hypoglycemic and/or angina symptoms.
7. Exercise with a partner.

Data from American College of Sports Medicine: *Guidelines for Exercise Testing and Prescription,* 4th ed. Philadelphia, Lea & Febiger, 1991.

diabetics who engage in exercise training. The risk of a hypoglycemic reaction is particularly high either during or within 24 to 48 hours of high-intensity, long-duration exercise. The American College of Sports Medicine has provided guidelines for avoiding hypoglycemic episodes in diabetics (Table 13).

Daily exercise is recommended for both type I and type II diabetics. Regularly scheduled exercise sessions with consistent durations and intensities help to maintain proper glucose control despite an increased level of physical activity.

Many diabetics are capable of an exercise intensity from 40% to 85%. Low-to-moderate intensity (40% to 60%) with extended durations (initially 20 min/session with gradual increase to 40 to 60 minutes) is a reasonable goal for the overweight diabetic.

Exercise intensity can be prescribed on the basis of heart rate. In diabetics with autonomic neuropathy and chronotropic insufficiency, however, use of RPE is favored because the heart rate may be misleading. Diabetics with retinopathy should not engage in exercise or sports that involve high-velocity and/or high-amplitude movements, jumping activities, or contact sports of any kind. Resistive exercises that increase blood pressure should also be avoided.

OBESITY

Compliance may be one of the primary challenges in prescribing exercise activity for the overweight patient. Thus, it is particularly important that exercise programs allow a gradually progressive increase in intensity and duration. Weight appears to be best controlled with exercise and sports activity of low-to-moderate intensity and longer duration. Such a program is also likely to be better tolerated and accepted by obese patients on a long-term basis than highly vigorous physical activity.

The preliminary goal in the obese person is to develop the habit of exercise. The physical activity is gradually increased to a level of caloric expenditure expected to result in gradual weight loss. Typically the goal is to exercise at sufficient intensity and duration to expend 200 to 300 kcal/session. Obviously, careful attention to controlling caloric intake is balanced with increase in physical activity. Anecdotal experience indicates that attempting diet control simultaneously with initiation of an exercise program may be overly stressful and result in failure. Once a regular exercise program is established, however, the overweight patient is more likely to comply with a weight-reducing, nutritionally sound diet. After a regular exercise program and appropriate caloric expenditure per exercise session are achieved, one can then focus on cardiovascular training, with a goal based on the patient's target heart range. Because many patients quit exercise if it becomes too taxing, it is important to individualize the program to achieve desired results without compromising compliance.

Low-impact or non–weight-bearing activities, particularly at the initiation of an exercise program, are recommended to reduce the risk of joint and soft-tissue injury. Walking, swimming, stationary bicycling, stair-climbing (on stairclimber machines), and low-impact dancing are excellent modes of physical activity for most obese patients. Alternating these activities may minimize boredom and increase long-term adherence to an exercise regime.

HYPERLIPIDEMIA

Exercise and diet control augment pharmacologic measures to control hyperlipidemia. If no other limiting medical conditions are present, patients respond to conventional exercise testing and prescriptions. Adequate caloric expenditure per exercise session is a primary goal. Relatively low intensities of 40%

to 60% $\dot{V}O_{2max}$ and long durations of up to 60 minutes are recommended.

ARTHRITIS

The participation of arthritic patients in exercise and sport activity is limited by the nature and severity of joint pathology. Patients with rheumatoid arthritis typically experience intermittent exacerbations of joint inflammation, whereas patients with osteoarthritis complain of continuous discomfort. Accurate exercise testing is compromised because joint pathology rather than cardiovascular function may be the limiting factor. Non–weight-bearing activities are favored. Cycling, arm ergometry, and especially swimming are recommended for most patients. High-velocity, high-amplitude, jumping, and contact exercise and sports activities are not recommended. Adequate warm-up, cool-down, and stretching exercises are particularly important in this population. Because joint discomfort may limit activities of long duration, exercise may be broken up into more frequent, shorter sessions. Exercise intensity must be individualized and may vary from day to day based on the patient's pain tolerance.

It is important to maintain a minimal degree of physical activity during joint flare-ups in rheumatoid arthritis to minimize loss of joint range of motion and problems of immobility. However, it is imperative to reduce the intensity and duration of activity during active inflammation to avoid exacerbating joint pathology and pain. In particularly severe cases, it may be necessary to defer virtually all exercise activity for a period of time, but only for as long as absolutely necessary.

CANCER

Exercise has been prescribed in patients with cancer to avoid the detrimental effects of immobility, possibly to enhance their immune status, and to improve their sense of well-being. Prescriptions for physical activity must be individualized for patients with cancer because cancer presents in a myriad of ways. Patients are also subjected to a variety of therapeutic interventions, including surgery, radiotherapy, chemotherapy, and immunotherapy, which impact on their ability to

TABLE 14. Conditions that Require Decreasing or Discontinuing Exercise Activityin Patients with Cancer

Presence of intravenous devices for chemotherapy.
Fatigue, nausea, and/or malaise following chemotherapy or radiotherapy.
Muscle weakness, dehydration, peripheral neuropathy with loss of sensation or dysesthesias, and pain as a complication of therapy and/or cancer.
Thrombocytopenia, leukopenia, and/or anemia as a complication of the cancer and/or therapy.

undertake an exercise program. In general, peak exercise capacity is between 3 and 5 METs. Intensity is most appropriately maintained at the lower end of the heart rate reserve (40% to 65%), although higher intensities may be achieved if the exercise sessions are of shorter duration and increased frequency. Various limiting factors may require decreasing or discontinuing exercise activity (Table 14).

Special care should be taken in patients with documented or suspected bone metastases to avoid causing bone bruises or fractures. Only low-resistance and moderate-to-high repetitions, preferably with a machine rather than free weights, are recommended to maintain strength. In particularly severe cases, even low-resistance exercises may be contraindicated because of excessive pain and high risk of fractures. It is recommended that patients with low platelet counts (<50,000) avoid resistance training 36 hours prior to venipuncture for enzyme studies because the training may affect enzyme levels.[1]

RENAL DISEASE

Patients with end-stage renal disease may experience a host of problems (Table 15). Obviously, any or all of these factors impact significantly on the ability to tolerate a formal exercise regime. Nevertheless, carefully tailored exercise programs can improve functional activity tolerance and strength, as well as lipid profiles and blood pressure control in some patients. Exercise prescriptions should be limited to end-stage renal patients who are stabilized on dialysis and medications and who are on an appropriate diet. Such patients tolerate only low-intensity activities, starting at very short durations. Exercise is typically initiated with intervals of 3- to 4-minute duration, alternating with rest periods. The duration is

TABLE 15. Complications Associated with End-Stage Renal Disease

Marked fluid shifts
Electrolyte abnormalities
Baseline hypertension
Hypertensive response to exercise
Anemia
Left ventricular hypertrophy
Congestive heart failure
Renal osteodystrophy
Muscle weakness and cramping
Lipid abnormalities
Glucose intolerance
Depression
Sedentary lifestyle
Low peak exercise tolerance (usually < 5 METs)
Low average peak heart rates (only 70% of age-predicted levels)

gradually increased to a target of 30 to 45 minutes based on the patient's tolerance. Exercise intensity should be 12 to 13 on the RPE scale. Heart rate measures are too variable to be useful in these patients.

Although patients on hemodialysis may tolerate and respond most favorably to exercise on nondialysis days, in some cases exercise training, such as cycling, can be done during the hemodialysis treatment itself. This practice has been documented to be safe, offers the opportunity to monitor responses to exercise, and may improve compliance. It is reported that exercise performed during the first 2 hours of dialysis is well tolerated and does not interfere with the dialysis.[1]

OSTEOPOROSIS

Osteoporosis is defined as decreased bone mass per unit of bone volume and occurs as a complication of various conditions. Prolonged immobilization, hyperthyroidism, chronic obstructive pulmonary disease, Cushing's disease, malabsorption syndromes, renal disease, certain malignancies, and alcohol abuse have been associated with the development of osteoporosis. It also occurs as an adverse effect of certain medications, such as phenytoin, steroids, and heparin. Postmenopausal osteoporosis, however, remains the most common manifestation.[13]

Weight-bearing stress or similar intermittent compression-loading increases bone mass.[9,10,12,22] Weight-bearing exercise can be an effective adjunct in addressing osteoporosis. Optimal prevention of osteoporosis is achieved when a regular exercise regimen is coupled with appropriate daily calcium intake. Estrogen is also helpful in maintaining bone mass in women.

Regular aerobic, weight-bearing activity at least 3 times/week, gradually increased to 30 to 60 minutes/session, is recommended for patients with osteoporosis in whom such exercise is not otherwise contraindicated. Swimming is not an effective aerobic exercise for treating osteoporosis because it has no significant impact on bone mass.[12]

SUMMARY

Only recently have exercise and sport activities been documented to have both physiologic and psychological benefits for patients with selected medical problems, including cardiac disease, hypertension, diabetes mellitus, and renal disease, among others. A clear understanding of how to determine an appropriate exercise intensity for a given patient, as well as the absolute and relative contraindications to exercise associated with a particular medical condition, is imperative if an exercise program is to be prescribed safely and effectively. Properly prescribed exercise activity may improve an individual's strength, endurance, functional capacity, and/or sense of well-being despite the presence of the aforementioned medical illnesses or conditions.

REFERENCES

1. American College of Sports Medicine: *Guidelines for Exercise Testing and Prescription,* 4th ed. Philadelphia, Lea & Febiger, 1991.
2. Astrand P-O: Why exercise? *Med Sci Sports Exerc* 24(2):153–162, 1992.
3. Begey DB, Ribisl PM: Developing exercise prescriptions for cardiac patients. In Peterson JA, Bryant CX (eds): *The Stairmaster Fitness Handbook: A User's Guide to Exercise Testing and Prescription.* Indianapolis, Masters Press, 1992, pp 121–136.
4. Berlin JA, Colditz GA: A meta-analysis of physical activity in the prevention of coronary heart disease. *Am J Epidemiol* 132:612–628, 1990.
5. Blair SN, Kohl HW, Paffenbarger RS, et al: Physical fitness and all-cause mortality: A prospective study of healthy men and women. *JAMA* 262:2395–2401, 1989.
6. Blumqvist CG, Saltin B: Cardiovascular adaptations to physical training. *Annu Rev Physiol* 45:169–189, 1983.
7. Booth FW, Thomason DB: Molecular and cellular adaptations of muscle in response to exercise: Per-

spectives of various models. *Physiol Rev* 71:541–585, 1991.

8. Burnstein R, Polychronakos C, Toews CJ, et al: Acute reversal of the enhanced insulin action in trained athletes: Association with insulin receptor changes. *Diabetes* 34:756–760, 1985.

9. Buschbacher LP, Buschbacher R: Fitness for life: The role of exercise in treating and preventing illness. In Buschbacher R(ed): *Diagnosis and Rehabilitation of Musculoskeletal Disorders.* Andover, MD, Andover Medical Publishers, 1993.

10. Camay A, Tschantz P: Mechanical influences in bone remodeling. experimental research on Wolff's law. *J Biomechan* 5:173–180, 1972.

11. Carter R, Coast JR, and Idell S: Exercise training in patients with chronic obstructive pulmonary disease. *Med Sci Sports Exerc* 24(3):281–91, 1992.

12. Dalen N, Olsson E: Bone mineral content and physical activity. *Acta Orthop Scand* 45:170–174, 1975.

13. Davis RW: Current concepts in the management of low back pain. *Phys Med Rehabil State Art Rev* 5(3):597–608, 1991.

14. Effron MB: Effects of resistive training on left ventricular function. *Med Sci Sports Exerc* 21:694–697, 1989.

15. Goldberg AP: Aerobic and resistive exercise modify risk factors for coronary heart disease. *Med Sci Sports Exerc* 21:669–674, 1989.

16. Goodyear LJ, Hirshman MF, King PA, et al: Skeletal muscle plasma membrane glucose transport and glucose transporters after exercise. *J Appl Physiol* 68(1):193–198, 1990.

17. Haskell WL, Leon AS, Caspersen CJ, et al: Cardiovascular benefits and assessment of physical activity and physical fitness in adults. *Med Sci Sports Exerc* 24(6):S201–S215, 1992.

18. Heath GW, Hagberg JM, Ehsani AA, Hotloszy JO: A physiological comparison of younger and older athletes. *J Appl Physiol* 51:634–640, 1981.

19. Hirshman MF, Wardzala LJ, Goodyear LJ, et al: Exercise training increases the number of glucose transporters in rat adipose cells. *Am J Physiol* 257(4 pt 1):E520–530, 1989.

20. Horton ES: Prescription for exercise. *Diabetes Spectrum* 4(5):250–257, 1991.

21. Hurley BF: Effects of resistive training on lipoprotein-lipid profiles: A comparison to aerobic exercise training. *Med Sci Sports Exerc* 21:689–693, 1989.

22. Jones HH, Priest JD, Hayes WC, et al: Humeral hypertrophy in response to exercise. *J Bone Joint Surg* 59A:204–208, 1977.

23. Lenfant C: Physical activity and cardiovascular health: Special emphasis on women and youth. *Med Sci Sports Exerc* 24(6):S191, 1992.

24. Leon AS: Physical activity levels and coronary heart disease. *Med Clin North Am* 69:3–20, 1985.

25. Nesto RW, Phillips RT, Kett KG, et al: Angina and exertional myocardial ischemia in diabetic and nondiabetic patients: Assessment by exercise thallium scintigraphy. *Ann Intern Med* 108(2):170–175, 1988 (erratum *Ann Intern Med* 108(4):646, 1988).

26. Paffenbarger RS, Hale WE: Work activity and coronary heart mortality. *N Engl J Med* 292:545–550, 1975.

27. Rauramaa R: Relationship of physical activity, glucose tolerance, and weight management. *Prev Med* 13(1):37–46, 1984.

28. Rodin J, Plante T: The psychological effects of exercise. In Williams RS, Wallace AG (eds): *Biological Effects of Physical Activity.* Champaign, IL; Human Kinetics Books, 1989, pp 127–138.

29. Sopko G, Obarzanek E, Stone E: Overview of the National Heart, Lung, and Blood Institute workshop on physical and cardiovascular health. *Med Sci Sports Exerc* 24(6):S192–196, 1992.

30. Thompson GD, Franks BD: Developing a personalized exercise program: Prescription guidelines. In Peterson JA, Bryant CX (eds): *The Stairmaster Fitness Handbook: A User's Guide to Exercise Testing and Prescription.* Indianapolis, Masters Press, 1992, pp 109–120.

Chapter 21

EXERCISE FOR LIFE:
The Role of Sports in Preventing and Treating Medical Illness

R.P. Bonfiglio, MD

Better to hunt in fields, for health unbought,
Than fee the doctor for a nauseous draught.
The wise, for cure, on exercise depend;
God never made his work for man to mend.

John Dryden, 1631–1700

No exercise is especially beneficial which does not interest and amuse the mind as well as exert the muscles.

Henry Lyman, MD, 1899

Webster's defines sport as "any activity or experience that gives enjoyment or recreation." Individuals engage in sports for many reasons and at various levels of competition. Motivation toward performance may vary greatly between a recreational athlete and a professional athlete. However, the potential benefits of sports participation can go well beyond short-term accomplishments like winning events.[1] Regardless of the level of involvement, maintenance of health can be an important component.

ADVANTAGES OF LIFETIME EXERCISE

The exercise component of most sports activities is especially valuable in preventing disease and disability.[44,45] A lifestyle that incorporates regular exercise provides significant medical benefit.[27] An appropriate sports regimen can facilitate well-being and reduce the risk of many common serious medical conditions. Thus regular exercise can enhance lon-

gevity, reduce the likelihood of disease, decrease the effects of existing medical conditions, and prevent certain forms of disability.[1,2,4,11] The specific potential benefits of regular sports participation include increased strength and endurance, improved flexibility, and improved sense of well-being and quality of life. Regular exercise can reduce hypertension, improve cardiovascular conditioning, decrease the percentage of body fat, and enhance serum lipid profiles.

A life of sports participation can help to prevent cardiovascular disease, osteoporosis, and many other medical conditions. It can also help to reduce the progression of diseases such as diabetes and hypertension. The disability associated with many of these diseases can also be reduced.

For individuals with impairment from disease or trauma, exercise can be particularly important. Sports participation can prevent some of the secondary complications of the underlying disease or condition. Exercise can also help to improve remaining function, thereby reducing the degree of disability imposed by the impairment. For instance, upper-body strengthening for an individual with paraplegia can result in increased independence with activities of daily living and mobility.

GOALS OF AN EXERCISE PROGRAM

In attempting to redefine a lifestyle to include sports involvement, an individual should identify the goals of the program. Exercise can provide many beneficial effects, including improved cardiovascular fitness, reduced body fat composition, increased strength, improved endurance, and greater flexibility. Regular exercise can also lead to improved heat tolerance and may also help to reduce the effects of daily life stresses.

The exercise program should be designed according to the goals established. For example, a program that emphasizes cardiovascular conditioning is quite different from one that emphasizes striated muscle strengthening. Reducing body fat composition requires a different program as well. Enthusiasts today are frequently interested in multiple positive results. Appropriate cross-training programs can achieve such benefits. The program should be monitored to be certain that each of the specific goals has not been diluted in the process of developing a cross-training program.

DESIGNING A LIFETIME EXERCISE PROGRAM

Rehabilitation physicians (physiatrists) are uniquely qualified to aid patients in utilizing sports to develop a lifestyle of fitness via regular exercise. Knowledge regarding musculoskeletal anatomy and physiology, benefits of exercise, and other modalities allows the physiatrist to guide sports participation and to design appropriate exercise regimens. The prescription of exercise is similar to prescribing medication: both should be tailored to the specific needs of the individual. Body habitus, overall lifestyle, family medical history, and sports interests should be taken into account.

Designing a lifetime exercise regimen requires a knowledge of an individual's strengths and limitations. An exercise program that takes into account an individual's strengths and interests is more likely to be followed by the participant. An individual with poor body habitus and stamina may not be suited for sports activities requiring sudden bursts of activity, such as racquetball or handball. An individual with medical problems must have an adapted exercise regimen that accommodates resulting limitations, especially if disability accompanies the disease process (see chapter 20, "Exercise and Sports in Persons with Medical Illness").

Potential benefits of sports participation can be negated by choosing the wrong program of exercise and by not providing sufficient patient safeguards. For example, "weekend" athletes frequently develop musculoskeletal injuries during middle life because they periodically overexert themselves and ignore stretching exercises. During their youth such activities probably would not have caused injury.

Baseline Assessment

As discussed in chapter 1, "The Preparticipation Physical Examination," designing a lifetime exercise regimen for prevention of disease and disability should begin with a baseline medical and health assessment. The extent of the assessment is influenced by the patient's exercise needs and his or her commitment to a lifestyle change. The extent of the assessment may also be influenced by the level of the individual's planned sports competition. Individual risk factors must be assessed, especially for potentially unstable medical conditions such as coronary artery disease.

In an individual with a family history of early mortality due to insulin-dependent diabetes or cardiovascular disease, a thorough initial assessment is especially important. Treadmill testing is particularly important to assess cardiovascular fitness, especially prior to initiating an exercise regimen that stresses the cardiovascular system. A patient with a personal past history of coronary artery disease may need to undergo more extensive diagnostic testing prior to the initiation of an intensive exercise regimen. Dialogue with the patient's cardiologist is important to design the most appropriate and safest exercise regimen.

In an individual with a chronic sedentary lifestyle it is also important to perform a thorough initial medical evaluation. Musculoskeletal injuries can limit performance of an exercise regimen in poorly conditioned participants. Muscles crossing two joints are particularly prone to injury. Flexibility assessment is imperative prior to initiation of an exercise regimen in an individual with a previously sedentary lifestyle. An individual with occupational demands of prolonged periods of sitting, such as an executive or secretary, may be particularly prone to abnormal lumbosacral motion due to prolonged flexed positioning.

In obese individuals, measurement of the percentage of body fat is useful. Underwater weighing is the most precise way to determine percentage of body fat, but caliper measurements can give an estimate acceptable for most purposes. The obese patient may benefit from exercise that improves cardiovascular fitness, endurance, and improved body composition, even if significant weight change does not occur. A specialized program of prolonged endurance training (longer than needed for cardiovascular benefits) is required to cause significant weight loss.

Osteoporosis

Osteoporosis is a common medical condition in the elderly, especially in women. More than 1.2 million fractures occur in the United States each year as a result of osteoporosis. Of these, around 44% involve the spinal column, 19% the hip, and 14% the wrist. By 90 years of age, 32% of women and 17% of men will have sustained osteoporotic hip fracture. Within a year after hip fracture, 12% to 20% will have died.[32,54]

In young adults skeletal maturation continued even after linear bone growth stops. Peak bone mass is achieved around the third decade of life.[39] Exercise prior to this peak helps to build bone mass and may reduce and delay osteoporosis and its secondary complications.[5,14] The level of physical exertion is a significant determinant of peak bone mass, subsequent maintenance of bone mass, and skeletal integrity. However, exercise cannot completely eliminate or prevent the osteoporosis associated with aging and hormonal status.[30]

The exercise program to prevent osteoporosis must be designed for the individual's needs and limitations. Weight-bearing exercise appears particularly useful for producing an increased bone mass. Therefore, practitioners of sports medicine should recommend weight-bearing exercise such as walking, golf,

or tennis for individuals prone to osteoporosis. A regular, vigorous walking program is therefore more helpful for prevention of osteoporosis than a swimming or bicycling program. Aerobic exercise programs designed for cardiovascular fitness may not be beneficial for preventing osteoporosis if they do not incorporate a weight-bearing component. Regional exercise may provide only limited effectiveness in preventing generalized osteoporosis. For example, lower-limb weight-bearing exercises have little effect on upper-body bone content.

Whereas exercise, in general, is beneficial in preventing osteoporosis, excessive exercise in young women may be harmful. Such women may develop amenorrhea and reduced blood levels of estrogen, which in turn reduce calcium absorption and maintenance of bone mass. Thus, women who are experiencing hormonal imbalances due to exercise should be warned of this potential hazard (*see* chapter 18, ''The Active Woman'').

Diabetes Mellitus

In patients with type II diabetes insulin requirements for glucose metabolism are reduced by exercise because of the increased sensitivity of skeletal and adipose tissue to insulin during and after exercise.[53,57] Hepatic glucose production is also reduced by exercise. Therefore, regular exercise can reduce oral hypoglycemic or insulin requirements in patients with type II diabetes. Regular sports participation also seems to reduce the incidence, or at least to delay the onset, of type II diabetes mellitus.[41]

In patients with type I diabetes, exercise also reduces insulin requirements because of the increased utilization of energy stores. In both type I and II diabetes, practitioners and participants should carefully monitor serum glucose levels when regular exercise programs are initiated. This helps to detect exercise-induced hypoglycemia so that medication doses can be adjusted as needed. Hypoglycemia can occur either during or after exercise in persons taking insulin or oral hypoglycemics. Late-afternoon or evening exercise is particularly problematic because of the risk of nocturnal hypoglycemia.

Strenuous exercise in a diabetic individual can precipitate symptoms from undiagnosed cardiac pathology. The effects can include angina, cardiac arrhythmia, and cardiac ischemia. Sometimes such symptoms are absent (silent ischemia) even in the presence of cardiac disease. A thorough cardiac evaluation should be undertaken before diabetic individual initiates a regular exercise program.

A lifetime of exercise can reduce diabetic complications later in life. Cardiovascular fitness is especially important. Maintaining weight close to lean body weight reduces the impact of diabetes on multiple organ systems. A regimen of endurance exercise performed for at least 30 minutes, 3 times/week, at 50% to 70% of maximal aerobic capacity is recommended.[53,57]

Designing an exercise regimen for an individual with secondary complications of diabetes can be more difficult. For example, an individual with severe diabetic neuropathy would be more prone to lower-limb joint trauma from an aerobic exercise program. An alternative program, such as an aquatic exercise program, is preferable. The buoyancy of the water reduces the joint trauma for such an individual. An individual with diabetic nephropathy is prone to increased proteinuria with excessive physical exertion. A moderate exercise program is therefore recommended.

Obesity

Obesity is best managed by the combination of an appropriate exercise program and a weight-reduction diet.[37,63] The optimal goal for prevention or treatment of obesity should be to decrease the percentage of body fat and correspondingly increase the proportion of lean body mass. Short-term diets are often used for weight control but are generally insufficient to accomplish long-term reduction of obesity. Rebounding frequently occurs with diet cessation and can make each succeeding diet more difficult. During dieting, the body seems to attempt to preserve fat-cell size. Homeostatic ''set points'' are established to prevent loss of fat and lead to a reduction in basal metabolic rate in an apparent attempt to maintain the abnormal state of obesity. Exercise can aid in breaking through these set points.

Many individuals attempt to lose weight by exercising close to maximal aerobic capacity for short periods of time. This type of exercise utilizes carbohydrate energy stores (which are later replaced) and is not the most effective way to reduce fat. A more moderate exercise regimen at about 60% to 70% of maximal aerobic capacity, performed for 60 minutes/day, is much more effective in burning fat. Regular aerobic exercise also helps to improve the serum lipid profile. Physical training is associated with a reduction in serum triglycerides and very low-density lipoproteins and an increase in high-density lipoproteins.[42]

In designing an exercise program for obesity, the clinician must recognize that many obese patients tend to underestimate their caloric intake and to overestimate their physical activity.[38]

Cardiovascular Disease

For an individual with a family history of early-onset cardiovascular disease, a regular exercise regimen is of particular importance in reducing the likelihood of cardiovascular and stroke events. A life-long commitment to regular exercise is especially important. The exercise must produce sustained cardiac levels of at least 60% to 70% of maximal aerobic capacity.[44] Episodic cardiac stress that occurs with mixed doubles tennis, for example, is therefore not as effective as a brisk walking or swimming program.

Regular sports participation is helpful from a cardiovascular standpoint for many reasons. Improved cardiac functioning results in a reduced resting pulse rate, increased maximal cardiac output, increased maximal rate of oxygen consumption, and decreased cardiac work for a given level of activity. As previously mentioned, regular exercise improves the serum lipid profile. Regular exercise can also reduce mild-to-moderate hypertension.[8,22,40] The antihypertensive effect of exercise is independent of weight loss or change in body composition.[20,23]

The level of physical exertion required to improve cardiovascular fitness is based on a determination of the person's maximal aerobic capacity. The target range for exercise should elevate the pulse rate to 60% to 80% of the predicted or measured maximal heart rate. Formulas for predicting maximal heart rate are available[30]:

For males: heart rate maximum = 206-0.80 x age (yrs)

For females: heart rate maximum = 198 - 0.63 x age (yrs)

Selecting the optimal program for an individual participant depends on current cardiovascular status, level of fitness, and avocational interests.[7] The exercise program should result in a sustained heart rate within the target range. The exercise regimen should be performed 3 to 5 times/week for 30 minutes to an hour. The individual participant may have to work up to this level gradually. Exercise stress testing may be indicated to guide the level of exertion, especially for individuals taking medications that limit maximal heart rate.

Pain Management

Exercise frequently produces musculoskeletal pain, which is usually transient in nature. Because of this, individuals with chronic pain are often likely to avoid exercise, adhering instead to the philosophy, "if it hurts, don't do it."

Exercise provides the stimulus for improving the strength and fitness needed to avoid injury. An individual with trunk weakness relative to lifting demands has an increased incidence of injury. Even an individual with decreased cardiovascular fitness has a higher incidence of back pain–related disability.[15] Many studies have demonstrated that persons with chronic low back pain have reduced spine extensor and abdominal muscle strength and endurance. Neck flexor muscle strength is also reduced in individuals with chronic neck pain.[52]

Exercise is the single most effective physical modality for pain modulation and improved functional capacity.[55] Exercise is usually an important component of any treatment program for an individual with chronic pain. Assuming that the underlying condition is medically stable, exercise can result in improved physiologic functioning of the involved body part.[6] Increasing paraspinal and abdominal muscle strength, endurance, and coordination is an important component of any treatment program for an individual with lower back pain. Improving spine flexibility is also important. Even more important, however, is the potential benefit of overall general conditioning. Exercise can also help an individual with chronic pain to reduce the effects of daily stresses and may help to modulate the central pain pathways by releasing endogenous opiates. Exercise and improved fitness also help to improve low self-esteem, a common problem in patients with chronic pain.

Designing an exercise regimen for treatment of chronic pain can be a challenge, especially when the patient does not appear particularly motivated to improve functional status.[50,61,62] Other physical modalities or medication may aid the patient with chronic pain to perform an exercise regimen more effectively. Exercise regimens for patients with chronic pain must be individualized. Factors to take into account include the body habitus, specific pain generators, overall musculoskeletal condition, stability of the medical condition, baseline cardiovascular status, and level of motivation to improve functional status. Exercise to improve flexibility in the painful area is a common starting point. Endurance-enhancing and strengthening exercises can be added as the patient gains confidence in the regimen. Exercise for cardiovascular conditioning should be part of every regimen for patients with chronic pain.

Exercise and Pregnancy

Exercise is an important component of a health maintenance program during pregnancy (see chapter 18, "The Active Woman"). Ideally, an exercise program should be initiated even before conception. Prenatal exercise is helpful for increasing and maintaining muscle strength and flexibility.[25] Spinal stabilization exercises can help to reduce back pain associated with the weight gain and center of gravity shifts secondary to pregnancy.[16,34] During pregnancy, the target heart rate during exercise should be set around 25% lower than for the general population (not to exceed 140 bpm). Walking, swimming, and low-impact aerobic exercise are frequently recommended during pregnancy.

Exercise for pregnant women with gestational diabetes is particularly useful for increasing insulin-receptor sensitivity.[29] It may also be a useful adjunct in preventing or reducing excessive weight gain. Exercise during pregnancy may help to reduce gestational hypertension and hyperlipidemia.[13]

Physical Fitness and Aging

Normal aging produces many physiologic effects associated with declining function, but maintaining physical fitness can delay or reduce their impact.[26,35,36,58] Normal aging results in a loss of muscle strength and muscle mass and a reduction in the number of muscle fibers.[24] Muscle mass typically decreases by 30% between the ages of 30 and 70 years. After age 70, further fiber atrophy occurs, predominantly affecting type II fibers.[45] Cardiac and pulmonary functioning also deteriorate with advancing age,[48] with a steady decrease in aerobic capacity and maximal work capacity. The percentage of body fat tends to increase and is associated with a corresponding decrease in proportion of lean body mass.

A lifetime of exercise can slow the loss of —and even enhance[19]—muscle function. In addition, exercise by older individuals, even those with a previously sedentary lifestyle, can enhance performance and overall health.[17,18] Regular exercise can help to decrease resting heart rate as well as systolic and diastolic blood pressure. Aerobic capacity and maximal cardiac work output can be significantly enhanced in older individuals, particularly in those with a previously sedentary lifestyle.[28]

Gait abnormalities are a common component of disability among older individuals and often limit functional mobility.[31] Normal gait depends on normal functioning of the neuromuscular, cardiopulmonary, and skeletal systems in a coordinated and integrated pattern. Injury or disease can disrupt normal gait, and because such conditions are more common among the elderly, the prevalence of gait abnormality is increased.[46] This may be prevented to some extent by a lifetime of regular exercise involving strength, flexibility, and coordination activity.

Falling is a common problem among the elderly. From 20% to 30% of community-living individuals over age 65 years fall each year; one-half suffer multiple falls.[60] Impaired gait and balance contribute to falling.[56] Poor muscle strength is also a significant factor, especially in the major muscle groups of the lower limbs. Walking is an effective conditioning stimulus for older individuals and may prevent the loss of strength that leads to falls. Walking at 3 to 3.5 miles/hour for 40 to 60 minutes several times per week is an appropriate exercise regimen for most healthy individuals over 60 years of age. For those who have been sedentary, this should be the eventual goal of training.

Exercise training can result in increased strength for older individuals. The strengthening effect appears to be largely due to a neuronal effect rather than to significant muscle hypertrophy. Regular exercise also appears to slow the progression of strength loss with aging.[11,59]

Sports Participation for Individuals with Disabilities

Between 35 and 43 million Americans have a disability.[51] Sports participation for individuals with disabilities is especially important for preventing the secondary complications that frequently follow disabling conditions.[21,33] In addition, exercise can lead to greater independence in activities of daily living, mobility, and vocational activities.

A personalized exercise program is vitally important for all individuals, including those with disabilities.[9,47] Again, depending on the goals and the existing condition, the sports medicine clinician can recommend an appropriate program. Individuals with medical conditions such as cerebrovascular accidents and myocardial infarctions can potentially reduce the likelihood of recurrence by a cardiovascular program. For individuals with spinal cord injuries, regular exercise can result in improved cardiovascular and pulmonary functioning. Wheelchair athletes have also been found to have fewer skin and bladder complications.[33]

PROGRAM PRESCRIPTION

Prescribing an exercise regimen should be as specific as prescribing medication.[10] There should be clear-cut goals. The potential benefits of the program must be weighed against potential complications. The intensity and duration of the program should be calculated. Excessive exercise can be as injurious as inactivity. Because exercise can have a myriad of effects, the emphasis on a particular type of exercise depends on the goals of the program.

The practitioner should help participants to design the most appropriate program on an individualized basis. A baseline assessment of the individual's interests, body composition, exercise potential, and preexisting conditions is essential. Determining the individual's exercise interests and abilities also facilitates program development.

The most appropriate lifetime exercise program varies considerably among individuals.

An exercise program that provides cardiovascular fitness and sufficient flexibility to reduce the likelihood of musculoskeletal injuries is important for persons of all ages.

SUMMARY

A lifetime of sports participation results in an improved level of physical fitness. Physical fitness can delay, reduce, or prevent disease and disability related to cardiovascular disease, osteoporosis, diabetes, obesity, and hypertension. Regular exercise is also important in reducing the impact of aging and in enhancing quality of life. Regular exercise for an individual with an impairment is likewise beneficial.

REFERENCES

1. Albright CL, King AC, et al: Effect of a six-month aerobic exercise training program on cardiovascular responsivity in healthy middle-aged adults. *J Psychosom Res* 36:25–36, 1992.
2. Arbeit ML, Johnson CC, Mott DS, et al: The heart smart cardiovascular school health promotion: Behavior correlates of risk factor change. *Prev Med* 21:18–32, 1992.
3. Arden MR, Schebendach J, Jacobson MS: Prevention of atherosclerosis in children. *Compr Ther* 15(10):69–74, 1989.
4. Berenson GS, Arbeit ML, et al: Cardiovascular health promotion for elementary school children: The heart smart program. *Ann NY Acad Sci* 623:299–313, 1991.
5. Birge SJ, Dalsky G: The role of exercise in preventing osteoporosis. *Public Health Rep* 104:54–58, 1989.
6. Bonfiglio RP: Musculoskeletal pain in the workplace. *Phys Med Rehabil State Art Rev* 5:553–563, 1991.
7. Butler RM, Goldberg L: Exercise and prevention of coronary heart disease. *Prim Care* 16:99–114, 1989.
8. Carlsson A, Britton M: Blood pressure after stroke. A one-year follow-up study. *Stroke* 24:195–199, 1993.
9. Clark GS, Blue B, Bearer JB: Rehabilitation of the elderly amputee. *J Am Geriatr Soc* 31:439–448, 1983.
10. Clifford PA, Tan SY, Gorsuch RL: Efficacy of a self-directed behavioral health change program: Weight, body composition, cardiovascular fitness, blood pressure, health risk, and psychosocial mediating variables. *J Behav Med* 14:303–323, 1991.
11. de Lateur BJ: Exercise for strength and endurance. In Basmajian JV (ed): *Therapeutic Exercise.* Baltimore, Williams & Wilkins, 1984, pp 88–109.
12. deVries HA: Physiological effects of an exercise training regimen upon men aged 52 to 88. *J Gerontol* 25:325–336, 1970.
13. Durak EP, Jovanovic-Peterson L, Peterson CM: Physical and glycemic responses of women with gestational diabetes to a moderately intense exercise program. *Diabetes Educ* 16:309–312, 1990.
14. Eisman J: OsteoPPPorosis—prevention, prevention and prevention. *Aust NZ J Med* 21:205–209, 1991.
15. Fast A: Low back disorders: Conservative management. *Arch Phys Med Rehabil* 69:880–891, 1988.
16. Fast A, Shapiro D, Ducommun EJ, et al: Low-back pain in pregnancy. *Spine* 12:368–371, 1986.
17. Felsenthal G: Rehabilitating older patients: Primary care evaluation, treatment, and resources. *Geriatrics* 44:81–90, 1989.
18. Fisher NM, Pendergast DR, Calkins E: Muscle rehabilitation in impaired elderly nursing home residents. *Arch Phys Med Rehabil* 72:181–185, 1991.
19. Frontera WR, Meredith CN, O'Reilly KP, et al: Strength conditioning in older men: Skeletal muscle hypertrophy and improved function. *J Appl Physiol* 64:1038–1044, 1988.
20. Ginsberg GM, et al: Resource savings from nonpharmacological control of hypertension. *J Hum Hypertens* 4:375–378, 1990.
21. Goldberg G, Berger GG: Secondary prevention in stroke: A primary rehabilitation concern. *Arch Phys Med Rehabil* 69:32–40, 1988.
22. Gorden NF, Scott, CB: Exercise and mild essential hypertention. *Prim Care* 18:683–694, 1991.
23. Gordon NF, Scott CB, et al: Exercise and mild essential hypertension: Recommendation for adults. *Sports Med* 10:390–404, 1990.
24. Greig CA, Botella J, Young A: The quadriceps strength of healthy elderly people remeasured after eight years. *Muscle Nerve* 16:6–10, 1993.
25. Heckman JD: Managing musculoskeletal problems in pregnant patients. *J Musculoskel Med* 7(8):29–41, 1990.
26. Heyneman CA, Premo DE: A 'water walkers' exercise program for the elderly. *Public Health Rep* 107:213–217, 1992.
27. Hodgson JL, Buskirk ER: Physical fitness and age, with emphasis on cardiovascular function in the elderly. *J Am Geriatr* 25:385–392, 1977.
28. Hoffmeister JM, Grüntzig AR, Wenger NK: Long-term management of patients following successful percutaneous transluminal coronary angioplasty and coronary artery bypass grafting. *Cardiology* 73:323–332, 1986.
29. Horton ES: Exercise in the treatment of NIDDM. Applications for GDM? *Diabetes* 40:175–178, 1991.
30. Idiculla AA, Goldberg G: Physical fitness for the mature woman. *Med Clin North Am* 71:135–148, 1987.
31. Imms FJ, Edholm OG: Studies of gait and mobility in the elderly. *Age Ageing* 10:147–156, 1981.
32. Judd HL: Prevention of osteoporosis. In Solomon DH (moderator): New issues in geriatric care. *Ann Intern Med* 108:718–732, 1988.
33. Knutsson E, Lewenhaupt-Olsson E, Thorsen M: Physical work capacity and physical conditioning in paraplegic patients. *Paraplegia* 11:205–216, 1973.
34. LaBan MM, Perrin JCS, Latimer FR: Pregnancy and the herniated lumbar disc. *Arch Phys Med Rehabil* 64:319–321, 1983.
35. Landin RJ, Linnemeier TJ, Rothbaum DA, et al: Exercise testing and training of the elderly patient. *Cardiovasc Clin* 15:201–218, 1985.
36. Larson EB, Bruce RA: Health benefits of exercise in an aging society. *Arch Intern Med* 147:353–356, 1987.
37. Lasco RA, Curry RH, Dickson VJ, et al: Participation

rates, weight loss, and blood pressure changes among obese women in a nutrition-exercise program. *Public Health Rep* 104:640–646, 1989.

38. Lichtman SW, Pisarska K, Raynes Berman E, et al: Discrepancy between self-reported and actual caloric intake and exercise in obese subjects. *N Engl J Med* 327:1893–1898, 1992.

39. Luckert BP: Osteoporosis: Prevention and treatment. *Compr Ther* 16(4):36–42, 1990.

40. Maiorano G, Contursi V, et al: Physical exercise and hypertension: New insights and clinical implications. *Am J Hypertens* 2:60S–64S, 1989.

41. Manson JE, Rimm EB, et al: Physical activity and incidence of non-insulin-dependent diabetes mellitus in women. *Lancet* 338:774–778, 1991.

42. Mendoza SG, Carrasco H, Zerpa A, et al: Effect of physical training on lipids, lipoproteins, apolipoproteins, lipases, and endogenous sex hormones in men with premature myocardial infarction. *Metabolism* 40:368–377, 1991.

43. Moritani T, deVries HA: Potential for gross muscle hypertrophy in older men. *J Gerontol* 35:672–682, 1980.

44. Morris JN, Everitt MG, et al: Vigorous exercise in leisuretime: Protection against coronary heart disease. *Lancet* II:1207–1210,1980.

45. Paffenbarger RS, Hyde RT, Wing AL, Hsieh C: Physical activity, all-cause mortality, and longevity of college alumni. *N Engl J Med* 314:605–613, 1986.

46. Penington GR: Benefits of rehabilitation in the presence of advanced age or severe disability. *Med J Aust* 157:865–866, 1992.

47. Pollock ML, Miller HS, Linnerud AC, et al: Arm pedaling as an endurance training regimen for the disabled. *Arch Phys Med Rehabil* 55:418–424, 1974.

48. Posner JD, Gorman KM, et al: Exercise capacity in the elderly. *Am J Cardiol* 57:52C–58C, 1986.

49. Reed RL, Gerety MB, Winograd CH: Expanded access to rehabilitation services for older people. *J Am Geriatr Soc* 38:1055–1056, 1990.

50. Reilly K, Lovejoy B, Williams R, et al. Differences between a supervised and independent strength and conditioning program with chronic low back syndromes. *J Occup Med* 31:547–550, 1989.

51. Report of the task force on medical rehabilitation research, June 28–29, 1990, Hunt Valley, MD.

52. Rodriguez AA, Bilkey WJ, Agre JC: Therapeutic exercise in chronic neck and back pain. *Arch Phys Med Rehabil* 73:870–875, 1992.

53. Ruderman N, Apelian AZ, Schneider SH: Exercise in therapy and prevention of type II diabetes. *Diabetes Care* 13:1163–1168, 1990.

54. Rudy DR: Osteoporosis: Overcoming a costly and debilitating disease. *Postgrad Med* 86:151–158, 1989.

55. Saal JA, Saal JS: Nonoperative treatment of herniated lumbar intervertebral disc with radiculopathy: An outcome study. *Spine* 14:431–437, 1989.

56. Sabin TD: Biologic aspects of falls and mobility limitations in the elderly. *J Am Geriatr Soc* 30:51–58, 1982.

57. Sonnenberg GE, Kemmer FW, Berger M: Exercise in type 1 (insulin-dependent) diabetic patients treated with continuous subcutaneous insulin infusion. *Diabetologia* 33:696–703, 1990.

58. Steinberg FU, Dean BZ: Physiatric therapeutics. 7. Geriatric rehabilitation. *Arch Phys Med Rehabil* 71:S278–S280, 1990.

59. Tallis R: Rehabilitation of the elderly in the 21st century. *J R Coll Physician Lond* 26:413–422, 1992.

60. Tinetti ME, Liu WL, Claus EB: Predictors and prognosis of inability to get up after falls among elderly persons. *JAMA* 269:65–70, 1993.

61. Weinstein SM, Herring SA, Shelton JL: The injured worker: Assessment and treatment. *Phys Med Rehabil State Art Rev* 4:361–377, 1990.

62. Weinstein SM, Shervey JW: Assessment and management of the injured worker with low back pain. *Phys Med Rehabil Clin North Am* 2:145–156, 1991.

63. Wilson MA: Southwestern internal medicine conference: treatment of obesity. *Am J Med Sci* 299:62–68, 1990.

Chapter 22

AQUA RUNNING FOR ATHLETIC REHABILITATION

Robert P. Wilder, MD, and David Brennan, MEd

Deep-water exercise is currently being incorporated into the treatment and conditioning programs of a number of rehabilitative populations, especially in sports medicine. Aqua running serves as an effective form of cardiovascular conditioning for the injured athlete as well as others who desire a low-impact aerobic workout. It consists of simulated running in the deep end of a pool aided by a flotation device (vest or belt) that maintains the head above water. The form of aqua running follows closely the patterns used on land. The participant may be held in one location by a tether cord, essentially running in place, or may actually run through the water the width of the pool. The tether may serve to increase resistance as well as facilitate monitoring of exercise by a physician, therapist, or coach. Because no contact is made with the bottom of the pool, impact is eliminated. The elimination of weight-bearing makes aqua running an ideal method for rehabilitating or conditioning the injured athlete, particularly those with foot, ankle, or knee injuries for whom running on land is contraindicated.

An understanding of the biomechanic principles of the aquatic environment, proper technique, and methods of exercise prescription assists practioners in incorporating aqua running into the rehabilitation and training programs of injured athletes.

Principles of Hydrotherapy

Several properties of water make it an ideal environment for exercise.[11]

Buoyancy: As a result of buoyancy, a body submerged in water is supported by a counter-force that acts against the downward pull of gravity. The submerged body seems to lose weight equal to the weight of the displaced water; the result is less stress and pressure on bone, muscle, and connective tissue.

Drag force: Due to viscosity and drag forces, water provides a resistance that is proportional to the effort exerted, much like running into a stiff wind. This resistance adds to the cardiovascular challenge of aquatic exercise without the stress of impact on joints and soft tissue.

Hydrostatic pressure: Hydrostatic pressure—the pressure exerted by water on a submerged body—is proportional to depth and equal in all directions. Hydrostatic pressure is postulated to aid cardiovascular function by promoting venous return.

Specific heat: Specific heat is the amount of heat needed to raise the temperature of a substance by 1°C. The specific heat of water is several times that of air; therefore, the rate of heat loss to water at moderate temperatures is much greater than the rate of heat loss to air at the same temperature. This difference is especially important in warmer climates, where heat illness is a significant source of morbidity, and in the training of the injured athlete who is deconditioned and not acclimated to exercise in warm environments.

Temperature: The aquatic environment allows regulation of the temperature during exercise. The ideal range appears to be 82° to 86°F (28° to 30°C) because little heat is stored and performance is not impaired. Competitive athletes typically prefer a slightly cooler environment.

BIOMECHANICS OF AQUA RUNNING

The form of running in water closely patterns the form used on land. For the runner or any athlete whose sport requires running, aqua running represents a biomechanically specific means of conditioning during a rehabilitation program or for supplementing regular training. The effects of training include improvement in cardiopulmonary performance as well as in the exercised muscle groups, which undergo changes in enzymes and capillary density, among others. The elimination of weight bearing and the addition of resistance change the relative contribution of each muscle group compared with land-based running. Every effort is made, therefore, to reproduce the running form used on land and to ensure the incorporation of the muscle groups used in land-based running. The following guidelines assist in maintaining proper form during aqua running[6]:

1. The waterline should be at the shoulder level. The mouth should be comfortably out of the water without having to tilt the head back. The head should be looking straight ahead, not down.
2. The body should assume a position slightly forward of the vertical, with the spine maintained in a neutral position.
3. Arm motion is identical to that used on land with primary motion at the shoulder (Fig. 1A). The elbows are bent and the hands lightly clenched with the thumbs on top. Arm flexion brings the hands to just below the waterline approximately 8 to 12 inches from the chest. Extension brings the hands to just below the hip. The elbow undergoes a slight degree of flexion and extension. Sprinters tend to extend the elbow to a greater degree than distance runners.
4. Leg motion requires great attention to detail to ensure proper stride mechanics (Figs. 1B and 1C). Hip flexion should reach approximately 60 to 80°. As the hip is flexed, the leg extends at the knee from the flexed position. When end hip flexion is reached, the lower leg should be perpendicular to the horizontal. The hip and knee are then extended together, with the knee reaching full extension when the hip

is in neutral (0° of flexion). As the hip is hyperextended, the leg is flexed at the knee. The cycle then repeats itself. The foot undergoes dorsiflexion and plantarflexion at the ankle throughout cycle. The ankle is in a position of dorsiflexion when the hip is in neutral and the leg is extended at the knee. Plantarflexion is assumed as the hip is hyperextended and the leg flexed. Dorsiflexion is reassumed as the hip is flexed and the leg extends. Underwater viewing has shown that inversion and eversion accompany dorsiflexion and plantarflexion, as it does land-based running.

Greater physiologic response in terms of maximal oxygen uptake and heart rate can be obtained by strict adherence to proper technique.

EXERCISE RESPONSE TO AQUA RUNNING

Studies have demonstrated significant differences in metabolic response between aqua running and land-based running.[2,5,7,8,13,14,17,18] Despite these differences, however, aqua running has been shown to elicit sufficient cardiovascular response to result in a training effect, which supports anecdotal evidence of its usefulness in rehabilitation of the athlete. According to the American College of Sports Medicine *Guidelines for Exercise Testing and Prescription*,[1] a training effect depends on maintenance of exercise at an intensity level between 40% and 85% of maximal $\dot{V}O_2$ or 55% to 90% of maximal heart rate for 15 to 60 minutes 3 to 5 times/week.[1] Studies have demonstrated the aqua running elicits responses well within the suggested ranges.

Several studies have examined maximal oxygen uptake and heart rate responses to both aqua running and land-based treadmill running.[7,8,14,17] These studies demonstrate that maximal oxygen uptakes during aqua running range from 83% to 89.3% of the values obtained during treadmill running and maximal heart rates from 88.9% to 95.1% of the values obtained on land. For submaximal exercise, Bishop[2] found that aqua running at a comfortable perceived exertion elicited mean $\dot{V}O_2$ levels of 73.4% and mean heart rates of 78% of the values during submaximal treadmill exercise. He notes that the ability to distinguish perceived exertion levels during the different forms of exercise may have affected the outcome of the study. Navia[14] noted that

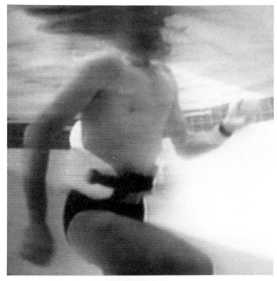

FIGURE 1. The form of running in water closely patterns the form used on land. Experience has shown that a greater physiologic response in terms of maximal oxygen uptake and heart rate can be obtained by strict adherence to proper technique. In the lateral view (close-up, top panel), note that the arm carry is identical to that used with land-based running.

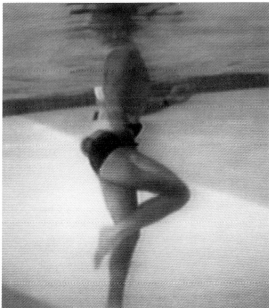
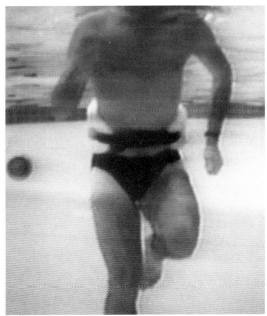

at higher workloads a particular heart rate corresponded to a higher submaximal oxygen uptake during aqua running than during treadmill running, suggesting that an aerobic training effect may occur at lower heart rates during aqua running than during treadmill running. Svendenhag and Seger[17] demonstrated a similar relationship between heart rate and submaximal oxygen uptake.

In a pilot study 10 subjects who underwent an 8-week training program of aqua running showed improvements in maximal oxygen uptake during both water-based and land-based graded exercise testing (19.6% and 10.7%, respectively), thus demonstrating a training effect as well as a crossover effect to land-based exercise.[5,13]

Several possible explanations exist for the differences in metabolic response to aqua running and treadmill running. Differences in patterns of muscle use and activation contribute to the differences in exercise response. Hydrostatic pressure is postulated to assist cardiac performance by promoting venous return; thus the heart rate does not have to be as fast to maintain cardiac output. Temperature has been demonstrated to have an effect on heart rate during exercise, with higher temperatures correlating with higher heart rates. Familiarity with aqua running also appears to be an important factor in maximizing physiologic response.

Despite the differences between aqua running and land-based running, aqua running elicits the physiologic responses necessary to promote a training effect. Higher oxygen uptake levels and heart rates can be obtained with adherence to proper technique. Aqua running also offers additional benefits, most notably the maintainance of quick turnover (rapid gait cycling) as well as coordinated movement between the arms and legs. These aspects facilitate return to land-based training.

EXERCISE PRESCRIPTION FOR AQUA RUNNING

Three methods are used for grading the intensity of aqua-running exercise: heart rate, perceived exertion, and cadence. Workout programs are typically designed to reproduce the work the athlete would do on land and to incorporate long runs as well as interval/speed training.

Heart rate. A high correlation exists between heart rate and oxygen uptake. According to the American College of Sports Medicine guidelines, a training effect depends on exercise at a level between 55% and 90% of the maximal heart rate (the target heart rate range).[1] The maximal heart rate can be estimated (220 − age) or based on heart rate levels attained during exercise of maximal effort. Although heart rate levels in the water tend to be lower than those attained on land, it is possible to approach land-based values by adherence to proper technique. Heart rate can be monitored by a waterproof heart rate monitor or by periodic palpation.

Rating of perceived exertion. Rating of perceived exertion (RPE) refers to a subjective grading of the intensity of exercise.[3,4,9,10,12,15,16] Thus, if one is jogging, perceived exertion is rated as low. Sprinting is rated with a high level of perceived exertion. The most commonly used scale of perceived exertion is the Borg scale, a 15-point scale with verbal descriptors ranging from very, very light to very, very hard (Table 1). We use the Brennan scale, a 5-point scale designed exclusively for aqua running with verbal descriptors ranging from very light to very hard (Table 2). We further instruct athletes that level 1 (very light) corresponds to a light jog or recovery run; level 2 (light), to a long, steady run; level 3 (somewhat hard), to 5- to 10-km road-race pace; level 4 (hard), to 400-800-m track speed; and level 5 (very hard), to sprinting (100- to 200-m speed). The Brennan scale facilitates the incorporation of both speed and distance work into workouts in a manner easily understood by both coach and athlete. A sample protocol is presented in (Fig. 2).

Cadence. Wilder, Brennan, and Schotte[18] demonstrated a very high correlation between cadence and heart rate with intraindividual correlations averaging 0.98. Competitive athletes in our program undergo a graded exercise test of aqua running following our standard protocol (Fig. 3). Cadence is controlled with an auditory metronome. By recording heart rate responses to varying levels of cadence, we can anticipate an expected physiologic response to particular cadence level. We can then design workouts with timed intervals at particular cadence levels.

When monitoring exercise intensity, the heart rate is used primarily during long runs—prolonged periods of exercise at a specified rate (the target heart rate). Rating of perceived exertion and cadence are most

TABLE 1. **Borg Scale of Perceived Exertion***

Level	Rate of Perceived Exertion
6	
7	Very, very light
8	
9	Very light
10	
11	Light
12	
13	Somewhat hard
14	
15	Hard
16	
17	Very hard
18	
19	Very, very hard
20	

Data from Borg G, Linderholm H: Perceived exertion and pulse rate during graded exercise in various age groups. *Acta Med Scand* 472:194–206, 1967.

TABLE 2. **Brennan Scale of Perceived Exertion***

Level	Rate of Perceived Exertion
1	Very light
2	Light
3	Somewhat hard
4	Hard
5	Very hard

*From Brennan DK, Wilder RP: *Aqua Running: An Instructor's Manual.* Houston, Houston International Running Center, 1990.

Total Workout Time and Workout No.	No. of Repetitions	×	Duration of Repetitions (min:s)	@	Exertion Level		(Recovery Period, s)
(37:00) 1	5	×	2:00	@	RPE	SH	(:30)
	8	×	1:00	@	RPE	H	(:30)
	5	×	2:00	@	RPE	SH	(:30)

Figure 2. Sample workout protocol. In this case, the workout protocol (no. 1) calls for 5 repetitions of 2-minute (2:00) duration each at a perceived exertion level of somewhat hard (SH), followed by 8 repetitions of 1-minute (1:00) duration each at a perceived exertion level of hard (H), followed by 5 repetitions of 2-minute (2:00) duration each at a perceived exertion level of somewhat hard. A 30-second (0:30) recovery period consisting of easy jogging follows each repetition. (From Brennan DK, Wilder RP: *Aqua Running: An Instructor's Manual.* Houston, Houston International Running Center, 1990, with permission.)

Name: _____					Date: _____
Predicted 90% Max Heart Rate: _____					Trial: _____
Stage	End Point	Cadence	Heart Rate	RPE	Comments
W	4:00	48			
1	6:00	66			
2	8:00	69			
3	10:00	72			
4	12:00	76			
5	14:00	80			
6	16:00	84			
7	18:00	88			
8	20:00	92			
9	22:00	96			
10	24:00	100			
11	26:00	104			
Post	27:00	48			
	28:00	48			
	29:00	48			

FIGURE 3. Data collection sheet in Wilder graded exercise test for aqua running. W = warm-up phase; post values = postexercise values during cool-down. © 1990 Houston International Running Center.

often used for interval sessions; RPE is most useful in group settings, whereas cadence is most appropriate for individual sessions.

Maintaining conditioning is a challenge for the injured athlete. Aqua running provides an effective means to continue training during rehabilitation. Aqua running may also be incorporated into a regular training program, providing a low-stress form of additional cardiovascular exercise.

REFERENCES

1. American College of Sports Medicine: *Guidelines for Exercise Testing and Prescription,* 4th ed. Philadelphia, Lea & Febiger, 1991, p 96.
2. Bishop PA, Frazier S, Smith J, et al: Physiologic responses to treadmill and water running. *Physician Sportsmed* 17:87–94, 1989.
3. Borg GV: Psychophysical basis of perceived exertion. *Med Sci Sports Exerc* 14:377–387, 1982.
4. Borg G, Linderholm H: Perceived exertion and pulse rate during graded exercise in various age groups. *Acta Med Scand* 472:194–206, 1967.
5. Brennan DK, Michaud TJ, Wilder RP, Sherman NW: Gains in aquarunning peak oxygen consumption after eight weeks of aquarun training [abstract]. *Med Sci Sports Exerc* 24 (suppl):S23, 1992.
6. Brennan DK, Wilder RP: *Aqua Running: An Instructor's Manual.* Houston, Houston International Running Center, 1990.
7. Butts NK, Tucker M, Smith R: Maximal responses to treadmill and deep water running in high school female cross country runners. *Res Q Exerc Sport* 62:236–239, 1991.
8. Butts NK, Tucker M, Greening C: Physiologic responses to maximal treadmill and deep water running in men and women. *Am J Sports Med* 19:612–614, 1991.
9. Carlton RL, Rhodes EC: Critical review of the literature on ratings scales for perceived exertion. *Sport Med* 2:198–22, 1985.

10. Dishman RK, Patton RW, Smith J, et al: Using perceived exertion to prescribe and monitor exercise training heart rate. *Int J Sports Med* 8:208–213, 1987.
11. Edlich RF, Towler MA, Goitz RJ, et al: Bioengineering principles of hydrotherapy. *J Burn Care Rehabil* 8:580–584, 1987.
12. Hetzler RK, Seip RL, Boutcher SH, et al: Effect of exercise modality on ratings of perceived exertion at various lactate concentrations. *Med Sci Sports Exerc* 23:88–92, 1991.
13. Michaud TJ, Brennan DK, Wilder RP, Sherman NW: Aquarun training and changes in treadmill running maximal oxygen consumption. *Med Sci Sports Exerc* 24 (suppl):S23, 1992.
14. Navia AM: Comparison of energy expenditure between treadmill running and water running [thesis]. Brimingham, University of Alabama Birmingham, 1986.
15. Seip RL, Snead D, Pierce EF, et al: Perceptual responses and blood lactate concentration: Effect of training state. *Med Sci Sports Exerc* 23:80–87, 1991.
16. Smutock MA, Skrinar GS, Pandolf KB: Exercise intensity: Subjective regulation by perceived exertion. *Arch Phys Med Rehabil* 61:569–574, 1980.
17. Svedenhag J, Seger J: Running on land and in water: comparative exercise physiology. *Med Sci Sports Exerc* 24:1155–1160, 1992.
18. Wilder RP, Brennan D, Schotte DE: A standard measure for exercise prescription for aqua running. *Am J Sports Med* 21:45–48, 1993.

INDEX

Page numbers in **boldface** type indicates complete chapters.